HOSPITALS IN TRANSITION

Everett A. Johnson
Director, Institute of Health Administration
Georgia State University

Richard L. Johnson
President, TriBrook Group, Inc.

AN ASPEN PUBLICATION®
Aspen Systems Corporation
Rockville, Maryland
London
1982

Library of Congress Cataloging in Publication Data

Johnson, Everett A.
Hospitals in transition.

Includes index.
1. Hospitals—Administration. 2. Hospitals—United
States—Administration. I. Johnson, Richard L.
II. Title.
RA971.J543   362.1'1'068   81-20634
ISBN: 0-89443-396-2   AACR2

Library of Congress Catalog Card Number: 81-20634
ISBN: 0-89443-396-2

Printed in the United States of America

1 2 3 4 5

Table of Contents

Foreword

If the decade of the 1960s were characterized as a decade of expanding horizons for hospitals in which all the problems in health care were solvable and if the decade of the 1970s were described as a decade of contracting horizons, defensiveness, regulations, and questions about the concept of the hospital, then the decade of the 1980s should be a decade of opportunity.

The opportunity, however, will have many risks. Cost problems for hospitals will get worse, and competition fiercer. The internal structure of hospitals will change; that is, traditional relationships between board, executive, and medical staff members will not stay the same. Corporate organizations will look completely different. Old hospitals, with old style management and medical staffs, will not survive the 1980s. For the first time in 25 years, there will be losers as well as winners. In 1990, the landscape will look entirely different.

Everett and Richard Johnson have seen and lived the last three decades in the hospital field. They have experience and insight into what is happening. This book, which reviews the past to learn for the future, is the guide needed to cross the difficult terrain of the 1980s.

The chapter titles signal that the views presented and the conclusions drawn are likely to be different from the past. For example, "Managing Physicians" is a phrase that would have been whispered in the 1960s and 1970s; "The Power Broker" is certainly not the traditional view of the hospital "administration" of the 1960s; and "Hospital Productivity" is a topic that in 1960 would have been seen as irrelevant to the hospital's true mission. In each topic discussed, management opportunities as well as dangers are presented.

This decade will provide both excitement and challenge. As this book shows, its going to be a lot of fun for those who live and work in hospitals.

John F. Horty
Horty, Springer & Mattern

Preface

When current affairs and issues in health care administration are contemplated, there seems to be no end to topics that might be addressed. Yet, the more experienced a person becomes, the easier it is to identify the common threads that affect all health care institutions.

If a person looks for a rationality of the whole, it will be missing. The grand design in health care is not found in its institutions or in its delivery. Rather, it is found in the process of integrating medical knowledge. The world of health care administration is an *ad hoc* response to the necessities of medical practice and the current state of integration of medical knowledge.

Administrators, like everyone else, seek a grand design in their work. Like any ideal, this can be pursued, but it cannot be achieved in the foreseeable future.

Because the common threads that can be perceived are limited, rationality in health care administration is needed. A way to comprehend and deal with the issues of the day should be defined. Elaborating on the common threads in health care management is the aim of this book. What they mean and how helpful they are to practicing health care executives depend on the executives' earlier experiences and the limits of their institutional freedom and personal courage.

An understanding of the major dimensions of how the field looks at its problems is important. How the questions are framed is more important than how they are answered. Unfortunately, the typical perspective of the field is restricted to the matters of the day that are up front in the operation of health care institutions. These kinds of issues include:

- What is the environment of administration?
- How are institutions governed?
- What are the restraints and regulations within which the field must operate in society?

- What roles are defined for chief executives?

- How can physicians be managed by organizations?

- How can health care institutions be evaluated and controlled?

- How can medical care services be financed?

- Where is modern day medical technology headed?

- How can institutional planning be made useful?

The roots of these questions can be traced back to five changes in our society that have occurred in the last decade:

1. rapid increases in medical technology
2. steady advances in medical knowledge
3. large-scale federal health care programs
4. higher rates of increase in costs of institutional operation
5. conservative and traditional thinking by hospital governance

From 50 years of unregulated institutional operation and freedom in decision making, the past decade has seen a move to excessive regulation of the field and restrictive payment for health care services. The clock cannot be turned back to the good old days. Much of the cumulative adverse effects of these changes could have been avoided by deeper insight, greater foresight, and institutional courage.

Change that comes gradually and is anticipated generally affects society in almost invisible ways and is accepted without noise and ruckus. When change is greeted with protests and limited abilities to recognize its inevitability, a desire for further repressive regulation is ignited.

Personal good health and quality health care is close to the heart of Americans. Without health in a modern society there is little opportunity to enjoy its benefits. One way or another, America's desires will be achieved. It doesn't matter how health care is regulated; what matters is the reasonable availability of quality medical care services. Whether or not its delivery is exciting, stimulating, and progressive to the people providing medical care is of little concern.

Through better understanding about the operation of health care institutions and willingness to strive for improvements, the field of health care administration can rebuild an environment for clinicians and professionals that reinforces their drive for excellence. We hope that this book will be one step along this road.

This volume is dedicated to all health care professionals who continue, under adverse conditions, to strive for the highest standards of health care knowing that they have already attained a level unsurpassed in the history of humankind.

Everett A. Johnson
Richard L. Johnson
March 1982

Part I

Environment of Administration

Part 7

Environment of Adjudication

Chapter 1

Changing Times

HISTORY

To look ahead, people must first look to see where they have been and understand what has already happened. Therefore, reviewing the hospital world in the United States from the 1920s to the present may be helpful.

During the decade of the twenties, many new hospitals were begun, particularly in the large cities. This was stimulated to a great extent by the general acceptance of surgery, laboratory medicine, and radiology as useful new developments in medical technology. By today's standards, patient bills were low, with average per patient charges of $10 per day or less.

The Depression of the thirties affected hospitals, as well as the rest of the country, and efforts at improvement and expansion plateaued. In the forties, World War II contributed to a demand for hospital expansion and improvement, with a great increase in fundamental medical research, and the medical armamentarium was significantly improved.

By the fifties, hospitals plunged headlong into major expansion, and a rural hospital system was developed with Hill-Burton funds. Major new medical knowledge was brought into daily use in most institutions.

The 1960s saw refinements in hospital operations and the development of ancillary health care services, such as social services, physical medicine, intensive care units, and pulmonary function departments.

By 1966, the hospital world changed, and most people did not recognize at the time by how much. When Titles XVIII and XIX of the Social Security Act were enacted by Congress, change came slowly at first and then increased each year into an annual torrent of new regulations.

By the early seventies, the economy came under wage and price controls, with hospitals and the construction industry the last parts of the economy to be freed from these restraints. Since early in 1975, the hospital industry has been growing and inflating at a rapid rate along with the rest of the economy.

3

FOUNDATION FOR THE 1980s

Between today and 1990, tumult and confusion will characterize coming events in the health care field. There will be personality clashes between institutions and government, ethics and financing, as well as between the concepts of decentralization versus centralization, as contrary views in society are sorted out and additional political support is found or lost.

Underlying all of these options are two fundamental choices. One opinion holds that behavioral science theory is sufficiently mature to provide guidance for solving the most complex of problems in health care delivery. The other opinion holds that the pragmatism and initiative of local people, exercised within broad review and control limits, will ultimately develop a more useful, responsive health care system.

A Drive for Federal Dominance

As these two broad viewpoints bob and weave against each other throughout the next decade, their wider implications in a philosophical context will be argued within the concepts of what freedom in America means. The true believers in institutional initiative and historical medical care traditions will point to past achievements within earlier freedoms of planning and operating that led to an expanding health care system.

However, there now exist three major forces that are, and will be, used in the 1980s to justify a drive for dominance of the health care industry by the federal government, in order to assure its hegemony in health care. The first major force is the assertion that all health care providers are not equal to but are the same as every other health care provider, that and equality between providers can only be achieved by reducing provider freedom to a common, standardized level. The second force affecting past freedoms of the health care system are the high levels of inflation in the economy. Inflation destroys a hospital's capital and diverts its diminished income from clinical to support service expenditures. Also, beggars cannot be choosers. The third force causing the loss of institutional freedoms is the effort to change the role of the hospital from providing health care services to being the force to secure change in health care delivery and becoming a provider of social services as well as health care services.

Missing in all of these present efforts is an understanding that the best results in health care are achieved when management is left to people who know something about it.

These forces portray the underlying foundation for the 1980s, which will cause pressures and limitations on the development of health care institutions.

Demise of Full Service Hospitals

Throughout the past three decades, hospitals in America believed and acted as if all but the smallest institutions could serve any and all health care needs in their service areas. To act in such a fashion today is to court financial disaster.

Restrictive reimbursement policies, rising costs of new medical technology, and high construction costs have made a full service hospital a thing of the past. In an era of growing professional specialization and increasing regulation, it is unrealistic not to rethink the modern day role of a hospital. It is no longer possible to be all things to all people for health care, except in rare circumstances.

What a hospital does, it should do well and with considerable humanity. To try to cover all the bases in acute medical care is to assume that it will either be done in a poor way or at such a high cost that the majority of the population will be excluded from its benefits.

Growth of Marketing Strategies

To survive as a valued medical resource in the 1980s, every hospital needs to examine carefully the health care needs of its community, decide which needs the hospital will serve, and how it will do so. Many hospitals roles are what they have always been. In providing meaningful leadership, hospital management must think through the community role of the hospital, whom it should serve, and the reasons for it. In other words, what are the marketing opportunities of the hospital?

Marketing concepts and jargon are useful ways to think about the services of a hospital, but are really not new. The goal of marketing activities in a service industry, as in the hospital field, is the same: improved convenience to the customer, new processes and systems, and lower costs. It is the supermarket versus the corner grocery store.

Historically, community hospitals had a marketing strategy, but wittingly or unwittingly, were limited by custom to supporting certain viewpoints and practices that limited aggressive marketing techniques. These limitations were:

- full support of the concept of fee-for-service medical practice, even when conditions were inappropriate for its application;
- equal economic treatment of all members of the medical staff, such as rotation of all internists for electrocardiogram (EKG) readings;
- providing services at just one location, the hospital site, and not competing economically with physician activities;

- competing only with each other, and then only in terms of the scope of clinical services.

Chaining and Commercial Ventures

During the 1970s, many hospitals in the United States recognized that these limitations on operations needed to be changed if hospitals were to prosper. Two basic types of hospitals evolved: the investor owned chains, such as Hospital Corporation of America and Hospital Affiliates, Inc., and the voluntary nonprofit chains, such as Good Samaritan and Inter-Mountain. Both types of chains are growing rapidly by the use of management contracts and ownership. The development of certificate-of-need legislation in states has further encouraged chaining, because these laws, in effect, operate as a franchising mechanism.

Voluntary hospitals that have broadened their operations to encompass the owning and operation of multiple sites for the delivery of medical care services have done so in the belief that survival in the current regulatory environment requires a redefinition of a hospital, from a center for acute care services offered at one site to a broader concept of being a provider of broad-gauged multihospital services as a conglomerate from prevention to rehabilitation.

Traditionally, hospitals have not commercially capitalized on the people traffic in their facilities, as other enterprises have done at the retail level, or on the large corporate capital base that they have accumulated in the last decade. Historically, the community health care market has been the domain of the physician. Today, all sorts of commercial ventures have entered the health care market, from rent-a-nurse companies to fly-away laboratory analysis. These companies have recognized that physicians' practices are essentially small businesses with low capital investment and that many small businesses in one industry will deter market domination by any one of the small firms.

As long as the entering large firm could afford the costs of a two-year market penetration effort and not have its major operations disrupted by local physician efforts, the market could ultimately be made profitable.

The outer limits of this kind of development are unknown. They have been undertaken by nonprofit hospitals, not on the basis that bigger is better, but because of a deep concern to protect a high quality and level of medicine in their institutions, and a recognition that restricted reimbursement practices would, sooner or later, deteriorate their present situation.

Growing Supply of Physicians

Another issue of the 1980s is the expanding supply of physicians. A major cause of this expansion has been the financial support provided by the federal government. Federal support expanded from $30 million in fiscal 1964 to about $1 billion annually in 1974, excluding biomedical research. The number of first-year medical students increased from 8,772 in 1964 to more than 17,000 in 1979.

About midway through the 1970s, the assumption of a physician shortage was replaced by a view that the supply of physicians was, or soon would be, adequate and that an oversupply of physicians was a possibility. As a result, the immigration of foreign medical graduates has largely ended. The major physician staffing issues now are maldistribution of both medical specialty and geography.

In 1978 there were 396,000 active physicians in the United States, more than a 30 percent increase since 1968. By 1990 the Department of Health and Human Services (HHS) estimates that there will be 549,000 physicians, an increase of about 60 percent from current levels. On a per capita basis, there were 177.3 physicians per 100,000 population in 1975, and it is projected to be 242.2 in 1990. During the 1980s, federal policy will probably be aimed at developing and implementing policies that will encourage the efficient utilization of physicians and a large reduction in the support of medical education.

Studies on factors influencing a physician's choice of specialty and location have shown that personal preferences about work content and the degree of professional stimulation in the work environment are major determinants of physicians' career choices. Although different medical schools consistently produce different specialty mixes of graduates, research so far has not identified specific medical school characteristics that account for these differences.

Considerable attention has been given to the relation between the location of residency training and subsequent practice location. Some studies have shown residency location to be an important influence on location choice; on the other hand, some have suggested that physicians probably select a residency training program in an area where they intend to practice. Interestingly, studies of the influence of economic factors, including incomes, have shown only a small relationship to both specialty choice and location.

Given a consensus that a greater proportion of primary care physicians is desirable, two major policy thrusts for the federal government have been put forward. One is to regulate the specialty distribution of residency positions directly in order to limit opportunities for training in other specialties.

Centralized regulation of residency positions was recommended by an Institute of Medicine Committee in 1976. Currently, HHS is considering using Medicare and Medicaid reimbursements to hospitals as sanctions for operating excess residency positions.

The use of third party reimbursement to physicians is also being considered as a mechanism for encouraging more primary care physicians. It has been proposed that third party payers should pay all physicians at the same level for the same primary care services irrespective of their specialty and to be more favorable to rural practice. Physician distribution problems will be of primary concern and emphasis during the 1980s.

Patient Expectations

A third area of concern will be patient expectations in health care during the 1980s. To try and think about a patient's individual expectations as a participant in the health care system is to wonder to what extent the patient will exercise greater control over personal behavior and actions in the future. To know what the patient of the 1980s expects in health care can be estimated by looking at the contrast between yesterday and today.

A hundred years ago, rather than living in a society with instant communications, rapid transportation, enjoyable creature comforts, and a cornucopia of food, an individual probably lived on a farm miles from neighbors and isolated from the world, and depended on the family for food, shelter, and heat, and on a horse for transportation.

In those times an illness meant that the family provided total care; a horseback trip would bring a physician a day or two later, carrying a black bag filled more with concerns and caring rather than a medical armamentarium of any usefulness. Patients knew they were responsible for their own health, its maintenance, treatment, and subsequent consequences.

Today an urgent illness means a telephone call on 911, transport to a hospital by a paramedic team in an ambulance equipped with telecommunications equipment, the prompt availability of a physician with comprehensive knowledge of human biology, an array of technical equipment, an improved set of probabilities for recovery, and a prolonged life with few limitations.

In 100 years personal responsibility for health has been transferred from the individual to the nation. Society is expected to bear the costs of poor health practices, when an individual's biological machinery fails under prolonged abuse. Personal good health seems to have become a responsibility of the nation and not a personal duty. Today the medical system is held responsible because it has failed to conquer all disease and the physical and mental outcomes from the many social maladies of our society. The past successes of reducing death rates, increasing life expectancy, and decreasing the health gap between rich and poor, black and white, and city and farm have created unrealizable health expectations. In the process, the medical demands of society have come to be reflected in the cliché of the "worried well," rather than of the "worried sick."

Today the prime determinants of health status are personal behavior, food, and the nature of the environment. Most people do not worry about their health until they lose it.

These thoughts are familiar ones in the world of medical care. The difference for the 1980s is that the largest single funder of health care, HHS, has accepted the concept that promotion of health care status should be extended through both individual and community action. This means that the research funding of HHS will shift during the 1980s from almost total emphasis on biological processes to major interest in social, behavioral, and environmental issues that affect health status.

Expanding Primary Care

In the 1980s, medical service at the primary care level will probably expand, and, rather than try to limit demand from patients, the government will focus restraints for rising costs on providers. The fundamental problem, however, is that the existing system provides irrational opportunities for health services to patients who rationally accept the offer. There are still many diseases that are untreatable but, because palliative support is provided in hospitals and health insurance covers the cost, patients use these services.

These diseases will remain incurable until new biological knowledge is developed. Therefore, if there is to be a trade-off between health care dollars, the bigger payoff is to use existing health care funds for expanding comprehensive medical research programs. Since the end of World War II when the federal government began substantial support of biomedical research, medical knowledge has expanded at a steady and, at times, spectacular rate. The most promising route for reduced health care costs is medical research, rather than expecting totally rational patient behavior.

CHALLENGES FOR THE 1980s

Seeking a Coherent Policy Perspective

What does all of this mean in terms of a challenge in the 1980s to American hospitals? As an American enterprise, hospitals are still seeking, with futility, a coherent perspective. To catalogue the current difficulties and problems is easily done. To provide good hospital care for all, that is pleasing to all providers of hospital services, may be impossible.

Within the past century one of the major health interests in our country should have worked out a plan for progress. Both the American Medical Association (AMA) and the American Hospital Association (AHA), however, are moving into the 1980s on a platform of doing better, what they have traditionally been doing for several decades. Congress and the administration are moving into the 1980s on the passé political notion of promising what will win elections but paying only what they must.

Pieces of a grand design for hospital care have been floated near the Potomac River, off and on, since the late 1950s. Occasionally a member of Congress or of the Senate has believed there is political mileage in a new shot at national health insurance, cost containment for hospitals, or a continuing potpourri of special interest programs.

The Department of Health and Human Services has been promulgating statements and papers on national hospital policy that have read more like an idealistic novel than a realistic appraisal of the future capabilities of the field.

In essence, despite the profuse rhetoric of the past decade, the current shortcomings in hospital care have never been faced in a coherent realistic way. Nor is it probable that a balanced policy perspective is likely to be forthcoming from any major source of health care leadership to guide developments in the 1980s.

Quality of Care

What should be the goal of the hospital field in American society for 1990? What are reasonable limits for the acceptance of change in ten years by patients, physicians, hospitals, trustees, nurses, bureaucrats, Blue Cross representatives, and politicians? In the past, statements of national hospital policy have too frequently been expressed in terms of soaring idealism that only discouraged knowledgeable health professionals.

Pursuit of medical excellence in the quality of care of patients, regardless of any other consideration, can no longer be a sole goal; nor can it be replaced by a conscienceless concept of cost control at the expense of quality.

The physician's adherence to the concept of doing everything useful for patients as the basic test of the quality of care is rooted in medicine's original approach as a scientific study. Medicine began to be scientific when anatomy became the framework of its study, which led to understandings of various parts of the human body, their interrelationships, and the internal causes of disease. As a result of pursuing medical knowledge within this paradigm, scores of specialized areas from molecular biology to plastic surgery have been established. All are still focusing at a better understanding of the internal workings of the human body.

In the last century, a fundamental dimension was added to the paradigm through the development of infectious disease knowledge and the practice specialty of public health. This additional element meant that factors external to the human body, affecting its internal functioning, were included in a concept of medical care. Environmental hazards from food, smoking, and pollution and concepts about wellness have become visible, but have yet to be incorporated into the physician's test of quality of care. That is to say, in daily practice, the typical physician tells a patient to stop smoking, but the physician does not develop the skills to help the patient modify behavior. The struggle of the 1970s, as a result of the sophistication of modern medical technology and its high cost for marginal improvements in diagnosis and therapy, raised the new test of economic justification in caring for a patient.

As a result of these exogenous elements affecting medical care, the historical definition of quality of care has finally come apart and now needs redefinition within an expanded framework. Quality of care can no longer be judged against the criteria of the maximum use of diagnostic and therapeutic measures that are appropriate to the provisional diagnosis. The key point in the medical care field, the contact between patient and physician, has not yet been affected by these exogenous elements, despite Professional Standards Review Organization (PSRO) efforts.

The historical medical viewpoint of the test of care assumes that patients want to improve and will passively accept the medical care prescribed; however, a major shift has occurred in the quality-of-life thinking of patients in the last two decades. Until recently, a physician was the only educated person in the medical care setting. Today a growing percentage of health care personnel and patients have education and experience equal to that of the physician. These patients are exercising their personal rights to set upper limits on the medical care they receive. The quality of life prospect beyond the acute phase of illness is frequently measured by patient and family and, if believed to be severely limiting, often results in restrictions being placed on physicians in their choices of therapies.

The ultimate test of a workable national hospital perspective must be based on a definition of quality of care that is acceptable to physicians, patients, and hospitals. Viewpoints of politicians, bureaucrats, and insurance representatives are secondary because they will gradually adjust to those of the primary opinion makers. That is to say, any statement of national health perspective must reflect and incorporate an accepted definition of quality of care. This must be achieved if the statement is to be useful as a guide for specific policies. A perspective affecting an expanded concept of today's elements of quality of care would include these kinds of concepts.

GOALS FOR THE 1980s

Seven goals of hospital care to be achieved by 1990 in the United States should be:

1. reasonable access to necessary hospital care services
2. mechanisms for integrating medical care between individual and institutional providers
3. programs to encourage the concept of wellness and preventive medical practices
4. additional ways for patients to participate in their health care at all levels
5. economic incentives that encourage the appropriate use of hospital services for the state of illness of the patient
6. hospital care at a fair price and efficient practices by the providers of services
7. initiative and innovation in hospital services through the leadership of the individuals and institutions providing hospital care

These seven goals are contemporary and, if presented separately, would be generally supported. Collectively considered, it becomes obvious that the outer limits of a particular goal may impinge or overlap areas of interest of another goal, and thereby the goals become unacceptable to specific health interests. However, each of the seven goals represents to some extent a goal acceptable to every element in the health care system. To examine programs that implement these goals, they are individually discussed.

Reasonable Access

Historically, access to hospital medical care has been limited to the admission of patients through members of a medical staff. During the decade of the 1970s, many hospitals drastically altered this traditional practice. Rather than waiting for a smaller-sized medical staff to fill the hospital with patients or for physicians to apply for membership on their own initiative, many hospitals became recruiters. They built primary care centers, still often called outpatient clinics by some physicians; erected medical office buildings; and discounted rents as inducements to recruit physicians. They also created more parttime physician-director positions to attract and stabilize their medical staff, and added fulltime, well-paid physician coverage for emergency room services. In many hospitals, administrative efforts to implement these strategies were vigorously, and successfully, opposed by local physicians.

Most hospitals, in the decade of the 1970s, took significant measures to improve access to their facilities and programs. Where they were coerced or unwilling to face the displeasure of a medical staff, there was a flaw in governance. This flaw was placing institutional harmony ahead of the public good by avoiding the appointment of additional physicians or by establishing hospital-based physician positions.

The access issue is an example of the federal government going in opposite directions at the same time. Currently, efforts are being made to close hospital beds in areas where there are more than 4.0 beds per thousand and to have 1122 reviews reject computerized axial tomography (CAT) scanning units, while reducing patient financial barriers through Medicare, Medicaid, and expanding the charity definition under Hill-Burton.

Unreasonable access to hospital care on a day-to-day basis can only be controlled through medical judgments made in the patient-physician relationships. Access issues for institutions are limited to location of facilities, whether or not to begin or stop a clinical program, and the program's scope of operation.

The public's access to hospital care is basically determined by the amount and type of financing flowing into medical and hospital care activities. To hold hospitals accountable for all failure of access, however defined, is a public disservice and a way to obscure political and governmental failures.

During the decade of the 1970s, the hospital field performed exceptionally well in carrying out its access responsibilities to the public. In the 1980s there will be a further expansion into more primary care level programs, but pockets of underserved areas will remain.

Mechanisms for Integrating Medical Care

The most difficult geographical area in which to provide reasonable hospital care is rural America. Large land areas with low population densities make quality hospital care at any level approaching reasonable cost impossible. The only way to provide a reasonable level of care is through nurse practitioners; well-equipped, freestanding emergency units that are backed up by the maximum in electronics and by a base hospital; and a rapid, reliable transport service.

This concept leads into the second goal, mechanisms for integrating medical care between individual and institutional providers.

Because of the high level of mobility in American society and the general state of well-being of its population, systematic and periodic primary medical attention has been an unattained ideal for the majority of people. Both at the level of the physician's office and the hospital, there is a considerable amount of duplication and redundancy in diagnostic testing, trying out of different therapies, and aimless switching of drugs.

The need to integrate levels of medical care is more a matter of concern to reduce needless medical expenditures than to improve the quality of medical care.

Up to the present, hospitals have not been seriously concerned with becoming the local mechanism for facilitating storage and access to all patient medical care information. Because a hospital is typically the largest local health care organization and probably has the only sophisticated recordkeeping operation and retrieval system for medical data in the community, a potential exists for developing concepts and implementing plans to integrate individual patient care information from all points in the community providing medical care.

With the rapid improvements now being made in the electronic storage and transmission of data, what was an impossible dream yesterday is today a possibility, and tomorrow, it will be an inexpensive service.

Beginning in the late 1960s, a few people began to see and write about the possibilities of developing a large central computer system to store individual medical records. Such a system is expensive and raises issues of confidentiality and appropriate use. It is more reasonable to contemplate a hospital-based network of computers than one large system. Most medical data is only used locally; the servicing and training required to keep such a system up and running can only be accomplished at the local level.

The Concept of Wellness and Preventive Medicine

The third goal for the 1980s is to provide programs to encourage the concept of wellness and preventive medical practices.

Hospitals have traditionally been seen by others and by themselves as repair shops to maintain and improve the physical and mental functioning of the human body. Organized and funded health education departments in hospitals were rare in the later 1960s and have only slowly increased in numbers in the 1970s. Today the typical hospital effort, even in large institutions, is one or two nurses working informally with patients and putting on smoking cessation and obesity clinics, mostly for public relations purposes.

The responsibility for advising patients about good health practices has always rested with physicians. Members of the public who rarely visit physicians and who do not have periodic checkups, which is probably a majority of the population, have not had the opportunity to learn good health practices. Because a hospital is the best-equipped local health care organization, it is the only agency that can operate health education programs that will reach a large segment of the population.

The financing of patient education departments in hospitals has yet to be worked out. When these programs are focused on inpatients, the number of personnel and costs involved are modest. To develop organized, comprehensive, public service programs will substantially increase costs. New sources of funding for these programs must be found and cultivated. To do so will require direction and assistance from the federal level, such as an expansion of the first steps now being taken by HHS and the activities of the Center for Disease Control (CDC). Another step would be to allow a one or two percentile increase over the eightieth percentile when a hospital operates a formalized health education department.

Unless there are unexpected new findings in medical research, the best hope for moderating rising health care costs must come from modifying public behavior to want to use good health care practices.

Patient Participation in Health Care

A fourth goal, which is related to both wellness and the costs of hospital care, is to provide additional ways for patients to participate in their health care at all levels.

The acute care strategies of diagnosis and treatment are dominated by the physician. Patients are mostly involved only at the extremes of care, for example, allowing or preventing tests and procedures or managing chronic disease processes. In the internal workings of the system, patients are typically treated as nonparticipants.

Often moral and ethical matters that arise during hospital care reflect the basic question of the rights and limits of patients and family members to participate in the medical care decision process. The thrust of legal and social changes in the past decade has been toward greater patient rights in determining their medical care. Along with this change has been a quiet shift in attitudes of physicians to accept and encourage an enlarged patient role. The more scientific and surefooted medicine becomes, the greater are the possibilities for joint patient-physician participation in hospital care.

The ways a patient can participate in hospital care in an economic sense have been well discussed for at least a decade with the use of outpatient ancillary services and ambulatory surgery. With five and six days being the average length of stay in several parts of the country, there is no need for additional economic incentives. The use of coinsurance and deductibles to control inpatient services and length of stay has lost its attractiveness to modify hospital costs.

The meaningful economic control point is no longer the hospital, despite political protests; rather, it is at the primary care level, between patient and physician. Discussing monopoly positions of hospitals is chasing butterflies; the working monopolies are between physicians, with the cartel director the primary care physician. Any price or service shopping by patients between physicians is an anathema to the profession.

The remaining choice is either to have the third party carrier shop on a group basis, such as closed and open panel health maintenance organizations (HMOs), or to reinforce wellness behavior through economic incentives directly bearing on the public.

In any event, hospitals need to reinforce and be part of a movement to bring the public and patients into optimal participation in their medical and health care, even though this is a secondary role to that of the medical profession.

Economic Incentives for Appropriate Use of Services

A fifth goal is to provide economic incentives that encourage the appropriate use of hospital services for the state of illness of the patient.

In light of the previous discussion—that appropriate use of hospital services has been by and large accomplished—there is little left to be done. This may be so in terms of absolute hospital costs generated by inappropriate utilization of its services. This does not deny, however, inappropriate hospital pricing policies, deliberate institutional abuse, and maverick patient-physician behavior. Monitoring of the system to avoid these outcomes will probably always be needed.

Hospitals, as informed and keystone health care organizations, must use their insights and influence on the whole range of provider services, as well as on insurance and government reimbursement, to see that each element is properly used in terms of patient needs.

The litany of abuses is long: inadequate outpatient reimbursement; inept application of certificates of need and section 1122; poor PSRO utilization review; gross underfunding of long-term care; and an obese system of regulation.

To accomplish the goal of the proper use of medical care services, primary responsibility and power rests with reimbursement sources and the medical profession. However, the focus of skills necessary to understand how the parts interrelate and which economic incentives are most likely to achieve appropriate usage exists in the medical and administrative leadership of hospitals. Therefore, a crucial responsibility to study and recommend with persistence how this goal can best be achieved rests upon hospitals.

Health care institutions and the medical profession will pay a price for failing to accomplish this goal, but the most serious price will be paid by patients through a deteriorating quality of medical care.

Fair Prices and Efficient Practices

The sixth goal, hospital care at a fair price and efficient practices by the providers of service, developed into a running fight between government and hospitals during the 1970s. It will continue to do so throughout the 1980s.

Everyone familiar with hospital care is aware of opportunities for improving institutional efficiency. What is more in dispute are the causes and remedies. Protagonists rely heavily on myths rather than facts, simplistic problem definitions of complex processes, and proposed solutions that are sure to further complicate problems, because they do not have sufficient organizational understandings and breadth. The rhetoric of hospital critics gives the impression that it is possible to achieve a totally efficient institutional operation. What ought to be discussed is what is a reasonable level of efficiency to achieve. No organization is totally efficient.

Hospitals are particularly vulnerable to criticism about efficiency because of the limits they impose on themselves to respect life and suffering. Economists are good theoreticians and poor humanitarians, because efficient hospital practice is sometimes dangerous to patients. However, the administrative and governance leadership of hospitals too frequently rationalize indifferent operations on this basis and avoid as many hard decisions as possible.

Despite the increasing criticism of cost-based hospital reimbursement formulas, it is unlikely that any satisfactory federally sponsored prospective payment system will be adopted. A refined cost-based system, which is called prospective system, may replace existing formulas. The only possibility to develop a truly prospective reimbursement system rests with hospitals themselves. After that is completed, hospitals must convince the federal leadership of its usefulness.

Initiative and Innovation in Hospital Services

If this goal is to be approached to any degree in the next ten years then the seventh goal will be important: initiative and innovation in hospital services through the leadership of the individuals and institutions providing hospital care.

Physicians and administrators, by the nature of their work, are conservative and tilted toward the status quo. This is an appropriate posture in medical care, where adventurism can cause great damage to patients. Yet, this creates an attitude of unwillingness to experiment organizationally.

The past 12 years have seen more organizational changes than the preceding 50 years. This has occurred because the system's leverage was moved from the institutional level to Washington. If hospital care is to reach its potential in the next decade, local initiative must be regained.

The degree to which these seven goals are achieved in the next decade will bring Americans improved hospital care. The degree to which they are ignored and not vigorously pursued will increase external regulation, raise costs unnecessarily, and justify public criticism of hospital stewardship.

Chapter 2

The Health Field Today—an Iconoclast's Delight

During the 1970s, most administrators seemed certain about issues in the hospital field that now appear to be different than their traditional opinions. As their certainty decreases, the temptation to pick out a seat in the grandstands and observe the field of action is strong. This sideline view isn't satisfying, however, because many of today's proposals do not square with accumulated experiences and insights.

Today, the health field is going through change for change's sake, rather than to bring about a more equitable distribution of health care resources or to provide needed services at a lower cost. The traditional belief that an increasing standard of excellence is an unequivocal measure of quality performance in the health field is rapidly being swept away. This may be as it should be, but it provides little comfort to face the future.

The watchwords of today are adherence, control, and policing of activities; all aimed at modifying and shaping the health care field to the concepts of those wishing to bring about rapid change. No thoughtful administrator would disagree with the need for change since it is the essence of progress. Yet, many of the critics calling loudest for change are using words like "physicians shall" or "hospitals must" to force imposition and confrontation, rather than to urge change based on previous experience and arising out of preceding events. Riding roughshod over the hospital field may lead away from, rather than toward, an improved health care delivery system.

CHANGES TO CONSIDER

Blue Cross

While many of the proposed changes are needed, additional ones are not even being suggested that ought to be considered. First on the list is the traditional relationship between hospitals and Blue Cross. For years, the health field believed that Blue Cross was the financing mechanism for hospitals and part of its family. Yet, over the last decade Blue Cross has gradually moved into a position where it now controls hospitals and will be indispensable for the implementation of any national health insurance program. In its role as Medicare and Medicaid intermediary, Blue Cross serves the interests of those paying hospital bills and the federal government, and not hospitals.

Blue Cross's future is not tied to hospitals, but rather to the interests of the purchasers of hospital services. The only ones who do not seem to recognize this situation are some hospital administrations and governing boards who still sign less than full-cost reimbursement contracts and who even go a step further by purchasing Blue Cross coverage for their own employees. These hospital administrations must recognize what Blue Cross officials saw more than ten years ago: hospitals and Blue Cross plans have different objectives. Yet, there are still some hospital leaders who are willing to grant special considerations to Blue Cross, over and above other insurance companies.

There can be no mistake about it; Blue Cross has identical interests with other insurance carriers. Therefore, it should be regulated in the same manner as these carriers. Where Blue Cross exists because of a special enactment of a state legislature, state hospital associations would be prudent to lobby against its special category and have it treated like all other insurance carriers in the state who offer medical care insurance. The net result would be favorable for hospitals, because Blue Cross would be forced to move from below full-cost reimbursement formulas to a payment structure that is the same as commercial carriers.

Much of Blue Cross' advertising centers around the theme of how they are protecting the public's interest by holding down duplication of hospital services and their costs. This is an appropriate public posture for Blue Cross, but it indicates strikingly the distance hospitals and Blue Cross have moved away from each other. In simple terms, Blue Cross is in an adversary public position with hospitals. To survive, Blue Cross has to be competitive in the marketplace against its commercial insurance rivals. Blue Cross' survival depends on its ability to attract subscribers at a rate lower than, or equal to, those rates offered by other carriers. Thus, any advantage Blue Cross can gain over hospitals to bring about this result is tried. Hospitals need to recognize the legitimate interests of Blue Cross and treat these interests with the same consideration as other insurance plans with similar interests in hospitals.

Health Maintenance Organizations

In the past several years, the public limelight has been focused on health care delivery organizations that have locked physician services, prepayment, and hospitals into one structure. This has been federally promoted as a desirable form of delivering health care. In this arrangement, hospital utilization may be as low as one-half of what it is in the uncoordinated forms of delivery, and these savings justify pushing the health care field in this direction through federally supported planning grants for health maintenance organizations.

Locking together in one corporate entity the three elements—hospitals, physicians, and prepayment—puts at risk the quality of physician services and appropriate use of hospitalization, because prepayment concerns become the dominant element in a closed loop system. This is to be expected since this kind of system can operate and become financially successful only when sufficient numbers of subscriber groups enroll. A benefit package must be offered at a price that is competitive in the marketplace with that of other health insurance carriers.

If the contractual range of services offered is broader than believed necessary by a purchaser, the higher monthly premium will deter buying into the system. Or, if a broad range of services is to be offered, it must be offset by rigidly controlling hospital usage by offering economic incentives to physicians for limiting the use of hospitals. The cost of providing physician services must also be carefully controlled. Both hospital and physician costs must be kept within established budgetary perimeters if the monthly subscriber rate is to remain competitive. Stated another way, the quality and amount of physician services and the use of hospitals are the variables in the system. To the extent that increases in monthly subscriber rates do not impede enrollment of new subscribers or the loss of existing subscribers, costs can be permitted to increase.

When premium rates appear likely to rise, management usually will take whatever steps are necessary to protect its existing price structure by compromising physicians and hospitals service levels. In a closed loop system, economics inevitably puts the prepayment element in the driver's seat since a system will fail without sufficient numbers of subscribers. Two examples demonstrate how this works.

First, assume a physician's group loses its only subspecialist in a particular field. As interviewing for a replacement proceeds, it becomes obvious that the existing salary level will have to be raised significantly, and, in fact, will be out of step with the overall salary scale of the physician group. Two options are available: (a) recruit at the going market rate and violate the group's salary structure, or (b) maintain the integrity of the existing salary scale by filling the vacancy with a less than fully qualified subspecialist. Where higher premiums are required, the physician group will be tempted to bring in a less qualified physician, because it is easier to accept lower standards for one physician position than change the monthly premium rate.

Second, assume that in order to be attractive to a purchaser of a health insurance benefits package, a hospital utilization rate of 550 or 600 patient days per 1,000 members (about one-half the national average) will be required for purposes of pricing the package. Some advocates of a closed loop system take the stance that this result demonstrates the value of integrated health care systems. Looked at differently, this result may be caused by harsh marketing considerations that have little concern with the quality of medical care, but more concern about higher sales and lower marketing problems. It is easy to understand why government officials and Blue Cross representatives are advocates of HMOs.

A review of the past history of HMOs leads to some considerations that need to be remembered when a new program is contemplated.

HMO feasibility studies usually project enrollments at a rate of approximately 10,000 additional subscribers per year, so that by the end of the third year, there will be 25,000 to 30,000 members. Many HMOs that started three to five years ago have been far short of these projected levels, often having reached no more than 25 percent of the projected goal with little likelihood of enrolling significantly greater numbers in the future. When HMOs have been sponsored by large voluntary hospitals, often 50 percent or more of its members are hospital employees and their families. An error of this magnitude can lead to expenses outstripping revenues and to front-end capital requirements much greater than provided for in the feasibility study. This will also lead to higher marketing costs than originally anticipated.

HMO projections of hospital utilization rates for members must also be carefully estimated. Feasibility studies usually project a rate of 550 to 600 patient days per 1,000 members. In the United States as a whole, there are 1,250 patient days per 1,000 population. HMO utilization rates vary from 40 to 57 percent of this rate. Should the projection prove too optimistic, operating losses will mount at a rapid rate. For example, if the national utilization average of 1,250 is substituted as a utilization factor for a member population of 25,000, the additional cost for purchasing hospital services would be 2.8 million dollars, an average hospital cost of $250 per patient day.

This means that the assumptions made in an HMO feasibility study must be carefully derived and be right on target for the initial three or four years of operation if a breakeven point is to be reached at the end of that time. When the enrollment projection is overly optimistic, marketing costs are underestimated, and a projected utilization rate is not met, an HMO can be undone financially. Given the cost constraints now being applied to hospitals, HMOs must provide ways to handle unanticipated financial difficulties if they are to succeed.

Prospective Rate-Setting Systems

Another major problem for today's hospital administrations is the effort to control hospital costs by the establishment of prospective rate-setting systems in various states. Basically, this concept requires that a hospital submit its operating budget for the coming fiscal year to a designated agency of the state for approval. Rates of reimbursement by service or on a patient day basis are determined, and the hospital is notified of the level of rates approved for the next period of operation. On the surface, this appears to be a reasonable and logical approach.

When the experience of states having prospective rate systems is examined, such is not the case. In New York State, which has had several years experience with it, the results are approaching disaster. Many well-managed hospitals are running out of money and operating on three to five days of cash reserves. If the system had been performing as hoped, why has this happened?

When all of the jargon is cut through, it turns out that prospective rates are a new name for ceilings, an old nemesis for hospitals. The game is more complex now than it was 30 years ago, but the effect is the same. Some of its more interesting gambits include:

- Interest expenses on borrowed funds are not recognized at the rate a hospital must pay, even though hospitals borrow money at the going market rate.

- Bad debts are inadequately recognized.

- Increased salary costs that are not budgeted for in the original submissions, ordered by arbitration, or resulting from areawide negotiations, can't be passed through during the fiscal year.

- Arbitrary guidelines of percentages are applied from one year to the next without regard to percentage increases in salary costs.

- Missed deadlines of rate approving agencies force hospitals several months into the next fiscal year before learning whether or not their projected rates have been approved.

- The amount of funds that may be spent on educational programs, such as intern and resident training or a school of nursing, are decreased each year.

Given an innovative rate-making staff of an approval agency, the list can become lengthy. This can also financially strangulate hospitals caught up in this kind of bureaucratic maneuvering. Even though the experience of hospitals in states with prospective rates has, to date, largely been unsuccessful, there are state hospital associations who still actively are considering these programs.

The American Hospital Association has been taking an active part since the days of World War II in shaping national legislation on health care. By the mid-1960s, the association recognized that Washington controlled the destinies of hospitals; therefore, they have been paying increasing attention to federal health care legislation.

Though there now are a number of physicians who are skeptical of PSROs, nearly all have been willing to give it a try to see what could be accomplished. Only if they finally decide that the PSRO programs are interfering with clinical judgments will they withdraw from participation. A program destined to affect the physician-patient relationship to control the expenditure of health dollars simply cannot be successful if its implementation depends on co-opting physicians. If physicians decide neither they nor colleagues they respect, are free to make what they consider to be sound clinical decisions, the program will fail. Recriminations will be plentiful, with the government attempting to convince the public that physicians are at fault. The days ahead are going to be exciting. The changes that occur are bound to delight the heart of an iconoclast.

Back in 1936, Carl Sandburg, commenting on the times, made an observation that has equal force today. He said:

> People are what they are
> Because they have come out of what was
> Therefore, they should bow down before what was
> And take it and say its good
> Or should they?[1]

NOTE

1. Carl Sandburg. *The People, Yes* (New York: Harcourt, Brace & World Inc., © 1936, 1964), p. 187.

Chapter 3

Who Needs a Role and Mission Statement Anyhow?

The need for a role and mission statement may be better visualized by imagining a conversation between a carpenter building a house and the owner.

Carpenter: *Hey lady, how wide and deep do you want the foundation?*
Lady: *Well, I don't know anything about foundations; just do what you think is best.*
Carpenter: *Now that the foundation is in, where do I start laying out for the kitchen?*
Lady: *Oh, that's going to be on the second floor.*
Carpenter: *What second floor?*
Lady: *I've decided on a three-story home with a kitchen on the second floor.*
Carpenter: *You have to be kidding. The foundation was laid out for a one-story ranch house.*

The moral of the story is that before people start to build a house, they must agree on essentials such as its length and width, number of floors, windows, construction materials, and so on. Within these limits, home builders expect owners to move walls, doors, and trim around as the house is being built, even though the previously approved plans and specifications were different.

In building a large corporate organization, people face the same problem: there must be a plan. All houses are not alike, and different people have different ideas about making a house a home. All hospitals are not alike, even though the public tends to think about hospitals as if they were alike.

---

*Reprinted with permission from HOSPITAL PROGRESS, February 1978 © 1978 by the Catholic Health Association. (Portions of this article have been edited to conform with the publication format.)

25

DEVELOPMENT AND SPECIALIZATION EXPLOSION

Until the end of World War II, hospitals were indeed almost all the same. Medical care was severely restricted by existing knowledge and technology. Over the past generation, there has been an explosive development as new medical knowledge and technology substantially increased specialization.

The general hospital has become the center for implementing these new developments. Specialization has proceeded at a rapid pace and has increased the need for expensive buildings, instruments, and technical skills. Therefore, hospitals have had to sort out and decide what they can do, since it is too expensive to be all things to all people for hospital care.

This development has been similar to university changes in the last quarter of a century. The old notion of a group of scholars working together on a collegial basis using only classrooms, offices, field houses, and residence halls has been outdated by the need for high energy research devices, expensive computers, and technical assistants. Today, universities must also pick and choose what they do, because funds are inadequate to meet all of modern day demands and opportunities.

The hospital field has responded to these changes by splintering into extended care and self-care units at one end of the continuum, and by becoming primary, secondary, or tertiary care hospitals at the other end. As specialization has increased, the size of the population in the service area of the hospital has become a crucial number. The more specialized a service or program, the more limited is its demand, and the larger a population base is needed to provide an adequate number of patients.

Today, medical specialization has reached the point where, in some cases, a population base in excess of a million persons is necessary to provide a sufficient number of cases to justify initiating a highly specialized program. This is why hospitals now divide up radiation centers, transplant services, open heart work, and burn units. The trend is toward an increasing number of expensive specialized services for both inpatients and outpatients.

THE HOSPITAL ROLE AND MISSION

If a hospital does not have a role and mission statement, its chief executive officer is in the same situation as a Nautilus submarine commander under the polar icecap without an inertial guidance system. The commander does not know which way to go from the present position.

Two basic questions for any project a person undertakes in life are "What are you doing?" and "Why are you doing it?" The same questions apply to corporations and hospitals.

If a board of trustees doesn't establish ground rules, it has, in effect, written a blank check for the chief executive officer. Fundamental policy direction requires saying this is where the hospital is to go and this is why it should be accomplished. How the hospital gets there is the business of its administration, as long as the methods and procedures are ethical and legal.

Competition for Hospital Resources

Determining the role and mission of a hospital is the most complex issue the administration can confront because the hospital is, at the same time, a service organization, an agent of state government, and an arm of medical education and research.

There are competing demands for the use of hospital resources as users seek to further their own interests. Without a role and mission statement, the administration is placed in a position of picking and choosing the commitment of its resources without knowing how all of its missions are expected to fit together. Without a template or map, administrators are aware that their choices are subject to criticism because of their own value system.

When criticism comes, as it will, the administrators' only defense is that they thought they were doing right, and yes, perhaps their value system is different from that of the criticizer. Under these conditions, the board of trustees will probably opt for peace at any price and hold the administrative staff accountable for getting into trouble.

A hospital has several constituencies, and each has a different perception of what the hospital should be doing. Each group should not be faulted for a biased perspective. However, the board of trustees should have an all-encompassing view and is in a position to balance competing demands.

There are conflicts in the demands for use of the resources. They are not regularly visible; they cannot be touched; and they are invisible on a day-to-day basis. They are, however, sensed through conversation, discussion, argument, negotiation, and the acts of individuals and groups. When they arise, it is in the context of a specific decision or proposed change in operations, which are expressed under adverse conditions with emotions high and rationales low.

The Role and Mission Statement

A role and mission statement is a foundation on which a hospital's public image is built. It is a statement of the direction in which the hospital wishes to move and explains the logic of balancing the conflict in demands from its constituencies. For example, if the primary mission is to provide secondary and tertiary hospital care and the secondary mission is medical education, the administration would choose to spend a greater proportion of its funds for patient services and less on expanding the house staff. Patient convenience would receive greater attention than the number of house staff and residencies needed to provide more than basic medical care.

A mission statement sets the tone of a hospital. It limits the hospital's role by definition. It is a guide for choices that must be made in the future. It prevents an *ad hoc* development that gradually creates imbalances in programming.

The purpose of an institution is explained by a role statement. The earlier example of building a house is premised on an implied notion of what a home should be and on the values that underlie the desire to express a specific socioeconomic status and life style. This is true of a hospital in a more complex fashion, and a much larger family must be considered.

A role statement is a balancing act. If there were unlimited resources, this would not be so, but high quality hospital care must be balanced by the reasonableness of its cost. Judgment and experience are needed to arrive at trade-offs. Over time, the criteria for these decisions change. Twenty-five years ago, television was a rarity in a patient's room; today it is an expected convenience.

Administrators face dilemmas in the more complex and invisible aspects of hospital operation. The types of mechanical systems and medical instrumentation in the facility are important, and are frequently discussed by people in the hospital who know these decisions have future importance. However, they are seldom publicly visible, even to a board of trustees. A role statement provides guidance to the administrative staff in leading negotiations and for attaining acquiescence and support for new accomplishments by the hospital. It lays out the ground rules that people are expected to adhere to and defines reasonable expectations for the hospital. Unless the many publics of a hospital know differently, they are right in expecting a hospital to do what they define as appropriate functions.

A major choice must be made when a role and mission statement is written; a board must determine the level of specificity in which it will be cast. The more global the statements, the greater the choices and judgment; the more specific, the greater the chances for future error and the more limited its application.

A role and mission statement is not a master long-range plan for a hospital. Rather, it is a reflection of the philosophy and permanent interests of the organization. A long-range plan is a tool for expressing more concretely the specific steps to be taken to accomplish the purpose of the institution.

If an individual were responsible for preparing a long-range master plan for a hospital, how would that person begin? If it is the only community general hospital serving 80,000 people and if it has no medical education programs, its role statement would probably be to continue to develop within its existing framework. But what happens if that institution comes to believe that it should be responsible for all health care delivery? Does it mean eliminating private practice physicians and providing medical care by hospital-salaried physicians? What does this decision mean for office and clinic space, for medical records, or for the physician who wants to practice in the community but will not be employed by the hospital?

For a hospital to alter drastically its previous role in a community requires a lot of public explanation, because the public is affected. The role of a large teaching hospital is much more complex than this simple example. Whose interest is served first and at what price to the other interests?

This does not imply that each role is separate and distinct from every other role. There are countless overlaps, and more than one obligation can be served by meeting another obligation. How these get sorted out, compromised, expanded, or contracted is a function of administrative judgment.

GUIDELINES FOR POLICY MAKING

Pressured by competing demands, a board of trustees can easily get lost in the future as one situation after another is raised for a policy decision. What will be the guidelines? It surely will be more than a political decision, even though arm twisting will sometimes occur. Will it be based on which trustees are sitting at the time the issue is raised and decided by independent uncoordinated judgments on what would be the best programs?

If long-term policies are determined by waiting for a specific issue to force a matter, then policy making is occurring under the most difficult of circumstances. Perspective will be limited, and there will be an urgency that forces individuals to overlook hidden implications. To best establish the mission of a public service organization requires deliberative thinking with concern and awareness of the long-term needs and aspirations of a society. The heat of action creates pressures to solve problems immediately to remove these pressures, no matter what the long-term implications.

A role and mission statement is a ruler for a board of trustees to measure specific program recommendations in terms of the permanent goals of the hospital. Specificity in stating future goals lacks permanence. A sound new clinical program can frequently be justified by pointing out how many people will benefit from it and in what ways their lives will be better.

However, this line of reasoning does not deal with how the particular program fits in with the larger needs of society. It does not answer the question of whether or not the same commitment of resources would benefit society better if spent in some other way. It is a fundamental obligation of hospital governance to be concerned with that question. If they won't, who else cares?

Adoption of a role and mission statement is a step toward creating a permanent influence by a board of trustees upon a hospital's operation. It provides a way of being predictable to the staff and to the public. It tells the larger world that the members of the board of trustees propose to have their institution serve society in a particular way and that they will measure all existing operations and future programs by this standard. Their success as trustees is likewise measureable by the degree to which a particular role and mission statement is accomplished.

Even though a role and mission statement adds stability and perspective for a long period of time, it is not a perfect guess about the future. As society and medical care changes occur, it needs to be reviewed periodically, and new determinations need to be made.

Chapter 4

An Overview of Mergers and Shared Services

Before an administrator even considers formally studying the feasibility of a joint service venture with one or more other hospitals or health organizations, some internal soul searching must be done. The current operating philosophy of the institution must be the first consideration. Questions to be answered include:

- Has the hospital ever shared any services before?

- If so, what were they?

- Have they been successful ventures?

- Was the hospital required to give up any essential freedom of action to comply with a joint venture?

- If so, was the transition painful?

- Would the chief executive consider sharing other services based on their past experience?

- How much autonomy and control is the chief executive willing to give up in order to share services with another institution?

DIFFICULTY IN SHARED SERVICES

There is a recognizable hierarchy of difficulty in the sharing of hospital services. If a chief executive understands the degree of difficulty of a proposed shared service and has satisfactorily answered these questions, the chief executive will be able to determine the degree of acceptability

---

*Reprinted and adapted from "Hospital Mergers and Shared Services" by Richard L. Johnson in *Medical Records News* with permission of the American Medical Records Association, © 1975.

or nonacceptability of jointly exploring the feasibility of a *proposed* sharing arrangement with the other interested parties.

This hierarchy is built around the fact that the closer a service impinges on basic medical/surgical care and affects the institution's image, the harder it becomes to share a service with other organizations. Following are four separate levels of difficulty, listed in order of least difficult to most difficult, when services are to be shared:

1. services not directly related to patient care, having no effect on the hospital's image, and requiring little or no change in current operating systems or procedures
2. services not directly relating to patient care, having no effect on the hospital's image, but requiring some degree of uniformity and standardization
3. clearly defined specialized clinical services that carry no threat of compromising general acute care, but may affect a hospital's independent image
4. services involving basic medical/surgical care and directly bearing on a hospital's community image

First Level of Difficulty

The least difficult services to share do not directly relate to patient care; they do not affect a hospital's community image in any way, and they do not require any change in current operating policies or philosophies of a hospital. These are services that may be purchased from an outside organization with little, if any, effect on the internal organization of a hospital. Steam, electricity, laundry, and purchasing (to some extent) are examples of services found at this level of organizational difficulty. In this category, the decision to provide the service internally, share with others, or purchase these services usually depends solely on economic factors.

Second Level of Difficulty

Services at the second level of difficulty likewise do not relate to patient care or hospital image issues. These services, however, do require some changes in a hospital's scope of operations. Examples of services falling into this category or level of difficulty are:

Financial Area

- electronic data processing of financially-based hospital systems
- collections

- negotiations of hospital charges with third party payers
- payrolls
- financial and operating statistics
- patient insurance checking

Personnel Area

- job description preparation
- employee placement service (recruitment)
- wage negotiations
- employee health
- inservice education programs for professionals, paramedicals, and others.

Operating Areas

- purchasing
- central storeroom
- maintenance
- housekeeping

Other Areas

- sharing medical specialists
- ambulance service
- parking facilities
- dietary planning
- security

Third Level of Difficulty

Services at the third level of difficulty do impinge on patient and medical staff functions, but carry no potential threat of compromising general acute care. Specialized clinical services that are clearly defined and function as a self-contained unit are the majority of applications at this level of difficulty.

Ancillary Services

- radiology (diagnostic and therapeutic)
- radiation therapy
- nuclear medicine
- clinical and surgical pathology
- inhalation therapy
- physical therapy
- occupational therapy
- pharmacy
- central supply

Patient Services

- obstetrics
- pediatrics
- psychiatry
- extended care
- rehabilitation
- long-term chronic care
- outpatient department (excluding emergency room)
- home care

Other Services and/or Programs

- residency training programs
- nursing education
- dietary
- medical records

In order to share these services successfully, there must be a standardization of inputs and outputs, joint appointments of some or even all of the medical staff, a willingness on the part of the hospitals to no longer be stand-alone institutions, a limited degree of economic dependence on other participating hospitals, and an attempt at joint long-range planning. These are necessary in order to reduce unnecessary duplication of already existing facilities and capabilities.

Economic factors play a secondary role in the decision-making process for the third level activities. More important to the practicability of these services are political and quality of care factors. The successful coordination of these functions requires an acceptance by the board of trustees, as well as by the administrative staff and medical staff. When the sharing or trading of inpatient services is considered, community acceptance of the program is a must for successful implementation.

Fourth Level of Difficulty

The activities involved in the fourth level of shared systems are those dealing with basic medical/surgical patient care and directly bearing on a hospital's image.

Patient Services

- medical inpatient care units

- surgical inpatient care units

- intensive care unit

- coronary care unit

- emergency service

Ancillary Services

- operating rooms

- recovery room

- patient transportation

Other Services

- patient billing and accounts receivable

- cashiering

- admissions

The determining factors in the feasibility of sharing these services have little to do with economic considerations. Quality of care and politics are the primary parameters in the sharing of services at this level.

SYNOPSIS OF SHARED SERVICES

A sharing of services may include the common utilization of personnel, the common utilization of equipment and facilities, or both simultaneously. There are three general models that can be used to describe the organizational types of shared service agreements in use. (See Figure 4–1.)

Figure 4–1 Three Models of Shared Service Agreements in Use

Third Party Entity

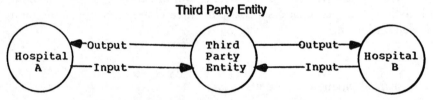

Examples: Data processing center, joint laundry

Purchased Service

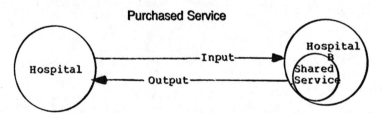

Examples: Power plant (steam, electricity), laundry, laboratory service, radiation therapy, physical therapy

Common Ownership and Operation

Examples: Multiple ramp parking facility, security service, joint laboratory, power plant

Affiliations are also a limited type of shared service. In addition to the sharing of personnel, equipment, planning, and management, other organizational intangibles are also shared among affiliates. Unlike total merger, however, the relationship of affiliated institutions is one in which two or more independent institutions neither lose organizational identity nor do they totally combine facilities.

The trading of services between institutions should not be construed as a hospital shared service. When two hospitals jointly agree that one will maintain a pediatric unit and the other will maintain an obstetrical, this is a trading of services, not a sharing of services.

The successful negotiation of an equitable shared service agreement often requires months, or even years, of discussions between participants. Four factors that must be considered by each of the possible participants who ultimately shape the extent and characteristics of a joint venture are:

1. past performance and current operating policies with regard to sharing;
2. location and size of each hospital with relation to its problems and overall goals;
3. organizational strengths and weaknesses;
4. level of involvement with other institutions.

Once feasibility has been determined, the five final criteria for operating successful shared service programs are:

1. Hospitals intending to share should be reasonably balanced and have some commonality of interest.
2. Hospitals should start with the least difficult and noncontroversial service for joint ventures, because they must learn first to live together in a simple relationship before trying more extensive involvement.
3. Organizational independence should be preserved as a critical factor in the design of a shared service governing document.
4. The top leadership of each institution should participate in the governance of the shared service.
5. Responsibility for daily management should be assigned to one of the participating institutions unless a third party entity is going to be established. The purpose of a shared service is to augment a hospital's service capability to its community, not to control or govern the new operation.

There are actually two generally accepted methods through which mergers take place. One is called "Pooling of Assets," and the second is called "Takeover" or "Acquisition."

POOLING OF ASSETS

Conceptual models for a pooling of assets method involve the emergence of a new corporate entity. The new corporate entity may be formed by dissolving the existing corporate structures, or it may be a "supercorporate structure" that has both existing entities reporting to it.

The pooling concept model often used is where both facilities and corporations are dissolved, and a new corporation is formed along with new facilities being built. (See Figure 4–2.) This model represents an ultimate goal in organization, not as a merger itself, but to provide immediate availability of a new facility to house a new organization.

In reality, most mergers of the "pooling of assets" type usually maintain their old physical plants with a completely new one planned for some time in the future. This was the case in a merger of the Mary Fletcher Hospital and the DeGoisbriand Hospital in Burlington, Vermont, in 1967. Both were teaching institutions affiliated with the College of Medicine of the University of Vermont. On January 17, 1967, the two hospitals were merged into a single corporate entity named the Medical Center Hospital of Vermont. During the latter part of 1968, a new facility was opened with an ability to care for an average of 509 patients per day.

Another example of this particular model is the Tri-Hospital Development Corporation, whose members are the Memorial Hospital of Warren,

Figure 4–2 Pooling Concept Model Using New Facilities

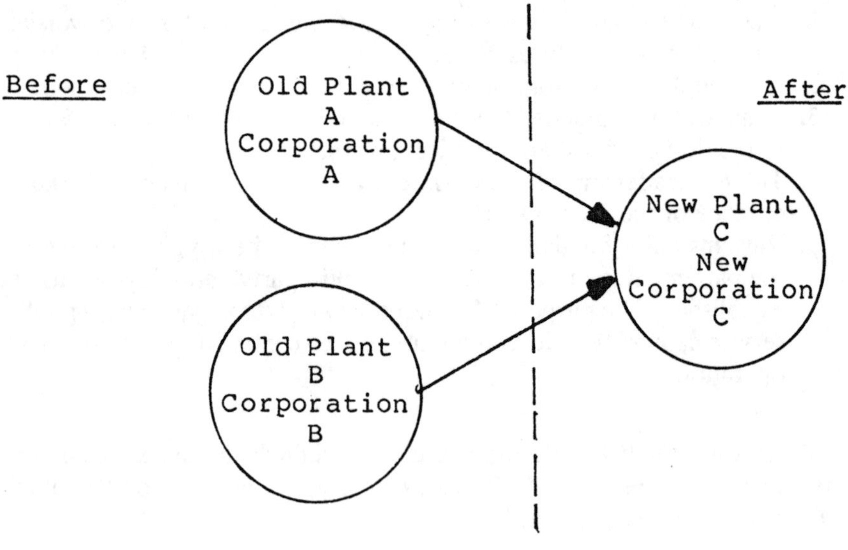

the Patrick V. McNamara Community Hospital, and the Ardmore Hospital, all in Pennsylvania. Until a new facility is built to consolidate the three physical plants, each hospital continues to function as a separate entity. Meanwhile, the merger effort is controlled by the corporation that has been superimposed on the existing hospitals.

A second model under the "pooling of assets" concept is one in which a new corporation evolves, but the facilities remain the same. (See Figure 4–3.) This model, while it may be an end in itself, also acts as an interim step in mergers like the Medical Center Hospital of Vermont. Between the time of the corporate merger in January 1967 and the opening of the consolidated facility in late 1968, this second model actually illustrated the real organization.

There is another possible variation of this concept that is seen from time to time. This is the case where one of the hospitals is abandoned, while the other undergoes complete renovation and enlargement to accommodate the total organization. (See Figure 4–4.)

The Norton-Children's Hospitals, Inc., (Louisville, Kentucky) merger followed this type of organizational pattern. The Children's Division, because of the availability of land and its location within the medical center area, was renovated and became a portion of the overall new structure. The Norton Division, on the other hand, because of its age and distance from the desired location, was sold upon completion of the consolidated facility in 1973.

Figure 4–3 Pooling Concept Model Using Existing Facilities

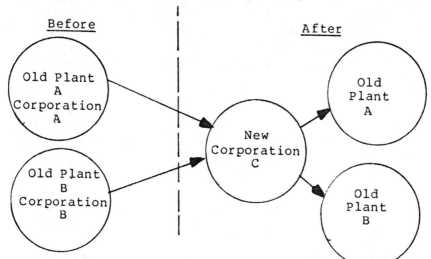

Figure 4–4 Pooling Concept Model Using One Facility After Renovation and Enlargement

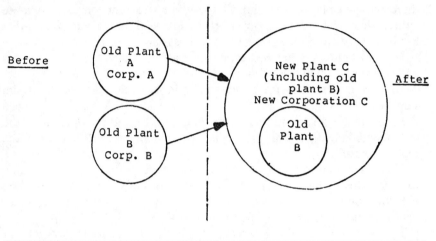

TAKEOVER OR ACQUISITION

The "acquisition or takeover" concept requires that one of the already existing corporations survive, while the other existing corporation is dissolved or completely subjugated to a secondary or supporting role.

The first model is one where both physical plants are disposed of, and new facilities are built. (See Figure 4–5.) This model, as in the case of the first pooling of assets model, may also represent the ultimate goal of a merger. The alternative interim step might be an immediate shutdown of one of the physical plants until a new consolidated facility is built, or both current facilities may remain operational until the completion of a new facility.

The second model under the "acquisition or takeover" concept is where one of the hospitals goes out of existence, while the surviving institution has the capacity to provide adequate health care without building any new facilities or with limited additions to its present physical plant. (See Figure 4–6.) This model represents situations where unnecessary duplication of facilities is readily apparent. The merger may be performed by Hospital B requesting to buy out Hospital A in order to eliminate or reduce competition in order to survive. The other alternative is that Hospital A decides to go out of business on its own and requests that Hospital B buy it out. This may merely be a token transaction on Hospital B's part. The actual physical assets of Hospital A may be sold to outside parties after its formal closing. Hospital A may end up as a plaque in a hallway in Hospital B.

Figure 4–5 Acquisition Concept Model Using New Facilities

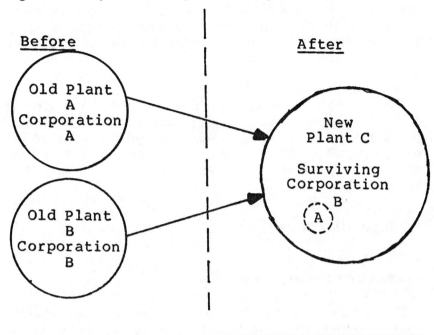

Figure 4–6 Acquisition Concept Model Using Existing Hospitals and Existing Corporate Structure

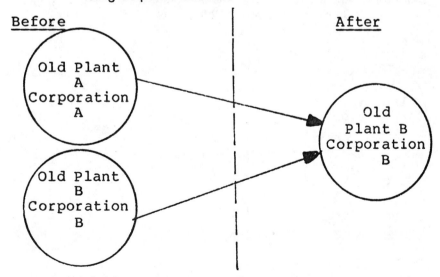

While this model may seem to be an extreme case, it is happening in many rural communities where the hospital's daily census in the service area is decreasing due to the emigration of a younger population group. Eventually, the decreasing population, with its reduced need for both medical facilities, applies fiscal pressures for consolidation. It may do this in an indirect manner by refusing to support fund-raising campaigns of either institution until one finally sells out.

The third model under this acquisition concept is where a surviving corporation continues to operate both physical plants. (See Figure 4–7.) For example, in January 1966, the West Jersey Hospital, a 360-bed, voluntary nonprofit hospital in Camden, New Jersey, purchased the Edgeworth Hospital, a 100-bed proprietary hospital located in Berlin, New Jersey.

DECIDING ON MERGER

Conduct a Preliminary Investigation

There are several essential differences in the unique characteristics of a voluntary hospital system that cause the merger of health care institutions to be an exceedingly difficult and traumatic experience. A decision to

Figure 4–7 Acquisition Concept Model Where a Surviving Corporation Continues to Operate Both Plants

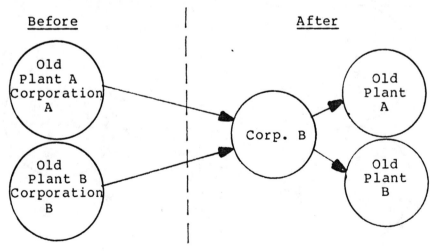

explore merger opportunities is a major policy matter. Before reaching such a decision a hospital should perform a self-analysis of its position. This analysis should include:

- a thorough review of the hospital's short- and long-range plans and goals;

- an examination of the motives leading up to the merger inquiry;

- an evaluation of the hospital's current organization with regard to its capability of merging with another organization and its ability to adapt readily to change;

- a self-determination of what hospitals should be considered as possible candidates for merger;

- determination of what type of organization would easily mesh and be compatible with the existing hospital organization.

A hospital considering the possibility of merger must be ready to cope with arguments that are based on community pride, religious preference, tradition, physicians' privileges, misplaced loyalties, and so on. One of the most frequently occurring problems is that no hospital wants to lose its identity, particularly when that identity is rooted in the historical foundations of the community it serves.

Within a hospital there are a number of major intrahospital challenges that must be resolved. Among these are:

- loyalty of trustees, auxiliaries, and other volunteers

- personal autonomy and security of existing medical staff relationships

- job security sought by employees

- disruption of the existing management system and its ability to be integrated into a new organization

- the initial costs of merger with regard to losses of medical staff, loss of patients, and loss of key personnel

- overextension of management resources

- overestimation of the ability of an existing hospital to provide expanded services

- underestimating the difficulties of integrating incompatible institutions

General integration problems often become monumental when there are difficult personnel problems. Marked differences between hospitals in executive or department director ages, backgrounds, and education can create negative reactions. Differences in salaries and fringe benefits can result in a large number of resignations and must be anticipated.

During the initial period of investigation, all conceivable problems that might threaten the merging organizations must be defined and then carefully documented. These problems should be ranked by their importance, and then studied, from the viewpoint of the new corporation for possible remedies.

Draw up a Formal Agreement

Once a preliminary investigation is completed and the possibility of merger is found to exist, the next step is for the trustees of both institutions to draw up a formal agreement of exactly what they plan to agree upon for merger to take place. In other words, the boards must agree to agree.

Merger proceedings should have as their starting point trustee recognition of the potential benefits to the community for accomplishing a merger.

The initial agreement between the boards of trustees about what they will eventually have to agree to should contain the following areas:

- common goals and shared responsibilities
- separate functions and interests
- corporate organization or contractual affiliation
- composition and representation of trusteeship
- units of administration
- procedure for changing the initial agreement

Getting these kinds of decisions is a long and tedious project. Few direct pressures can be applied because of the lack of financial leverage that is commonly used in business mergers.

There are two other essentials that should occur early in the negotiating process. The first is the choice of administrative leadership for the merged organization. The second essential is at least a tentative choice of a name for the new organization.

Legal Considerations

Since most hospitals are operated as community nonprofit entities, control cannot be gained by an exchange of stock, or by outright purchase for cash. Successful hospital mergers must take place through an agreement of governing boards that places primary concern on whether both communities will be mutually benefited. A successful plan must also protect the interests of the trustees, physicians, employees, and auxiliary members.

Some of the legal considerations that must be taken care of prior to merger are:

- examination of certificates of incorporation and amendments of each hospital in order to determine what restrictions, if any, would hamper merger of the institution;

- examination of the bylaws and amendments of each hospital for the same reasons as the articles of incorporation;

- audit of financial statements of the merging institutions;

- examination of wills, trusts, assignment of incomes, and other similar documents showing gifts to each hospital.

Finally, there are two additional jobs for the hospitals' attorneys in the premerger stage. The first is an examination of state laws to determine whether a merger between nonprofit institutions is legal in that state. Second, the attorneys must determine how many votes must be taken by each board; what is to be voted on; and the pluralities needed to authorize a merger.

With regard to the first item, when Norton Memorial Hospital and Children's Hospital decided to merge, the pertinent state laws in Kentucky prevented a legal merger. These laws were subsequently amended by the general assembly and the hospitals were then merged.

There were two votes required by each board of trustees in the Wilmington Medical Center Incorporated merger. First, both boards of trustees voted on whether to accept the merger "in principle." This vote required a simple majority to pass. The second vote was for the acceptance of the agreement for merger. Passage of this vote required a two-thirds majority.

Accounting Considerations

Premerger accounting considerations must be evaluated because they are concerned with how a merger will be accomplished. If a merger is a "pooling of interests," then the balance sheet items can merely be consolidated by adding the two separate corporation figures together. In this type of merger there is no need for a reevaluation of fixed assets.

If a merger takes the form of an acquisition, then a reevaluation of fixed assets may be necessary before a consolidated statement can be prepared. If, for example, an acquired hospital is bought for a fraction of its book value, the surviving corporation will then have to reevaluate fixed assets on a substantially reduced scale. This reduction would not only affect the depreciation schedules of the hospital, but also its cost reimbursement contracts as well.

Attitudinal Considerations

Attitudinal problems in hospital mergers are typically the most critical problem upon which success of merger negotiations will rest. While the ultimate decision for merger rests with the governing boards of each hospital, their final decision will be influenced by physicians, patients, employed personnel, and community leadership. In turn, each of these groups' attitudes are shaped by factors of importance to them.

Once board members are convinced of the desirability of merger, they in turn must develop this understanding in the medical staff, patients, employees, and community. In many cases, however, medical staff members are ahead of board members in their attitude for merger.

A particular medical staff issue in merger negotiations occurs when hospitals are not uniform in the delineation of clinical privileges for physicians. If the two hospitals considering merger have significantly different criteria for establishing physician privileges, opposition can be anticipated from one or the other medical staffs. Generally, the more restrictive set of criteria is adopted as the surviving delineation of clinical privileges. Medical staff members who are already restricted within the constraints of the wider range of privileges will be even more restricted as the result of a merger.

Under these conditions, a board of trustees can expect some loss in medical staff members. These anticipated losses should not be overlooked in identifying the anticipated cost of mergers.

The probability of this kind of medical staff problem occurring can be determined early in a merger study by examining the ratio of board certified specialists to general practitioners. For example, if Hospital A's staff is made up of 70 percent specialists and 30 percent general practitioners and Hospital B's staff has just the opposite composition, the probabilities of this problem occurring are high.

Management of merged hospitals requires successful application of innovative and highly developed management skills. In essence, managers and department directors at all organizational levels are going to have to be capable of accepting the challenges of a new organization, or they will fall by the side. The process of merger is often confusing to middle-management employees.

A good first step in the managerial consolidation process is to centralize staff management functions and decentralize line responsibilities for patient care. The anticipated results of such a move will be to raise the decentralized decision-making authority to its highest functional level. This will increase a sense of security at the middle-management level and provide a broader, firmer, more cooperative base for further departmental consolidation moves.

In summary, good premerger planning can take some of the edge off postmerger problems. Awareness of pitfalls provides an opportunity to circumvent many problems and to be prepared for the issues that must inevitably be faced and resolved.

Chapter 5

Mergers and Consolidations

When PL 93–641 was enacted, it expanded the scope of hospital reviews of health systems agencies (HSAs), as well as the authority for carrying out these responsibilities. This law made it clear that these agencies have the authority to ensure that applications brought before them have thoroughly examined the potential for multihospital arrangements. Section 1502 of that act provides for ten national priorities, three of which deal directly with developing services through multi-institutional planning.

In essence, the law emphasizes the concept of areawide needs versus institutional needs as seen by a hospital. As part of its communitywide focus in health care, it implicitly assumes that cooperative planning and its logical extension to cooperative institutional efforts will lead to consolidations or mergers. It further assumes that when a merger takes place, the results will be more satisfactory than if two institutions remained independent. This may or may not be the case in a specific community.

THE CONCEPT OF MERGER AND HOSPITALS

Whenever two hospitals discuss the possibility of consolidation or merger, there are usually one or more of the following factors at work:

- potential patient volumes of service that justify only one service rather than two .

- inability of one or the other hospital, or both, to secure planning agency approval for projected programs of service

- restrictive reimbursement from third party agencies

- obsolete facilities and major equipment

- escalating construction costs

- chronic low occupancy in one or more major hospital services
- inability to attract new physicians to the medical staff
- a decreasing market share within a hospital's service area
- inability to secure long-term debt
- a desire to take advantage of physical proximity of the two institutions
- reduced time commitments of physicians for participation in activities of the organized medical staff when combined
- existing roles and programs in both hospitals that complement each other
- a perception that continued competition is counter-productive to a community's best interest and cost containment efforts
- a desire to beat competing hospitals

A hospital that is not aware of any of these problems is not a candidate for a consolidation, but may be one for a takeover merger if it is to be the surviving corporation.

The popularity of the concept of merger is relatively new to hospitals, though over the last few decades they have occurred from time to time. As conglomerates have developed in industry, the mergering of individual businesses into conglomerates has been reported with increasing frequency and led to the use of the same concept in the health field. The use of the term "merger" refers to the turning over of one corporation's assets and liabilities to another corporation. Essentially it is a takeover, with one of the corporations surviving. The model adopted by the Samaritan Health Service in Phoenix, Arizona, and Foote Hospital in Jackson, Michigan, are examples of this type of hospital merger.

In the health field the most frequent form of a merger has been consolidation. In this approach two or more hospitals deed over their assets and liabilities to a newly formed corporation that may continue to operate the existing hospitals. Hospital examples of consolidation include Orange Memorial Hospital and Holiday Hospital in Orlando, Florida, and Childrens Hospital and the Norton Infirmary in Louisville, Kentucky.

A variation from the typical consolidation and merger pattern is where two corporations are left intact, but a governing board with identical membership on both boards is created. Here decision making is centralized, but, because of restricted endowments and trust funds, it is deemed appropriate to retain two corporate structures. This model has been used by the Ear, Eyes, Nose, and Throat (EENT) Hospital and Ochsner Hospital in New Orleans, Louisiana.

Because of interest in the use of the holding company form of organization by business firms, hospitals frequently consider this model. Fairview Hospital in Minneapolis is often regarded as a prototype for hospitals interested in this type of organization. What is meant by this term in the hospital field is a takeover merger in which the institutions absorbed are permitted to retain considerable control over their operations. From an organizational standpoint, they become operating divisions of a single corporation although they have separate legal identities.

GENERAL OBSERVATIONS

A number of conclusions about consolidations and mergers can be drawn: the reasons for undertaking them; the role of the joint committee; anticipated capital and operating cost results; and their success or failure.

Capital Expenditure

Before discussing each of these aspects in greater detail, some general observations are in order. By and large, the results achieved have not been in keeping with the expectations of those who supported consolidations or mergers. When first considered, it usually seems obvious that substantial operating savings can accrue to a community if merger can be accomplished. The opinion is expressed that by combining a number of hospital activities, significant operational savings can be achieved. The necessity for capital expenditures to make an effective combined operation is ignored. In only rare instances does a hospital have sufficient unused capacity to take on an additional volume of service without having to rearrange or add square footage, purchase new equipment, or change workflows. When these elements are added in, costs usually go up and not down on a per patient day as had been anticipated. The capital costs that must be incurred usually more than offset any operational savings. This is seldom known or appreciated at the time consolidation discussions commence or are urged by an HSA board.

Also, there is a tendency to make an employee count of which positions can be eliminated, total up the dollar amount of savings, and jump to the conclusion that a merger or consolidation is feasible. Overlooked are capital expenditure factors and the percentage of revenues from different cost reimbursement programs. When cost-based reimbursement is between 80 to 90 percent of a hospital's revenue, there is little opportunity to achieve additional operational savings since only 10 to 20 percent of a hospital's revenue is generated from noncost reimbursed programs. As the percentage of cost reimbursement declines, the greater the likelihood that operational savings can be developed as the result of a merger. Thus, an individual should expect to find higher levels of interest in mergers where hospitals have low levels of reimbursement from cost-based programs.

Autonomy

A second observation about mergers is that they usually cannot be accomplished when two hospitals are approximately equal in terms of financial strength. If both hospitals are in strong financial positions, discussions between the two may break down over the issue of giving up individual autonomy. This was the case of St. Luke's Hospital and Mercy Hospital in Davenport, Iowa, where negotiations proceeded for three years, up to the point of actual transfer of assets and liabilities to a new corporation and, at the last moment, it was decided not to merge. In this instance, both hospitals were financially stable and could see no advantage in giving up their institutional autonomy.

Public Interest

A third observation is that governing board members usually underestimate the amount of time and difficulty involved in consummating a merger or a consolidation. Because of their personal experience in industrial mergers, they tend to believe that a hospital merger can be decided on a similar basis where a comparison can be made between the stock market value of corporation A and corporation B, and that a decision can be reached about the purchase price using these guidelines. This is not the case, however, because whatever is done is accomplished in the interest of the public good. Both parties must approach merger negotiations from the sole desire to benefit patient care and the community-at-large. This is subject to a wide variation in what is thought to be the public interest. Physicians tend to judge proposed hospital mergers on the basis of how it affects them. Obstetricians want to know whether or not obstetrical units are to be combined, and if so, at which institution. Pathologists and radiologists are interested in knowing who is going to be appointed to direct these professional services. If one hospital's medical staff is predominantly physicians who are specialists and subspecialists and the other staff is primarily family practitioners, the nonspecialty medical staff will inevitably be concerned with restrictions that might be applied to their existing clinical privileges.

The same kinds of fears are found in management. Which administrator will become the chief executive and which director of nurses will survive are the kinds of questions that motivate the behavior of administrative personnel.

Other factors are important to the board of directors. Some trustees will want the proportion of board seats allocated to each of the existing boards to be based on the share of assets contributed by each hospital to the merged organization. Others think that bed size should be used to determine allocation of trustee positions. Where one hospital or both are religious, the distribution of board seats is often based on religious affiliations of the trustees. In yet other cases the decision is made on a geographical representation basis.

STEPS TOWARD MERGER

Getting the Parties Talking

Most hospital merger discussions begin with economic factors as the primary concern of trustees. A typical pattern is for a key trustee to arrive at the conclusion that the community would save money if merger possibilities were explored. Usually the trustee's mind turns to the nearest geographically related hospital because it has been used over the years as the basis of comparison to his own hospital. The trustee then cautiously suggests to other key board members that it might be fruitful to explore a merger possibility. Because he does not want to be considered an advocate of the other hospital by his own trustees, the trustee may not permit his actions to go beyond the point of arranging a highly informal, unstructured meeting between trustees of the two institutions. This meeting usually does not have a formal agenda and is regarded by both parties as quite tentative in nature, imposing no obligations on either side. This climate of "let's discuss but not commit ourselves" leads to a lack of formal planning once the conversations become serious and often to an inadequate basis for proceeding to the next steps toward merger.

In some instances board members may agree to request the two chief executives to pursue this possibility and outline a course of action to be followed. When this device is used, it is unusual to reach meaningful results. Administrators easily recognize the sensitive areas that are possible sources of disagreement, such as appointments to a combined medical staff or strongly-held attitudes of individual governing board members. The result is often a stalemate, with the two chief executives unwilling to report back to their own boards and return the problem to them. The best that can usually be hoped for are two administrators who can reach agreement on minor trade-offs or sharing of services that do not directly affect or impinge on patient care. The lesson to be learned from experience is that merger is a governing board matter that cannot be delegated to others. Trustees represent ownership in the nonprofit setting, and owners must deal with owners if a merger is to be accomplished.

Discussing All Alternatives

Once both parties to a merger decide to examine inter-institutional possibilities carefully, they usually reach a conclusion that all alternatives, such as trade-offs of clinical services, sharing of selected services, or merger or consolidation, should be explored without establishing any priorities. This is understandable from trustees' points of view. They want to be able to be assured ahead of time that the time spent on the project will lead to results. But by failing to establish priorities between the potential major roadblocks, they create difficulties that go unrecognized at that stage of development.

Should the joint merger committee start at a point of discussing possible trade-offs, such as hospital A taking all obstetrics and hospital B all pediatrics, the door to consolidation or merger is quickly closed. Obstetricians using the hospital that will lose its obstetrical service and the pediatricians using the hospital that will lose its pediatric service are going to be inconvenienced, so it is to be expected that they will be against such a move. In this situation trustees quickly come to appreciate the fact that merger can be achieved only when they are willing to override the objections of particular physicians. To do so creates a degree of ill-will that leads away from, not toward merger.

The sharing of hospital services, such as the laundry, a computer, joint purchasing and stores, or a common print shop do not affect medical staff members because they are not involved. However, administrators have interests in these operations, and they may agree to such a step because of the belief that the results will meet their early expectations of improved efficiency and quality of service. Frequently, however, these results are not achieved, and often sharing services leads to administrative friction. Anything less than achieving the optimum becomes a reason for not going any further in sharing additional services. Because this result almost inevitably occurs, the joint shared service is not a step toward a merger or consolidation, but rather acts as a deterrent to it.

Many governing boards believe that if a merger cannot be accomplished within a reasonable period of time, the joint sharing of hospital support services may create a climate for merger some time in the future. They fail to appreciate organization dynamics that subsequently take place.

Setting Priorities

If the objective is to bring about a hospital consolidation, it is wiser to examine the subject openly and candidly, rather than act as if trade-offs or sharing are acceptable as steps toward a merger. At the same time laying a merger proposal on the bargaining table too quickly is apt to result in a quick termination of negotiations. Both parties have to be ready and willing to enter into discussions. If one side is willing to move and the other side is not, the issue cannot be forced. Put in different terms, the two parties should not sit down at the negotiating table until the "grapevine" has clearly indicated that both are receptive to discussion. All too often there is a rush to get the two parties talking before they are of an equal mind about where they may be headed.

Knowing that few hospitals are aware of this hazard, how to deal with it after the fact is important. When negotiating parties recognize that they may have moved forward too rapidly in a negotiation, the chairman may be placed in an uncomfortable position. He may find that some participants have thought about a possible merger, that other trustees have been giving first priority to sharing services, and that still others may have considered trade-offs. Even an adroit chairman may be caught in an awkward situation.

To avoid this predicament, a chairman must make sure that trade-offs, sharing, and merger are ranked in priority for investigation. Even though trade-offs and joint sharing of services do not lead to merger, it is possible to aim for consolidation or merger, and then back off to sharing or selected trade-offs.

When first priority is given to consideration of consolidation, where both hospitals pool their assets and liabilities into a newly created corporation, and with the goal of building one new hospital by replacing the two existing ones, care must be exercised to prevent the selection of a site before the successful completion of negotiations. To permit a new site to become part of the negotiations almost always leads to a breakdown of negotiations since some of the participants will focus on that issue as a primary issue rather than the concept of consolidation. This can be avoided by deferring this decision to the new governing board. Similarly, the issue of medical staff bylaws is better left for decision making after consolidation.

THE ROLE OF THE JOINT STEERING COMMITTEE

Because of these typical reactions to merger or consolidation, an organizational tool that will operate effectively must be selected. The creation of a steering committee is a logical outgrowth of informal conversations between two hospitals. Typically each hospital is represented by selected trustees, chief executive officers, and physicians, who are the acknowledged leaders of their medical staffs. In appointing these persons, thought must be given to those persons who may have conflicts of interest with the planned goal. Ideally, steering committee membership should be limited to individuals who can maintain objectivity throughout the process.

Persons with clear-cut vested interests in the decisions reached often lose objectivity under the pressures that inevitably arise in steering committee deliberations. For this reason it may be desirable to exclude not only the chief executives as voting members, but also physicians practicing in the two institutions. Physicians who vote on steering committee matters often find themselves uncomfortable with their medical staff colleagues when they support steering committee decisions that adversely affect selected specialists. Both administrative and medical staff inputs are essential to the process, but present conflicts of interest when voting gets under way.

Phase One: Review Programs and Facilities

The activities of a steering committee may be divided into two phases. The first phase is to review existing and planned programs and facilities of the two hospitals. When this is completed, economic justification can be explored for merger or consolidation. In addition, this phase needs to be concerned with an assessment of existing attitudes of key trustees, physicians, administrative personnel, and knowledgeable community leaders. Attitudinal factors are the single most important aspect in determining merger.

Once these assessments have been made, a decision must be reached: either push for merger or consolidation, or back off to joint sharing or trade-offs. If the decision is to proceed on consolidation or merger, then phase two is entered.

Phase Two: Develop a Strategy for Consensus

This second phase centers on the development of a strategy to arrive at a consensus by both governing boards so that they are in agreement with the position of the steering committee. Phase two requires frank and candid discussion by the steering committee and needs to be conducted in private. At this stage, key persons with vested interests in the first decision should be excluded, unless they represent ownership interests. Participants may become uncomfortable at this stage since they are privy to a great deal of information that simply cannot be shared with those persons not directly involved. Caution has to be exercised to be sure that the information being discussed remains confidential. Objectivity in dealing with information is a crucial ingredient for all who participate.

In order to function effectively throughout both phases of the process, six considerations need to be kept in mind:

1. Both hospital governing boards should provide their steering committee representatives with a clear mandate that delineates their authority through the adoption of a formal resolution. At the time of adoption, all board members need to understand that they will not be kept informed of the discussions in a detailed way as they take place.
2. Persons with vested interests need to consider carefully how they may jeopardize their personal interests if they serve on the steering committee.
3. For an effective decision-making process, the size of the steering committee should be small, preferably in the range of six to ten with one-half from each hospital.
4. The chair should not be rotated on the steering committee, since stability and continuity in this position is needed.
5. Each hospital should be willing to submit its recommendations for steering committee membership to the other institution for concurrence.
6. All steering committee members need to recognize that decisions reached by that body, once adopted, become an individual responsibility to accept and support among their constituents.

Selecting a Corporate Structure

With the quantitative data and attitudinal factors identified, the ground rules for steering committee participation accepted, and a decision for pursuing consolidation or merger accepted, the focus of negotiations shifts from "Should we do it?" to "How shall we do it?" Primary concern then centers on selecting an appropriate corporate structure. Should one hospital corporation survive? If so, which one? If neither, should a new corporation be formed?

Answering these questions and related issues involves hospital attorneys, who need to examine carefully the conditions and restrictions on gifts and endowments, discussions with holders of outstanding long-term debt, anticipated adjustments from cost reimbursement sources, the costs of reconciling differences in personnel fringe benefits between the two hospitals, and the size and composition of the governing board. A wide variety of these subjects will find their way to the agenda of the steering committee. As problems unfold, steering committee members may push to hurry up, consummate the merger, and deal with the problems of reconciliation afterwards.

Getting the Two-Thirds Vote

At this point, the knowledge and sophistication of steering committee members in merger negotiations often create a different viewpoint than prevailing trustee viewpoints among the nonsteering committee board members. This is often overlooked. Since approval of a merger requires a vote by both full boards of trustees, the kinds of questions that will be asked and the kinds of replies that will be acceptable in full board meetings must be considered. A tactical judgment must be made between the hurry-up approach or the "let's get answers to all reasonable questions before we put the questions to both governing boards" approach. In either event, sound strategy dictates that two votes be taken by both boards. The first vote may occur as early as the completion of phase one, or it may be held when nearing the end of phase two. In either case, the full boards of both hospitals are usually asked to adopt a resolution stating that they agree in principle with the merger. This requires a majority vote when a quorum is present. Such a vote has no legal standing but merely signifies the intent of both parties. The form of the merger is known and discussed. If hospital A is to take over hospital B or if hospital A and hospital B are to form a new corporation is usually clarified at this point.

At some later date, usually measured in weeks or months, the governing boards will again be asked to vote on the matter. The second time, a two-thirds approval is required as specified in most states under their laws governing the acts of corporations. The objective of the second phase is to assure a successful two-thirds vote by both hospital governing boards.

No timetable can be developed for phase two. The amount of time required depends on how long it takes to secure agreement on the type and form of the merger; and more importantly, how long it takes to answer every individual steering committee member's questions as fully as possible. Until there is informal unanimous agreement among all members, there is no point in going to both boards of trustees to seek a two-thirds approval. The difference in personal attitudes has to be reconciled, because the steering committee's support of the merger is needed in a successful vote. If necessary to secure support from all participants, the steering committee may informally come to agreement on the names of the trustees for the new corporation and the filling of the key corporate positions. Because of their involvement in merger discussions, it is not unusual for a steering committee to agree to appoint its members as the trustees of the surviving or new corporation.

In the event consolidation is the chosen route, a steering committee is faced with appointing an attorney to file for incorporation and to construct a new charter and bylaws. The two hospitals also need to employ an accounting firm to prepare consolidated financial statements and to work with the attorneys on a way to deal with the holders of any outstanding long-term debt. In a takeover merger it is particularly important to use an outside auditing firm to assure a full disclosure of existing and potential liabilities of the hospital being acquired. Both the attorneys and accountants should be new to the scene and clear of any charge of potential conflict of interest from either side.

When a steering committee has agreed on an appropriate organizational structure and has worked with the attorneys and accountants to resolve problems in their respective areas of concern, the committee then should come to grips with the need to develop a plan that assures a successful vote by two-thirds of both boards and quick dissemination of information to hospital personnel, medical staff, and the mass media. This can be accomplished by completing the following five steps within one day:

1. Conduct a joint meeting of both governing boards to explain the recommendations of the steering committee.
2. Conduct separate board meetings to act on the steering committee recommendations.
3. If approved by both boards of trustees, hold an early afternoon meeting of hospital department directors to inform them of the decisions reached.
4. Conduct a late afternoon meeting with the separate medical staffs to inform them of the decisions.
5. Hold a press conference the following morning to inform the mass media of the decision about merging or consolidating, and to answer any questions they might have about the matter.

If the two boards do not agree, then it is not necessary to hold meetings with department directors, medical staff members, or the mass media. During the latter stages of phase two, the key members of the steering committee are often requested to have one-on-one interviews with the other trustees so that the majority of their questions and concerns can be resolved before taking action at separate board meetings.

Even when all of the steps outlined are carried out, there still is no assurance that a steering committee's recommendations will be accepted at separate board meetings. If the recommendations fail to be approved by either board of trustees, the steering committee is faced with a decision of whether to try again or to cease operation. This determination should be postponed for a week or two after any final board action so that an objective reappraisal can be made about the desirability of a second effort.

The process of merging hospitals is a unique experience that depends on putting community interest before institutional pride. Those who have participated in this kind of activity have come to appreciate just how wide the gap is between the idea and reality. Oliver Wendell Holmes knew this when he wrote, "Every real thought on every real subject knocks the wind out of somebody or other."[1]

NOTE

1. Oliver Wendell Holmes, Sr. *The Autocrat of the Breakfast Table.* (New York: The Heritage Press, © 1955), p. 100.

Chapter 6

Rural Hospitals Face Change for a Bright Future

Of the whole spectrum of acute hospitals, those serving rural areas are least likely to be adversely affected in the coming years. This will be the case even though they have traditionally had the lowest occupancy rates, the greatest number of general practitioners, the most limited range of services, the lowest average costs per patient day, and often the greatest difficulty in balancing their books.

Before looking at their future, a few facts are needed to put into perspective the difference between nonmetropolitan hospitals and metropolitan ones, since this is the closest distinction which can be made because of the way data on the hospital field is collected. Of the 5,875 community hospitals in the United States, 49.9 percent are nonmetropolitan, while 51.1 percent are in the SMSA's (Standard Metropolitan Statistical Areas). In terms of the 941,844 beds in operation, 26 percent are nonmetro and 74 percent are in the cities and their suburbs. The average size of hospitals is 236 beds in the cities and 84 beds in smaller communities. Average length of stay is 7.1 days in rural America and 7.9 days in cities, a difference of 11.3 percent.

When all types of beds are included, rural hospitals average 13.5 surgical operations per bed per year, while the larger metropolitan institutions average 19.2 operations per bed per year. The smaller hospitals average 65.2 visits per bed per year in the emergency room and city hospitals 76.0 visits annually. The average occupancy is 68.2 percent for rural hospitals and 77.4 percent in the city.

The conclusions that can be drawn represent a mixed bag of effects. Nonmetropolitan hospitals are one-half of all U. S. community hospitals,

---

*Reprinted with permission from *Hospitals*, published by the American Hospital Association, © January 16, 1978, Vol. 52, No. 2.

but have only one-third of the beds, have lower occupancy rates, are less intensively used, and have a shorter average length of stay.

As complexity has been heaped upon complexity through increasing regulation, the small rural hospital chief executive has found that he daily deals with physicians, employees, patients, and visitors who behave in about the same way they did last month or last year. Yet, every time he opens his mail and reads trade association newsletters, professional periodicals, and communications from government agencies, he inevitably concludes that the hospital system has deepening problems. When he thinks about hospitals in terms of the small, rural hospital he is usually left somewhat bewildered because the outcry seems out of proportion to what he can observe at home. He appreciates that the hospital he manages is providing the same needed community service it did yesterday, last year, and a decade ago.

As a frame of reference consider what is likely to be the circumstances of a typical eighty-four bed hospital in a town of 13,000 serving a trading area population of 21,000. Such a hospital usually has at least one physician who has accepted a personal responsibility of working towards the improvement of the hospital care. This physician is probably the only boarded general surgeon in the community who has a reputation which is secure, and who acts as a confidant of the other physicians, and the administrator as well. In all likelihood, he arrived in town twenty or twenty-five years ago with no fanfare, few friends, and a new bride. He made up his mind that the most desirable qualities of living could be found in a small town and that, in such a setting, this could be combined with his drive for professional competence without being compromised. Having made such a choice, and lived by it for two or three decades, such a physician inevitably becomes the clinical leader of the community. In reviewing his performance, one is likely to find he has been the prime mover in eliminating fee-splitting, bringing younger, competent physicians to town, and that he has been progressive both clinically and socially: reacting positively to changing times and government regulations. He probably has established close personal ties with the leading figures at the state university medical school and is known throughout the medical community of the state.

Most rural areas throughout the country have this kind of physician, one who represents the very best that can be found in private practice. As government regulations grow, and there is talk in congressional circles of attempting to control physicians' incomes, one wonders if these leaders in rural medicine will continue to give as much of themselves in the future if there is an imposed system of medical controls, or if they will join the ranks of those physicians who have become forty-hour a week clinicians. Will such physicians be willing to substitute PSRO criteria for their own clinical judgements in coming years? These are the imponderables to be faced in the next decade.

Prospectively determined hospital rate schedules are likely to have a far greater impact on urban hospitals than rural ones. Rural hospitals are less apt to be targets of union activity than their city brethren, and therefore will not get caught in a squeeze between an approved rate structure and subsequent concessions made at the bargaining table with organized labor.

A small rural hospital is not likely to be required to justify to the same degree proposed building projects that will be required of urban hospitals when submitting a certificate of need application. Many of the criteria now being applied by HSA's are based on an assumption that there are several hospitals in the same service area and that the comprehensiveness of available services should be rationalized.

Because many rural hospitals have limited, or no other hospital competition, they may find the certificate-of-need application has sections in it that are not pertinent to their situation. For example, most of the HSA project application forms have a section requesting documentation from other hospitals in the area indicating their agreement to support the application. If the application is for routine laboratory equipment and the nearest hospital is 45 miles away, the securing of a letter of support hardly seems worthwhile. Yet it doesn't seem prudent to take a casual approach to filling out such a form, knowing that those reviewing them are doing it for both urban and rural hospitals. Giving these forms a "lick-and-a-promise" runs the risk of being turned down for lack of completeness, even though there is no question about need.

Assuming careful documentation, a rural hospital may find itself trying to justify its application for new laboratory equipment with an inadequate hospital occupancy rate in terms of HSA standards. A rural hospital may be running an occupancy rate in the sixty to seventy percent range and worry about this factor being used to deny a request for laboratory equipment. The administrator may find himself in a Catch-22 situation. To protect the hospital's interest he may consider making a big production of the required public hearing, by taking two or three physicians, the part-time pathologist, and three or four trustees to such a hearing. If the meeting is seventy to eighty miles away, he is faced with asking these people to make a 150 mile round trip, for what may turn out to be a routine approval that takes five minutes. On the other hand, if someone on the board of directors of the HSA raises a question, the rural hospital may well need the presence of its representatives.

Turning from the HSA problems of rural hospitals, the basic question they face as an essential part of the health delivery system is "What is a substitute for the small, rural freestanding hospital?" Thanks to television, and the show M*A*S*H, the helicopter has moved to the forefront in thinking about the rapid transportation of patients. Would a small town be willing to replace its hospital with "The Eagle of Mercy" or "The Winged Caduceus"? From a cost standpoint, it could easily be justified. A new "chopper" would require a capital investment of no more than five to ten new beds, based on project costs of recent construction. From a logistical standpoint, it would not be an insurmountable hurdle to handle eight to nine admissions per day.

On the other hand, a modern hospital is no longer an institution of beds with ancillary services attached, but rather, has become a collection of diagnostic and treatment facilities with beds attached. A helicopter service doesn't provide answers for the problems of the need for an emergency room, stat orders, and a growing volume of tests and procedures provided by the ancillary services. It must be concluded that helicopters are no answer, even if cost justified.

If the rural hospital can't be replaced, can it be organized differently for greater efficiency and effectiveness? There are some possibilities to be considered, including:

1. Sell out to an investor-owned chain.
2. Sign a management contract with an investor-owned chain.
3. Sign a management contract with a nonprofit chain.
4. Form a consortium of rural hospitals within the state.
5. Buy out, and own and operate several rural hospitals in the same area.
6. Become a satellite of a large voluntary hospital in the metropolitan area.
7. Stay as is.

Thinking along these lines, the problems are not too hard to identify, perhaps being easier to spot than they would be in a large city with many hospitals and related health care institutions. But the solutions are no easier and might even be more difficult to come by, because of the growing restrictions on resources. Not only are dollars being stretched further and further to cover the necessities of operating a hospital, but the lack of well trained personnel in some of the key positions means that cross training and sending employees out for this purpose is a never-ending chore. As part of a large system, this problem would be ameliorated.

Yet, to be part of a larger system may have some drawbacks as well as advantages. Local HSA's are strong in their insistence on cooperative planning among hospitals. This is not a serious problem, though many of the guidelines don't have much applicability to a rural hospital. The obstetrical department is a particularly thorny problem. Even though the department may have maintained an average occupancy of between fifty-five and sixty percent, the guidelines call for seventy percent; and its applicability to a rural hospital can be questioned. Even if an enthusiastic junior HSA staff member tried to apply such a guideline, a rural hospital could probably marshall sufficient support through community leaders, such as a mayor, chief of the medical staff, president of the chamber of commerce, and chairman of the hospital board. Through their efforts, a public hearing could be packed, and in a practical sense, it would be virtually impossible for HSA board members to vote to decertify an obstetrical service.

In hospital circles it is frequently heard that the future of small rural institutions is more shaky than that of larger, urban hospitals. Measured only by the usual statistics, it appears this would be a conclusion one might reach. But those people who have lived in a rural community know that a hospital will continue, no matter what regulations agencies might adopt. A rural hospital belongs to its community, and the people who live in the area. This is unlike an urban area, where people feel differently about hospitals. In cities hospitals are not apt to be regarded with the same warm feelings. There is little, if any, feeling one way or the other. The hospital is impersonal; like the fire department, it is there if needed, but isn't considered a part of daily life. In a rural community though, everyone reads the daily newspaper and its list of admissions and discharges; and visitors are always dropping in for a five-minute chat with a patient during their lunch, or on their way home from work. This can be demonstrated by the abuse of official visiting hours in rural hospitals. In cities, visiting hours can be strictly enforced, but attempt to do so in a rural community and the public image of the hospital will immediately suffer. Being part of the life of the community means that there is a feeling of goodwill towards the hospital which is its greatest strength in the coming years of adversity. This is an asset every rural hospital administrator appreciates.

A single hospital in a small town is the least vulnerable of all hospitals, but the same is not equally true for two hospitals in one small town. In all likelihood, they will find it necessary to consider consolidation, particularly if both hospitals experience an average occupancy below HSA guideline levels. Reimbursement formulas will sooner or later automatically force the issue by paying costs at an arbitrary occupancy level of 80 percent. Where both hospitals are running in the sixty to seventy percent range, it will only be a question of time before the cash flow will decrease to the point where the two governing boards will have to sit down and seriously discuss consolidation. Once a merger is accomplished, a much stronger position will result, because the issue before the public will no longer be one hospital or two, but one hospital or none at all: quite a different community equation. Looking ahead, it can be concluded that the number of two-hospital towns will be sharply reduced in the next decade, but this will eventually lead to a politically strengthened rural hospital system.

It can be asked if that outcome is really a total answer, or if there is still something missing. The missing part has to do with the increased complexity of dealing with regulatory agencies. While this represents an ultimate strength of a rural hospital, external demands for documentation and justification of its continued existence cannot be ignored.

These factors can swamp the existing capabilities of a rural hospital management information system. Report forms for post audit reviews, OSHA standards, PSRO data on a wide variety and type of cases, patient origin data, inventory records, departmental cost information with appropriate apportionment of indirect expenses, and on and on, are now part of daily activities. A rural hospital is at a disadvantage in this kind of regulatory environment because they need access to a wide range of highly qualified specialists to competently handle these problems. But these specialists are not needed full-time, only when another legal-looking form comes to the administrator's desk. This now seems to be occurring at the rate of one per week.

The information requested often goes well beyond the needs of a hospital for internal management control, yet agencies seem to be unconcerned with this problem. Agencies have a way of making it plain that the information requested is vital to proper consideration by a consumer-dominated board of directors who would never understand a lack of compliance with what they consider to be a reasonable request for information. The fact that data may be misleading is beyond the control of the rural hospital. What would be helpful would be to have in-house legal talent to look after such problems. Unfortunately local attorneys used by rural hospitals on corporate matters are seldom attuned to agency regulations. The kind of expertise now needed may not even be available locally, but if it is available, it is probably in a large investor-owned chain hospital.

There are other kinds of services that are already, or may soon become, out of reach of a rural, freestanding, small hospital: deep therapy, complicated laboratory examinations requiring highly sophisticated equipment or personnel, ultrasound, neurosurgery, CAT scanners, cardiovascular surgery, sophisticated orthopedic procedures, or neurological disorders. Beyond these services, it may be difficult to come up with any additional services. The increased local availability of both specialists and better trained family practitioners is leading to fewer and fewer patient referrals away from a community.

Of the 323 diagnostic groupings for live discharges, excluding deliveries and newborns among the top fifty hospital diagnoses, 15 percent of the total, account for 51.5 percent of the discharges.[1] Of these top 50, with the exception of one or two, all diagnoses are routinely admitted to most hospitals. In a review of the same classifications, but using patient days rather than live discharges, has shown that the leading fifty diagnoses account for 35.7 percent of all patient days.[2] Since an average length of stay in metropolitan hospitals runs 11.3 percent greater than in rural hospitals, it means that the more difficult and complicated work is being referred from rural to metropolitan institutions. Direct patient care in the future will be handled more and more at the local level as well qualified family practice physicians move to small towns. Those requiring specialty care not available in town will continue to be referred out, but this volume of referrals will likely decline in the future.

The role of a small rural hospital is bound to grow in spite of all the dire predictions about the upcoming demise of these institutions. Recognizing that mergers and consolidations are bound to occur, a shake-up seems inevitable. The remaining hospitals will provide better quality patient care, which is all to the public's benefit.

In spite of this medical trend, the growing need for specialized management skills in rural hospitals will not keep pace. With a stable population base and the possibility of a decreasing average length of stay, the need for additional beds in rural areas will be lessened over the next decade. However, governing boards will still expect an administrator to somehow come up with a management information and control system that readily answers the questions that outside agencies are posing.

Reviewing the list of seven options, it is clear that any one of them, except staying as is, can be considered. None of these options will probably affect the clinical situation, since referral patterns are well established; but the management issues will be the difficult ones to hurdle. To keep management reporting systems up to the level required will cost dollars not now being spent. If the option chosen is to become part of a chain operation, whether it be operated as an investor-owned corporation or by a large voluntary, nonprofit hospital in a metropolitan area, the additional cost for supervision by the parent organization will find its way into the operating costs of a rural hospital.

Becoming part of a larger system is not the only reasonable option. Instead of entering into an arrangement on someone else's terms, some hospitals will start a system of their own, either buying other hospitals in the same general area, or forming a consortium of rural hospitals.

The consortium approach will probably have the greatest appeal to other institutions, but has the weakest organizational structure, similar to those used in shared service programs. In most cases, the expectations of hospitals which have entered them are never fulfilled. Hospitals in consortiums are not only users of shared services, but also are typically represented on its governing board; which put its management in an untenable position since they were often forced to respond to the interests of each board member, rather than to the governing board as a whole. Other consortiums are of a purely voluntary type where a member can withdraw at any time. These tend to work effectively only as long as the consortium never has to say no to one of the members. Having no means of mandating group decisions, they usually fall apart, or wind up being only paper organizations. Consortiums are not a sound avenue to pursue if a hospital is really serious about obtaining better operating efficiencies.

Shared services are similar to consortiums, unless they are operated as a purchased service. Hospitals need a clearly defined relationship to a shared services organization. Filling two roles, one as a trustee for the service, as well as one of its major consumers, puts an administrator in a difficult position when he wants to raise cain over performance.

The strategy for the next several years is discernible. On the clinical side, a rural hospital needs the flexibility that comes with private practice of medicine. Should physician income be regulated, or physicians compensated for their services on some other basis, the rural populations will be the first to be adversely affected. On the other hand, if left relatively unregulated, the prospects for rural physicians in the years ahead are better than at any time in the past. Whether the rural hospital is freestanding, part of a chain, or operates a system of its own, physicians will not be much affected one way or another. Yet they probably will not realize this and may be the major stumbling block when these possibilities are seriously explored in a rural community.

The management question is really the tough problem. Professional administrators know what looms ahead for hospitals, but how to get trustees to share these concerns and be willing to act on them is much more difficult. Starting to build a system of hospitals in a surrounding area takes several years, but being taken over by a chain can be accomplished in a short period of time. Yet if a hospital doesn't start an acquisition program of its own in the next few years, it might very well be left with the only alternative of being signed up itself. The need for reimbursement specialists, industrial engineers, in-house attorneys, risk management, advice on long term loans, certificate of need expertise, improved training programs and facilities, and an electronics specialist, is going to become obvious. Without these services, the rural hospital will muddle through, but will drift from crisis to crisis. This can be avoided if enough hospitals get into the same corporate structure so that these services can be provided to all its hospitals.

Hospital visitors are similar to trustees in their outlook on a hospital. Typically, they, like the hospital, physicians, and personnel, will have a difficult time believing that this might change or be forced to change at some future date. Not that they aren't tuned in to what is going on in the rest of their country, but rather their hospital is so much a part of their community they will have great difficulty in believing that outside forces could be felt so close to home.

How to overcome this feeling that rural hospitals will not be caught up in the rising tide of events, until it is too late, is probably the most difficult problem of all. If an administrator approaches the governing board about acquiring other hospitals, no matter how carefully he lays the ground work, some of the trustees will conclude that he is an empire builder and has found a convenient way of justifying it. Others will see the future, but will not be willing to move on it because they believe the hospital should wait until a financial noose is really tightened by regulating agencies.

Coping with an uncertain future starts with an appreciation that hospital problems will continue to require the kind of dedication found among three or four key trustees in every hospital. As in the past, an administrator will need this group who in turn will lead the rest of the board to make the tough decisions that rural hospitals will have to make if they are to continue to serve the public that depends on them for their patient care.

NOTES

1. *Length of Stay in PAS Hospitals, United States, 1974,* by the Commission on Professional and Hospital Activities, Ann Arbor, Michigan, October, 1975. [p. 109.]
2. Ibid.

Chapter 7

Revisiting the Wobbly Three-Legged Stool

Recognizing that the wobbly three-legged stool analogy for a hospital organization structure has sadly been in need of mending, the remedy often suggested has been to recommend organizational structure where the medical staff, governing board, and administration acted as parts of the whole and not as separate entities. This notion has been gaining acceptance in hospital administrative circles and has been increasingly known as the corporate structure model. To those who have had this idea, it became a meaningful step toward developing an organizational response to coping with external pressures that have been mounting at a faster rate than could be accommodated by the traditional organization model used by most hospitals.

REORGANIZING HOSPITALS INTO THE CORPORATE STRUCTURE MODEL

Because hospitals are complex management enterprises, it was easy to suggest adopting the familiar corporate model as the organization structure for a hospital. It seemed eminently sound that what had served American industry well would obviously be a useful model for an industry that is becoming a major technological business. Toward this end, hospital administrators have become presidents, and associate administrators have become executive vice-presidents. Measured in terms of responsibilities carried by senior executives in industry and the complexities of their assignments, hospital executive positions should be equivalent; titles would be identical. When the chief executive becomes president, then the leadership of the governing board should be titled chairman of the board.

To carry this logic another step in the corporate organization, those who manage major functional components, such as nursing and medical affairs, should be titled vice-presidents. In the case of finance, those individuals might be renamed treasurers, with controllers reporting to them. In addition, hospitals have developed a vice-president or director of marketing, as hospitals have come to recognize that they are offering services in a competitive marketplace.

In conjunction with these organizational rearrangements, boards of trustees have been exhorted to examine the meaning and contribution of their governance activities more closely. Trusteeship is no longer being measured by donations and gifts to a hospital, but by how much trustees contribute to organizational effectiveness. It is the quality of the decisions they reach in determining the guiding policies that is the crucial ingredient of their contribution.

As a result, those hospitals that have gone furthest in developing a corporate structure act and behave in a manner similar to their industrial counterparts. Boards of trustees of hospitals can be expected to handle matters in a fashion akin to a corporate board of directors, with both spending approximately the same amount of time on the discharge of their responsibilities.

DIFFERENCES BETWEEN THE HOSPITAL AND CORPORATE WORLDS

Yet, if this is true, why do hospital trustees act differently than corporate directors? Is there something that has not been taken fully into account that makes governance in a hospital different than in industry? If so, what are these differences?

Fiscal Performance

It might be useful to examine the legal and philosophical bases of the two types to identify the reason for any difference in performance. Industry is an economic enterprise with social overtones. The hospital, on the other hand, is a social enterprise with deepening economic overtones. This is recognized in the use of the term trustee. Trustees are persons who are legally responsible for organizational activities in an enterprise that they do not own or have an economic interest in, but they are accountable to the public for the conduct of the affairs of the institution. This is different from corporate directors, who have direct accountability to the shareholders and bondholders of the corporation.

This difference is profound and has ramifications that are felt throughout an organization in the way in which it operates. Corporate accountability to shareholders is measurable in terms of earnings per share and dividends paid. In addition, directors own anywhere from a few hundred shares to several hundred thousand shares of the corporation, so they have a personal interest in seeing that the focus of the enterprise remains primarily financial. At the end of each year when the financial results are in, shareholders, investment analysts, and stock exchanges have a fair indication of how well they performed their duties as directors.

When these same people become hospital trustees, they do not behave in the same way as when they slide into a director's chair in the boardroom of a corporation. Is this because the nature of the beast is different, or is it because tradition has become so deeply ingrained that it affects individual boardroom behavior? Perhaps it is both to some degree. When an industry has its historical roots in the donation of time to causes, as personified by religious groups who have dedicated their lives or in the donation of money for philanthropic purposes, the degree of accountability changes.

In the case of the for-profit corporation, if year-end results have been financially better than had been anticipated, the board of directors recognizes senior management performance by awarding bonuses. If, to the contrary, the results are subpar, bonuses are reduced, and the operations are reviewed in an effort to determine if management failed or if what occurred was beyond their control. The customers that purchased the products of the corporation are presumed to be satisfied if the profit and loss statement shows a large net profit.

Hospital trustees of nonprofit institutions find themselves in a different situation for a variety of reasons. As representatives of the community providing a public service, they use the year-end results of the profit and loss statement only to ascertain whether or not the hospital was in the red or black. If in the red, they become concerned, unless the hospital has a tradition of losing money on its operating expenses and covering it with nonoperating revenues, such as endowments and tax revenues. If in the black, they are interested in assuring themselves that the surplus from the year's operation is modest and will remain that way. As corporate directors, they would think the larger the black number, the more favorable the results. This is not so in the hospital because it would be regarded by trustees as taking advantage of the public. In either case, a black or red figure, the senior management is likely to be largely unaffected by financial results, unlike what occurs in the for-profit world.

An executive in a nonprofit hospital treads a thin financial line, not too much profit or too much red ink, but rather one that approximates a zero balance for the year's effort. Since there are no shareholders concerned about seeking to maximize return on their investment, there is no direct pressure on management to provide a year-end surplus. In fact, trustees most often see their role as requiring them to protect the public, which means an interest in the lowest possible surplus. Hospital trustees view their responsibilities from this perspective and give primary concern to it, as long as the hospital is not going bankrupt.

Often this attitude does not square with the perception of professionally trained administrators who see themselves as being as fiscally responsible as other corporate executives in the community. They likewise may expect that this ability should be highly regarded by their trustees. It is a way of demonstrating fiscal competency in carrying out the complex managerial responsibilities of a hospital. This idea is reinforced by prior experiences where a hospital had a staggering debt, was far behind on its accounts payable, or could not get a certified audit and was brought into the black within a period of two to three years. It then comes as a shock a couple of years later when a governing board does not remember what conditions had been like earlier and does not appreciate the administrator's role in reestablishing fiscal solvency.

Administrators see an interrelationship between fiscal matters and operating problems and are aware that a wrong course of action can reverse the financial state of affairs. Administrators who would not let the situation recur, are unlikely to appreciate the fact that a board of trustees is often willing to take this risk and deal with current problems without being unduly concerned about potential fiscal difficulties in the future.

At the base of the trustee attitude is adherence to the concept that a hospital is a social enterprise with economic overtones, but these are only overtones and are regarded as such by them.

Chief Executives

Because of both education and experience, a hospital chief executive often views a medical staff in a different light than do trustees. The organized medical staff is seen as part of the hospital operating structure to be dealt with cautiously and with great sensitivity. Administrators often would like to deal with a medical staff in the same manner that all of the other operating departments are handled.

The governing board usually sees a medical staff as an organizational anomaly not found in other forms of enterprises. They acknowledge that physicians have to meet certain standards for admission to a medical staff, but once the physicians have met these standards, they quickly come to see and treat physicians as surrogate customers. Consequently, when physicians express displeasure with administrators, governing boards listen carefully and are inclined to be responsive. If this dissatisfaction reaches a point where staff members collectively request the board to terminate a chief executive, a board more often than not accedes to their request. In these situations, there is little likelihood that being fair, weighing administrative performance over time, or determining the accuracy of a medical staff's position is apt to occur. In many cases a board of trustees accepts a medical staff's recommendation without carefully and critically examining the issues. Trustees react in this way because they recognize a hospital as a medical care institution; as a community activity; as a place where minimum standards for professional performance are enforced; where physicians choose whether or not to use the facilities; and where operating departments headed by the administrator provide the support systems that permit these other activities to occur. Trustees usually do not see a hospital chief executive as the person who leads and inspires the medical staff; instead they view the chief executive as guiding only hospital personnel.

In this sense hospital chief executives are different from their industry counterparts. In industry, chief executives are clearly responsible and accountable for providing leadership and for pushing toward higher and higher goals that use corporate resources for their attainment. They are expected to be out in front, challenging the organization to achieve increased performance. There are no boundary markers limiting their abilities, as long as they achieve the results in a sound economical manner. Growth in assets, net profits, units produced, and share of market are applauded.

Not so in the voluntary nonprofit hospitals. Even though chief executives in hospitals have all the management attributes of their counterparts in industry, they are constrained in the hospital setting. They are the leaders of a support system, one that is expected to do its job efficiently and responsively to medical care interests. They are expected to see that the adopted professional standards are enforced, and they are not expected or permitted to raise these standards, but only encourage their accomplishment. They are not free to consult with the medical staff, receive their advice, and then make decisions; they must secure the medical staff's approval before implementation.

Even though hospital executives are every bit as accomplished as their industry counterparts and are as versatile in their managerial skills, the executive role restrictions prevent them from exercising these skills to the same degree. They cannot get out too far in front of a medical staff. If they acquire too much influence in the community, push to develop a multihospital system at a rapid rate, control a medical staff too directly, achieve too large a financial surplus, or, in other words, if they behave as aggressive, brilliant, hard-working executives, they run a strong risk of courting personal organizational disaster. When a medical staff feels threatened by executive performance, their feelings often come from the belief that the hospital administrator is in charge of support activities, not the entire hospital, and that the physician's role of dispensing medical care must be protected. Medical staff members act on this belief when threatened by strong executive performance.

The Role of Physicians

Physicians see themselves in two ways with regard to their hospital professional activities. They accept, though sometimes grudgingly, that they are part of a larger system of medical care in the hospital and are willing to participate in medical staff activities, accepting the need to abide by professional standards of the institution. In their office practice they view themselves as individual entrepreneurs, solely responsible for the diagnosis and treatment of patients. They are aware through their education and training that a continuing concern for personal competence must be adhered to in their office as well as in the hospital. They believe the same quality of medical practice should be applied in both settings.

When caring for hospitalized patients, physicians believe they organizationally should be unencumbered to practice as they see fit, as long as their personal standards of performance exceed those required by an institution. They view a hospital as providing resources on a demand basis that are needed from them for treating patients. They do not see a hospital as a control mechanism that decides their hours, work schedule, income, or professional direction.

Any decisions taken by a hospital that can be interpreted, even remotely, as being in the direction of control are usually met with sharp reminders about their independence. Individually, physicians may inform either board members or administrators that they are free to take their patients to other hospitals and may well do so if matters are not righted to their satisfaction. This kind of statement is often heard when trying situations develop in a hospital. An administrator often views this physician behavior as a threat akin to blackmail, while physicians see these actions quite differently. To them it represents the exercise of a professional right they have earned, and they can take their business elsewhere as a matter of licensed freedom.

The dilemma today is that a hospital is now a large, heavily capitalized, technological enterprise operating in an increasingly complex social setting, but with attitudinal viewpoints of both trustees and physicians that do not square with the dynamics and flexibility required for institutional survival.

In the future, hospital chief executives are going to find themselves in the position of the messenger who brought bad news to the king and was rewarded for the effort by being decapitated.

Physicians may be a source of difficulty in the next decade with increasing federal regulation of health care institutions. By the nature of their profession, physicians can be expected to be proponents of the status quo about the role of hospitals. The fact that the health care system is under siege by HHS reimbursement practices, state rate review commissions, and HSAs does not concern most physicians. Unless these agencies directly affect the services and equipment they use in clinical activities, physicians will not be concerned. In this regulatory environment, physicians have difficulty understanding why housekeeping, maintenance, personnel, public relations, and the other service departments of a hospital cannot continue to receive less funds in order to protect the clinical services of the hospital, even when overall reimbursement is being restricted. Lacking organizational exposure to the need for balance between hospital operational activities, a medical staff is prone to arrive at conclusions that experienced health care managers recognize as something less than desirable.

In addition, the frustration levels of physicians increase with each passing year as they find their hospital activities curtailed in ways over which they have little control. Faced with higher rent for office space, higher malpractice premiums, the necessity for providing fringe benefits for their office staff, more insurance form paperwork, increased scrutiny of fees, greater accountability for clinical decisions, and a public doubting that their services are worth the prices charged, physicians feel a need to react. Unable to counter economic pressures and increased infringements on their own way of doing things, they may come to regard a hospital as the place where they will make their final stand to protect their professional rights.

The role of a physician in a hospital and the organizational relationship of the medical staff to the governing board and administration must be rigidly restricted and must remain the same. Even though the government is forcing hospitals to become the major control point in the health care delivery system, physicians who find themselves threatened will determine not to let it happen in a hospital where they view their role as being of considerable economic importance to the hospital and providing leverage to protect their institutional interests and attitudes.

Contracts

Given the disparity between a changing societal role for hospitals and inflexible physician attitudes, there are bound to be more forced terminations of chief executives in hospitals during the next decade. These actions will not be ameliorated by a corporate structure where there is increased authority for a chief executive officer. In terms of the external environment, expanded administrative authority is needed if a hospital is to protect itself from increasing government control; in terms of attitudes of physicians, timing could not be worse. Since governing boards recognize physicians as the hospital's customers, they will be careful not to adopt policies that alienate the medical staff.

Under existing circumstances, prudent chief executives of hospitals should seek employment contracts from their governing boards. In a highly charged social environment, a senior hospital executive needs to appreciate that there will be growing medical staff suspicion of administrators, and the changes in organizational structure and policies that were easily accomplished a few years ago may become rallying issues for medical staff members who are out to protect their traditional turf. Fair play, honesty of intent, and desirability of any proposed change in hospital policies are not sufficient protection for chief executives in this climate. What worked a few years ago as a way of accomplishing organizational change may not be relied upon in today's environment. Rationality, a sensing of the future, an approved long-range plan; none of these persuade a threatened medical profession. Yet these are the tools of management for coping with organizational problems.

Given this is a period when external factors dictate change and rapid decision making, but, if decisions must be made in an environment dominated by a desire to maintain the status quo, the chances of a chief executive's survival are questionable, even when competent and well trained. In these circumstances, a chief executive needs greater protection than has been necessary in the past. A contract will not prevent unrest, but it recognizes that the risks are now greater and provides a measure of protection in this uncertain climate.

To push for a single unified structure with all major functions reporting to the chief executive is not likely to be greeted with enthusiasm by today's medical staff. Chester I. Barnard put his finger on the reason why it cannot be easily accomplished.[1] He pointed out that executives' authority can be exercised only to the extent that those over whom they are exercising it accept their right to do so. Medical staff members usually deny this right of administrators. In fact, in many hospitals they deny the authority exists even for another physician who may be in an administrative position, such as a fulltime chief of staff or medical director. From the standpoint of organizational theory, having a person who can be held accountable to lead the medical staff activities seems like a good idea. Yet, this may not now be the situation. The emphasis now is on leadership rather than authority, on sensitivity rather than control, and on persuasion as the preferred administrative skills. Even though a single, unified, top level structure is certainly desirable, it seems to be unattainable for the majority of hospitals because of prevailing physician attitudes.

Social Responsibility

Rather than striving to adopt a corporate structure model totally, an adaptation in structure that recognizes the uniqueness of a hospital organization is more sensible. Governance must recognize that board members of hospitals have a degree of commitment that significantly differs from that of outside directors of industry and business corporations. Trustees willingly devote more time to board meetings, committee meetings, ceremonial functions, education sessions, and trips on behalf of the institution than their business counterparts. Involved trustees often may donate from 500 to 1,000 hours annually to hospital affairs, while by contrast an outside corporate director may annually spend 50 to 100 hours on corporate affairs.

This difference is not due to hospital management being weaker than industry management, but it springs from a public accountability responsibility that makes a trustee different from a director. In the future a corporate director may become more like the hospital trustee, rather than the other way around. At a meeting of 68 leaders of business, labor, education, legal, and accounting professions at Harrison, New York, under the auspices of the American Assembly, an affiliate of Columbia University, discussion of the issues of governance of private corporations were held.

This group reached a number of significant conclusions about corporate governance that included:

- Profit and social responsibility are compatible.

- Corporations can and should improve their responsiveness to emerging social and ethical questions.

- Boards have a primary role in interpreting society's expectations and standards for management and should not reflect the views and interests of a corporation management.

- The majority of board members should come from outside corporate management, and those representatives doing a significant amount of business with the corporation should not count as independent directors.

- There should be a separation of function between the chairman of the board and the chief executive officer.

- Corporations should hold open meetings with public groups to discuss social issues.

- Public issue committees should be established.

- Self-regulation of an industry should be encouraged, but to prevent self-serving, there should be a third party oversight to set standards and to monitor compliance.

- Corporate boards should recognize the value of a well-informed public.

On balance, the assembly recommended that corporate governance should represent a careful compromise between those seeking to preserve corporate autonomy and efficiency, and public groups seeking to control or guide corporate power to constructive social ends. Corporate policy should be a blend of inside and outside interests, and, while providing for greater public participation, it should not include worker representation as is found in European-style corporations.

These goals strike a responsive chord among hospitals. Industry is moving toward the goal of becoming less restrictive. Hospitals need to move to the same ground from the opposite direction of having been too liberal on the side of too much community interest. Both groups need to blend community interests with those of their corporate goals. It is a delicate balance that is not easily achieved.

For hospitals, the need to be able to cope with increasing government regulations dictates governing boards of a modest size because speedy decision making is a survival requirement in an evolving government-hospital relationship. However, there needs to be an appreciation that community interests should not be shut out from being a voice in the development of policy.

Caution should be exercised in restructuring the governance of hospitals. To adopt a corporate structure model blindly may well lead to undesirable results for hospitals. What is needed is to pick and choose among those aspects of a model that will permit the hospital to carry on its role in society without compromising the public's interest in health care.

A change in the hospital organizational structure to a corporate model is not going to be accepted readily by physicians if it requires an accountability to a chief executive officer, even if there is a medical director or chief of staff. The concept of a single, unified structure, given the prevailing attitudes of the medical profession, is a workable idea only as long as the decisions reached by a hospital do not trample over strongly held concerns of its more vocal members of the medical staff. In order to minimize this risk, policy development needs to involve appropriate physicians from the first steps to final approval by a governing board. The result may be no better and might not be as sound as if an administrative staff decided what to do, but once having determined policy, acceptance among the medical staff will be greater and the chance of successful implementation enhanced. This strategy is of particular importance for the near term, until physicians understand that additional constraints are being placed on them and come to realize that they are not hospital inspired, but arise from external factors. Until that time, internal organizational tensions will steadily increase, and decision making on shifts in programs, services, and organizational structure will have to be slowed down to the rate of acceptance of the medical staff.

In decision-making areas that are usually not of concern to physicians, such as compliance with civil rights regulations, methods to finance long-term debt, real estate and zoning problems, retroactive Medicare adjustments, and processing certificates of need, rapid decision making can be accomplished if a governing board is properly sized and structured. To this extent it can function like a corporate board without involving its membership in the details of the operation.

NOTE

1. Chester I. Barnard. *Functions of an Executive* (Cambridge, Mass: Harvard University, 1938), p. 109.

Part II

Governance

Chapter 8

Hospital Ownership and Governance in Transition

As hospitals have grown and become more complex and inhibited by increasing regulation, their governance has been in evolution. Four patterns have developed from the existing types of hospital ownership and trustee organization. A review of what has occurred will provide a perspective on previous developments and suggest trends that are likely to occur in the future.

GOVERNANCE HISTORY

Until the late 1930s, when the United States was just moving out of a major depression, governing boards typically exercised a detailed interest in hospital finances, physical plants, and personnel matters, but they knew little or nothing about clinical activities. Administrators had no training for this position, since none was available, and all members of the medical staff were medical generalists rather than specialists. Board meeting agendas were usually devoted to approving individual invoices for payment, reviewing each account receivable, and granting salary increases that were presented by the hospital superintendent.

Federal Hospitals

Depending on the type of ownership of a hospital, its governing structure varied. Hospitals operated by the federal government were governed by federal laws and administrative regulation. Instead of a governing board, the administrator reported to a central management office in Washington through a clearly delineated chain of command, whether the hospital was operated by the Veterans Administration, the Public Health Service, or the Armed Forces.

State Hospitals

Large state institutions for health care usually provided specialized services, such as treatment in psychiatry or tuberculosis; the administrative officer operated under similar governing mechanisms to those of the federal level.

County and City Hospitals

In hospitals owned and operated by county and city governments, the pattern of control was different. Governing boards emerged, and trustees were either elected by public ballot or appointed in one way or another by county commissioners, city councils, or local judges. The enabling resolutions that created these hospital entities defined a board's powers and quite often severely restricted them in the spending of capital funds, but were silent about quality of care matters. Through the years, decision-making authority at the local level remained largely unchanged in governmentally-owned and operated hospitals.

Proprietary Hospitals

In proprietary hospitals, a different pattern of governance was followed. Ownership and management were almost always identical. The governance function was mainly a paper organization that existed in order to comply with state laws governing formation of for-profit corporations used in business and industry. This pattern remained intact until the late 1960s and the advent of the investor-owned hospital chains.

Community Nonprofit Hospitals

Religious

Unlike government-owned or proprietary hospitals, community nonprofit institutions developed two related but distinct types of organization. When religious groups owned hospitals, the governance function usually rested solely in the hands of an order of sisters. Since the mission of a hospital was its dedication to both the ministry of healing and the evangelistic spirit, this type of structure was considered appropriate. Members of the board were usually also employed by the hospital in either an administrative or nursing position. Also, one or two representatives from the mother house often sat on the corporate board.

Nonreligious

The other type of hospital was nonreligious in mission but was regarded as a social agency of the community. Its roots arose from interested citizens of a local community who were willing to devote both their time and money to support the institution. From the beginning, appointments to this board were prestigious, because only the most financially successful persons were members. Since these hospitals were not considered to be business ventures and existed to take care of the sick, irrespective of ability to pay for the care received, a broad base of community interest was considered necessary. In order to focus these interests, associations were often formed with minimal requirements for participation, such as annual dues of five or ten dollars. Association meetings were held once a year, and hospital trustees were elected from among ranks of association members.

This type board structure is the one most often thought to be representative of a community and is used as a model for the voluntary nonprofit hospital. In reality, it is only one of several models that have been developed, though it still dominates the hospital scene. Because of its origins in a local community and its perception as a social agency that was formed to provide service without making a profit, these governing boards are often large, ranging from 12 to 15 members at the lower extreme and up to 50 or more members at the upper extreme.

In order to sustain interest in its hospital, the board leadership usually tried to create a sufficient number of committees so that each trustee had a specific assignment on one or more committees. Assuring individual trustee interest was believed to be of more importance to hospital leadership than a concern with whether or not this was an effective use of administrative time. This concern for continuing trustee interest stems from a belief that fund-raising projects undertaken by a hospital depend on trustee contributions for ultimate success. This belief has carried over to the present, even though the amount of funds raised is often less than one percent of an annual budget and has no significant impact on the operations of the modern hospital.

In the traditional model, chief executive officers are considered to be servants of the board and not leaders of its governing function, as is often the case in a freestanding proprietary or religious hospital. As administrators, they are expected to respond to the board's desire to attain the best possible care at the lowest possible cost. Today, because of the financial size of a hospital's operations, this usually means that they should manage the institution so that it does not incur an annual deficit on an accrual basis, but neither should they report a surplus. Preferably, they should reach as close as possible to a zero balance between income and expense.

In addition, administrators are expected to cooperate with the medical staff.

These two requirements, a zero annual financial balance and a directive to cooperate with the medical staff, are increasingly difficult to cope with from a chief executive's viewpoint, since the patient care institution of 40 years ago has now become a large, technology-oriented enterprise that is both labor and capital intensive. From a governance perspective, a hospital is still a social institution, though one with deep economic overtones.

Like trustees, physicians see the hospital mainly from a historical point of view. Medical staff members continue to believe that the administrative organization is there to provide support services for their diagnostic and therapeutic decisions, which physicians regard as the primary mission of an institution. Even though the environment in which the hospital now operates is highly regulated, with its income, allocation of expenses, capital expenditures, and new programs or substantial changes in service controlled, and even though the hospital is one of the major employers in town, chief executive officers are forced to manage in the traditional manner. This prevents them from bringing about organizational changes that will permit a freestanding voluntary hospital to respond effectively to a changing environment.

MULTI-INSTITUTIONAL SYSTEMS

As the vulnerability of the freestanding hospital increases, chief executive officers and a growing number of trustees have concluded that many of these conditions are intrinsic to the character of a health care institution and should remain so. This has led to a conclusion that the best way to survive in the future is through the formation of larger health care systems where individual hospitals become only one part of several related corporate activities. While there has been some acceptance of this approach in the hospital field and a need for multiple operations is perceived, four distinct kinds of multi-institutional systems have developed with separate and distinct characteristics in their ownership and governance. Each type of organization has led to identifiable differences that affect trustee behavior, administrative performance, and medical staff characteristics.

These four types are:

1. a chain of acute hospitals, geographically dispersed, operated on a for-profit basis;
2. several nonprofit hospitals in a local community operated by a centralized management;

3. a health care corporation operating a prepayment plan and providing physician and hospital services in multiple locations;
4. a health care system operating primarily in a local area through multiple corporations that may be a mixture of for-profit and nonprofit activities.

For-Profit Chains

An example of the for-profit chain of hospitals is the Hospital Corporation of America, where a corporate board is concerned with the operations of a large system of hospitals. In addition, each of its hospital units has an advisory board of seven to nine members, of which approximately two-thirds are practicing physicians in the individual hospital. This is a unique organizational structure that builds in several strengths.

A local board at the individual hospital level of the corporation concerns itself with two major responsibilities: (a) responsiveness to community health care needs; and (b) the quality of care rendered. A number of matters that ordinarily would be on the agenda of the board of a free-standing hospital are not considered by the board in this arrangement, but instead become transactions between the administrator and the corporate headquarters staff. Items, such as an annual operating budget, operational indicators of performance, planning of construction projects, personnel salaries and fringe benefits, zoning, purchasing, and productivity, are screened by corporate specialists and not by the local board. This speeds up the decision-making process of the individual hospital and enhances the quality of administrative decisions. A local board is then freed to concentrate on patient care considerations and medical staff interests. Since the local board is dominated by physicians, the complexities of reimbursement formulas and complicated financing arrangements are not discussed but are handled by specialists at the corporate level.

The corporation board in this type of institutional chained structure can concentrate on matters other than direct medical care and take on characteristics of a large industrial corporation. A typical hospital corporate board agenda deals with fiscal, organizational, marketing, and tax matters. Because the governing board of the chain is divorced from local institutions, its composition and size does not have to respond to the pressure for local representation. Since an investor-owned chain operates a system of hospitals throughout the country, no one institution is entitled to a board seat just because a hospital is part of the system. The number of board memberships is limited to a workable size and composed of persons of sufficient stature to engender confidence in national financial and business circles.

At the present stage of development, nearly all investor-owned chains of hospitals are examples of horizontal expansion with the multiple facilities performing essentially similar functions. As fewer and fewer hospitals become available for easy acquisition, these companies will start moving toward vertical integration by creating a series of subsidiary corporations to cope with specialized activities. These companies will probably form an insurance company to handle malpractice and liability policies, a capitation plan to handle prepayment health care, a purchasing company to buy large volumes of supplies, a subsidiary for nursing homes, a real estate company, a consulting firm, a company to provide hospice services, and other possibilities as they see an opportunity to provide a service and earn a reasonable rate of return. In time, successful investor-owned chains will be a mixture of horizontal and vertical integration.

Nonprofit Hospitals Operated by Centralized Management

The second major type of emerging ownership model is the large, free-standing, voluntary community hospital that acquires or manages by contract several local hospitals within its region. There will be a centralized management that provides specialists in finance, reimbursement and productivity improvement. Also, with a centralized management, costs of operation are spread across a broader financial base than would otherwise be possible.

Because of the local nature of this kind of multihospital system, the prevailing governing board structure is likely to become more cumbersome as additional facilities are added. When the first merger is attempted, the temptation is strong to include all trustees of both institutions on the surviving governing board in order to accomplish a merger. These same attitudes may prevail in a second merger. At some point, whether it is the second, third, or fourth merger, the governing board will become too large. When this point is reached, the real functions of governance are often delegated to an executive committee and the full board only fills a ceremonial role, meeting quarterly or annually to approve the actions of its executive committee.

As governing boards become too large, their size hampers speedy and effective decision making. Yet, given the conditions that surround the establishment of a centralized management, the governing function becomes more ineffective. Largely unrecognized is that initial corporate and governance structures are often likely to remain in place for many years and that it is difficult to bring about a reorganization later. Making the organization structure work has a lower priority than creating the new mechanism.

In situations where two hospital corporations consolidate but continue to operate at both existing sites, an alternative to adding both boards together may be employed. Where agreement has been reached on limiting the size of the new corporate board, there is likely to be proportionate representation on the new board that roughly approximates the previous "equity" position of each hospital. Often used as criteria are the number of beds in each hospital, the net value of assets minus liabilities, factors such as the fund-raising ability of one institution versus the other, or some intangible characteristic unique to the situation.

Where some method of determining proportionate representation is used, a danger exists that after consolidation the new governing board will be composed of two factions that may not see eye to eye on key issues. If, during the negotiation process, a number of important points were side-stepped to achieve harmony and consummate a consolidation, the unresolved, troublesome issues move to the agenda of the new governing board. There they become almost impossible to solve and a major effort is required to keep these issues from becoming insurmountable hurdles that will result in a demerger.

Another alternative is to use a corporation board as if it were a holding company and to have advisory boards for individual hospitals that have specific and clearly delineated responsibilities and authorities. In its pure form this is not a holding company; rather, it is a corporation with divisions that are permitted wide latitude in decision making. Within specified parameters, each institutional board is free to make its own decisions, even though there is only one corporation for all of the hospitals in the system.

A Corporation with a Prepayment Plan and Multiple Locations

A third model for multihospital systems is to create a mechanism for financing health care through a prepayment system that owns and operates a system of hospitals for its subscribers and also contracts with an organized group of physicians to provide medical care. By the use of financial incentives, a prepayment system can make it advantageous for physicians to use ambulatory approaches to patient care, and the system can obtain an economic advantage for keeping patients out of hospitals. This is a closed-loop system developed by the Kaiser-Permanente Foundation. When hospitals are not owned and operated by a prepayment system, but instead inpatient services are contractual and are arranged with individual hospital corporations, this becomes a typical HMO model. In both cases, a closed system or an open contract method, the goal is the same: to bring about the lowest possible hospital usage rates; to maintain quality of care; and to use economic incentives for physicians that encourage the use of ambulatory medical care services.

A Mixture of For-Profit and Nonprofit Corporations

A fourth approach in multihospital systems developed out of a different set of circumstances. When it was recognized that Medicare and Medicaid did not reimburse full cost to a hospital for services rendered and that those two segments of revenue continued to increase as a percentage of total revenues, some hospitals began to search for ways to close the widening gap between expenses and income. These hospitals concluded that what they knew best was health care and that any additional kinds of activities undertaken should be in this general field. They also appreciated that the degree of regulation that now exists for both hospitals and nursing homes did not offer a reasonable rate of return under present conditions. Yet, they knew that within the health field there were a number of health-related activities not controlled by regulation, and these were likely to remain uncontrolled for the foreseeable future.

To close the deficit gap and take advantage of the nonregulated activities, these hospitals created foundations, sold laboratory services to physician offices, sold laundry and selected administrative services to other hospitals, and began to buy and sell real estate in order to turn a profit that might be used for hospital purposes.

From the perspective of the next decade, aggressive, freestanding hospitals will be converted to health services corporations. In all likelihood, they will be a mixture of several for-profit and nonprofit corporations unified by the use of a holding company or by an interweaving of hospital trustees serving on various corporate boards. The major consideration in the mixture of activities and corporations will be the effects of tax laws and, in particular, the tax implications of unrelated business income. This will involve professional office buildings, revenues from providing services to outside physicians and institutions, and other money-making activities. In essence, vertical integration of health services will develop in communities containing a mixture of those activities that are in the tightly controlled and regulated sector of the industry (that is, hospitals, foundations, and nursing homes) and those that are in the uncontrolled sector (that is, physicians, office buildings, commercial ancillary services, prepayment, and primary care centers). Their central focus is likely to be either a foundation or a holding company, depending on state statutes.

As multiple corporations similar to this fourth model are formed, the governance function will expand. Since the purpose for initiating additional corporations is an undergirding of the financial strength of a hospital, selected trustees from hospital governing boards will be asked to serve as directors of these newly formed corporations. As the number of new corporations reaches four or five, the pool of available hospital trustees will have been depleted in terms of the amount of time they can devote to an unpaid activity. Some other form of control will then have to be devised to ensure that the original reasons for engaging in other businesses than direct patient care services are upheld.

Two possibilities may be considered: (a) adopting a holding company concept; or (b) resorting to a foundation, as the controlling corporate structure. In both models there will be problems that must be resolved.

The holding company model was initially conceived as a financial mechanism for use by for-profit organizations. The Internal Revenue Service (IRS) rules that have developed around this concept are based on the percentage of outstanding stock held by various interests in the subsidiary corporation. As the percentage of stock rises in a holding company, its authorities broaden with respect to control of the subsidiary corporation. When this principal is applied to multiple corporations in the nonprofit sector, and a foundation or a nonprofit corporation (501(C)3) is used as the holding company, it is argued that a seat on this governing board is the equivalent of stock. The same rationale can be invoked as used in the for-profit model.

In using this concept, care has to be exercised when the health care conglomerate is a mixture of nonprofit and for-profit corporations but has a nonprofit parent corporation. Controls must be established to assure that the total volume of all activities and the percentage coming from the for-profit corporations will not exceed IRS regulations for unrelated business income. This is to protect the continuation of a 501(C)3 status of the parent corporation as a nontaxable entity.

GOVERNANCE IN THE NEXT DECADE

No matter what form is adopted by multi-institutional corporations in coming years, the base of corporate operations has been significantly broadened, and its multiple locations will inevitably lead to changes in the governance structure. Individual hospital facilities will continue to have governing boards. If these hospitals are to be part of one large corporation, then its board will be advisory. When they are operated as subsidiary corporations, they will have their own boards. In both cases they will have carefully delineated authorities and responsibilities.

As new health-related corporations are developed that engage in other than acute bed care, the physician's influence at the level of the parent organization is going to diminish, as distance to the top lengthens and is more remote from direct patient care and as persons with financial experience dominate. Since there will be greater emphasis on the use of long-term debt for meeting the capital needs of the organization rather than fund raising, the number of members of a governing board will become smaller. At the local hospital level, boards can be expected to remain as they have been in the past, drawing on leading citizens and outstanding physicians. Where fund-raising interests have historically led to a large board, they will probably continue as long as a local hospital remains nonprofit and freestanding.

The growth of multihospital systems during the next decade will lead to both horizontal and vertical integration of the industry. Some hospitals will first move through horizontal growth and then into vertical integration patterns. Others will move directly into vertical patterns. The imperatives of growth will eventually be reflected in the composition and size of governing boards, but will lag behind operational changes that will take place. Complexity will increase and require the delegation of a larger scope of responsibility and authority to top management. Conversely, competent executives will have to continue to expand their management skills to keep up with the increasing requirements for corporate leadership.

Traditional ways of governing and managing hospitals will not be suitable for coping with the shifts that will be taking place as multihospital systems develop. Old ways will have to be discarded, philosophies modified, and thinking expanded to a larger scale to encompass increasing corporate complexity. At the same time, new organization structure will have to be initiated as more sophisticated management tools and techniques are used to keep pace with changing times.

Chapter 9

The Trustee Role in Maintaining a Hospital Service Tradition

To raise a question about maintaining the service tradition of hospitals suggests that there is a reasonable doubt that the hospital field is continuing to place patient interests ahead of bureaucratic concerns. In light of the effects of Medicare and Medicaid, this question is long overdue.

Has the industry changed its values about what is important in hospital care? To answer this question, earlier motivations and actions should be examined. Both need not be in agreement, because institutions and people often justify action on the basis of a true motivation, even when it appears inconsistent to outside observers.

HOSPITAL COSTS VS. SERVICE TRADITION

In some places in Washington, the hospital field is characterized as gluttonous and obese in economic terms, and wasteful of scarce resources. Whether this is true or not, there are a sufficient number of national leaders who believe so or who cannot find sufficient evidence to the contrary, and opinions, right or wrong in terms of the facts, often lead to action.

If the service tradition had been sufficiently believed in the recent past, the Hill-Burton charity allowance issue would never have surfaced. Obviously, a part of the public believes hospitals have begun to place money concerns ahead of service tradition.

Today, there is a steady drumbeat in state capitals and Washington to do something about hospital costs. From Talmadge to Kennedy to Carter, the message is to slow the rise in hospital expenses; this is based on a theory that quality care can continue, if hospitals would only strive for a reasonable amount of efficiency. Yet, no one has analyzed this hypothesis to determine its reasonableness. The way things are headed, soon everything in the hospital field will be under federal control.

Because there must be hospitals in a civilized society, an effort will always be made to keep them functioning, at all costs, including the downgrading of a belief that a service tradition is valuable. While people may rail against this kind of decision, the need for a functional hospital is more important than the hospital's ambiance, patient amenities, and personal concern for every patient. The choice ahead has been well phrased by Kahlil Gibran: "The most pitiful among men is he who turns his dreams into silver and gold."[1]

Unfortunately, the demands of society are now moving faster than the capacity to serve them. This may, however, be a symptom of a maturing industrial society and will be alleviated at some distant time, when the riches of technology have been maximized into productive capacity.

In the meantime, health, education, and social services will be shortchanged and forced to make the adjustments needed to close the gap. A price will be paid for nuclear-powered carriers, triton submarines, and defense expenditures that are needed, but are ultimately wasteful. This is the result of an unbalanced and inhuman world that does not practice American beliefs and philosophy.

Political processes and the realities of world leadership lead to hard choices in the commitment of scarce resources. In a democracy, where the national leadership must periodically face an electorate that wants to know what has been done for them lately, facing priorities is postponed and obfuscated for the sake of reelection.

If this is the real America, in the decade of the eighties, then the task is not to acquiesce on vital health care issues, but to have the strength, the articulate voice, and the courage to force rational choices in the way society expends its resources.

This is a new challenge for hospitals and their governance. The ways of the past have not been demanding; resources, if not plentiful, were adequate. Somehow, needed beds and services were added, although not always on schedule or to the extent desirable.

Now the service tradition of hospitals is being forced by restrictive reimbursement to make hidden compromises that are not in the best interests of patients, but are necessary for institutional survival.

This view, however, does not condone the waste of health care resources. If there are better ways to do the job, to get lower unit costs of operation, it is irresponsible not to do so. Health care institutions are rightly pilloried when their operations are extravagant.

Most hospitals are someplace between these two extremes. There are wasteful hospitals and medical practices, and there are sloppy hospital administrations and boards of trustees. The extent of their extravagance is not known on an industrywide basis. Is it three percent or ten percent or thirty percent? Is it logical to expect all hospitals to be maximally efficient, or what is an optimal or reasonable expectation? No industry, as yet, has achieved maximum efficiency. What then is acceptable for hospitals?

THE CHALLENGE CONFRONTING TRUSTEES

As boards of trustees learn to wrestle with these problems, the historical rationalizations for inadequate striving for optimal performance will no longer be acceptable. State and federal governments are now looking toward hospitals to provide the foundation on which major changes in the total health care system will take place. Given the historical independence of the practice of medicine and its antipathy toward hospital and institutional impingement on its traditional freedoms, these views promise to make the days ahead exciting.

Hospitals are a societal necessity, and they will be trapped between the forces of medicine and government as each strives to bend hospitals to their performance. This will be a time of testing hospital governance. If the service tradition is to be preserved, hospital trustees must make the case. No other health care voice is creditable. Physicians or hospital administrators who raise their voices will be interpreted as clever and self-serving, and of dubious motivation. The worst that could be alleged about hospital trustees is that they are naive and tools of more sophisticated interests, and this is, at best, a doubtful argument since trustees have experienced the struggles of a hospital boardroom.

If hospitals are to maintain a service tradition, there is no substitute for intelligent, knowledgeable trustee participation in the struggles with the bureaucracy and the legislators. If trustees don't have the courage or the time, why should physicians and administrators? Trusteeship has always meant guardianship, stewardship, and the conscience of the community.

Will trustees accept the challenge? The price individuals pay for daring to speak their minds and convictions can often be dear. The costs can be real in terms of reprisal and frequently appear unrelated at the surface. Businessmen are aware of these dangers, while many professionals and housewives are unaware of the practices of political "hardball."

Whenever people decide to tilt against political forces, they had better be sure their own shop is in order. Many hospitals and trustees cannot be so sure. Within the boardroom, subtle conflicts of interest, real and potential, are present. When a person argues for continuing the historical service traditions of hospitals, motivation is self-evident, until the day a newspaper reports how a board member has benefited or might benefit from hospital trusteeship.

What about a hospital that cannot demonstrate trustee participation in a quality assurance program when a member of the medical staff has committed a malpractice and when the community is alive with doubts about the quality of medical care in the institution? Every hospital must prepare for these eventualities by removing the possibilities of conflict of interest and initiating a meaningful quality assurance program.

In providing meaningful leadership for a hospital, trustees need to think through the role of their hospital in the community, that is, whom it should serve and why. In an environment of restrictive reimbursement, high cost, new medical technology, growing professional specialization, and increasing regulation, it is unrealistic not to rethink the role of a modern hospital.

When a hospital board expresses a desire to maintain its tradition of service and concern, it must also decide how its philosophy can be carried out. To hold to a philosophy without thinking about the resources needed is to practice will-of-the-wisp governance.

If these observations appear strained and too extreme, then the experiences in the northeastern part of the country, particularly in New York and Massachusetts should be reviewed. They are in a position of having had to compromise the service traditions of the hospital industry. They had no choice. This painful experience could happen elsewhere.

In the "good old days," an administration was able to identify an unmet medical need, prepare a program to meet the need, and proceed to provide a new service. The uncovered expenses could be somehow folded into the next annual budget.

Things are different now. No matter how serious the need, if the full amount of funding is not available, no program will be developed. Hospital trustees must rise to the challenge of reasserting local initiative in health care. Too frequently trustees have hovered dubiously between mute rebellion and prattling submission to directives from on high.

There are eight events now occurring across the hospital field that will affect the future role and responsibilities of governance. These events are:

1. Hospital administrators are becoming chief executive officers and presidents of the board.
2. Physician representatives of the medical staff are being elected as trustees.
3. Boards are decreasing in size and reorganizing their operations.
4. Consumerism in governance is on the wane.

5. Hospital associations, as such, are either being eliminated or their functions absorbed into a board of trustees.
6. Hospitals are developing multiple corporations and interlocking directorates.
7. Advisory boards are growing in popularity as more hospitals become part of chain operations.
8. Mergers of hospitals within a local community are reducing the total number of trustee positions.

Planning

Because of the familiarity of these events, it is more useful to comment on specific parts that may have a telling effect on the future of hospital governance. However, the process by which these eight events will be affected will arise out of the present and future planning authorities vested in governmental units and their regulatory activities today and tomorrow.

Much of the planning being done is on the basis of what ought to be, in terms of some improved model of a regionalized health care system that has been colored by unattainable objectives introduced by consumer elements in the decision process. Within the next 30 years, consumerism will be removed from the local level. It will be raised to the state and federal level and limited by broad policy decisions. The local planning agency will then become technically oriented and limited to approving programs that are consistent with national health policy and are cost effective.

This shift in planning authority will be forced by hospital boards as they seek accountability from planning agencies through the courts in the years ahead, when absurd demands are placed on proposed projects, and hundreds of thousands of institutional dollars are lost by ineptness of agency staffs and their boards. Sooner or later, people will realize that consumer politics and naive decisions are interfering with excellence in planning.

In the years ahead, hospital boards may lose their independent authorities to determine whether or not to replace existing facilities, to add new facilities and programs, or to reduce or eliminate programs and services if these trends continue.

Hospital boards of trustees will have to learn the value of routinely developing and periodically updating institutional role and mission statements. One of the persistent scrambles between trustees and planning agencies will be the issue of appropriate institutional roles and missions. It will probably be a serious point of contention between the two bodies, with no authority granted to the planning agencies to do much about how an institution defines its marketplace. They will have the power to say no, but never yes.

Regulation

Regulation of health care will follow a separate course, but will also affect hospital governance.

Within the decade, heavy reliance on regulatory activities will be accepted as counterproductive. The practice of issuing a steady, never-diminishing stream of new regulations will overload the system and reach a point of absurdity.

Federalization of the hospital system will be considered and rejected on a political basis, and gradually administrative regulations will be ameliorated.

Out of this process will arise new controls focused on clinical programs and services. It is not at all unlikely that the specialty composition of a medical staff will be determined by planning agencies, and the authority of a board will be limited to the appointment of physicians to fill the authorized slots. This authority will be exercised on the rationale of balancing hospital services against community needs and the optimal use of medical personnel.

The future thrust of planning and regulation will encourage most hospital governances to undertake one or more of the eight kind of changes now occurring in the organization of a board of trustees. The most clear-cut change that will occur is the massing of larger corporate groupings of physicians and of hospitals.

The driving force for change will be a continuing concern of trustees about the cost of hospital care. Federal pressure will remain on hospitals and physicians, including limitations on hospital revenues and medical practice incomes. The hospital response will be to develop more hospital-based medical practices and group practices. As this event occurs, physicians will find ways to increase further the number of trustee chairs filled by members of the medical staff. In some instances, the number of physician-trustees will approach a majority membership of the board.

Hospitals will respond to continuing cost control pressures by more mergers and consolidated services. Because free enterprise concepts are deeply rooted in American society, the investor-owned national chains will continue to expand, and a corollary chaining of religious hospitals and large nonprofit community hospitals will also take place.

These institutional mergers will reduce the total number of hospital trustees in a community by eliminating the merged corporation's board. However, they will probably be replaced by advisory boards if the merger is into a chain, and the emphasis will be limited to clinical matters.

With oppressive regulation and planning, continuing cost controls, and fewer bail-out choices for hospitals in financial deep water, consumerism will fade along with the old traditional hospital association. Restricted dollars will reduce the games people play, and there will be a recognition that the hospital boardroom is no longer a place for unabashed goodwill.

Other changes will take place in hospital governance, including major changes in the agendas of boards of trustees. The kinds of topics presented and the lengths of the discussions will shift.

In relative terms, procedural and financial activities will substantially decrease, while evaluation, policy, and informational activities will expand.

These shifts will occur because boards of trustees will be forced to deal at the policy level to keep their institutions afloat. At the same time, the financing of hospitals will become straitjacketed without much option for decision making in a financial sense.

At the present time, most boards of trustees operate as if the theories of organizational structure and behavior have been suspended and as if whatever they do will inevitably assist the administrator and the hospital to carry out its role and mission. The facts appear to be different.

Times have changed in hospital care. A new level of commitment in trusteeship is needed if the established and proven values of hospital care are to be meaningful in the days ahead. These values will only be continued if trustees participate in the larger health care system. If they fail, they will fail in daring to lead. The challenge ahead will be met only by a hospital governance that is enlightened and courageous. The goal is worthy of a trustee's best efforts.

NOTE

1. Kahlil Gibran, *Sand and Foam: A Book of Aphorisms* (New York: Alfred A. Knopf, 1926), p. 49.

Chapter 10

Cost Accountability for Health Care

The concept of accountability is widely used and often inappropriately applied. Ideally it should coincide with responsibility. The bigger the issue, the more likely its misuse. In a more than two hundred billion dollar health care industry, these two complementary notions are out of phase with each other.

George Bernard Shaw in *The Doctor's Dilemma* neatly framed the basic issue when he wrote:

"It is not the fault of our doctors that the medical service of a community, as at present provided for, is a murderous absurdity. That any sane nation, having observed that you could provide for the supply of bread by giving bakers a pecuniary interest in baking for you, should go on to give a surgeon a pecuniary interest in cutting off your leg, is enough to make one despair of political humanity. But that is precisely what we have done. And the more appalling the mutilation the more the mutilator is paid."[1]

When Shaw's observation is combined with the public myth that more medical care equals better health, the foundation for irresponsibility about health care costs has been well laid. As is known today, the marginal value of continually increasing medical care expenditures is rapidly decreasing.

Past medical successes have led to current medical failures. As life expectancy increases and as formerly fatal and disabling diseases are overcome, an older population faces diseases that are difficult to treat. The rapid expansion of nursing homes, high energy radiation centers, and transplant programs are all examples of a costly response with a low cost-benefit ratio.

When this situation is combined with the goal of equal access to health care, no one should wonder about the reasons for the high and increasing costs of health care.

WHO IS RESPONSIBLE FOR CONTROLLING COSTS?

Physicians

In a simpler time, responsibility in medical care was much clearer. The surgeon was the "captain of the ship" in the operating room, and a nurse took a risk in questioning or contravening a physician's order. Before the widespread use of hospital insurance, physicians cared about hospital rates.

Responsibility is now diffuse, and a much larger cast of people deliver health care services. The spate of regulations calling for PSROs, HSAs, HMOs, and utilization reviews are efforts to reinstitute a larger sense of personal responsibility. Along the way to reinstituting responsibilities, incentives for accountability have been warped.

The maximum allowable drug (MAX) regulation requiring the use of generic drugs is an example. The physician controls a patient's drug therapy, yet the penalty for selecting a higher cost brand name drug is on the hospital.

Another example of a dysfunction for cost accountability is malpractice insurance. At the visible level people are concerned about 500 percent and greater increases in premium costs. At the invisible level people wonder about the cost effect of malpractice as physicians protect themselves from legal uncertainty. Since there is always one more thing physicians can do— another x-ray, drug, laboratory test, consultation, or different treatment— they reduce risk by increasing the things they do to a patient. Physicians can do this because the patient does not usually pay directly for services.

Cost accountability flies out the window when averages or means are used as criteria for deciding how much is enough. An average connotes a range, with some elements higher and others lower. Even though general surgery is subdivided into categories such as appendectomy and cholecystostomy, the distributive issue remains. Medicine is an imprecise science with many variables in diagnosis and treatment. If more medicine equated reasonably well with a condition of health, there would at least be a chance of success with this approach. Since outputs of health care are unmeasurable, emphasis has centered on inputs. Again the thinking is that the more consumed the better.

An identical problem faces all social services, including education, government, and welfare. To a degree this is the reason that rising costs of these services encourage greater and greater regulation.

Control is implicit in the concept of accountability. Fairness means that persons should not be accountable for things over which they have no control. How much control do physicians have over patients? What happens if they honestly admit to a patient that he has an untreatable disease or condition? How long will they be in practice if they ignore the common cold?

Hospitals

Do hospitals control medical staffs and their hospital practice? Only an independently wealthy administrator would say yes. Most administrators know that the operation of PSROs will only control costs of care at the outer edges of the issue and will simply encourage physicians to be faster with a pen.

Equal access for medical care means either removal or a decrease in effectiveness of the traditional control device for rationing health care, that is, a patient's participation in the costs of the services consumed. The lesson of 1966 in the Medicare and Medicaid programs was that use of the medical system increased in response to lowering direct patient charges for service. Since the factors of production of medical care are limited in the short run, the inevitable occurred, that is, inflated medical care costs.

Until incentives to seek medical care are altered, cost containment ideas will only tilt with the fringes of medicine. When money is no barrier to medical care, the system cost can only be controlled by overcrowding. Discrimination of one type or another is inherent in all medical care. The poor are discriminated against by using money as the gatekeeping device.

Government

In the American system of mixing private and government expenditures for health care, no one is faced with the entire matter of cost. Partial accountability keeps escape routes open. A desire to maintain individuals' freedom of choice of physician and to reduce money as a barrier to medical care mandated a continuation of a mixed private public system for financing health care services.

Limited accountability is inescapable under these conditions as is a proliferation of regulations. The government has tried to decrease health care costs in vain. The most ambitious attempt so far was the National Health Planning and Resources Development Act of 1974 and its establishment of health systems agencies. The mandate is to reduce costs while improving the delivery of health services.

With the tools provided and no control over expenditures (either capital or operating) but with an authority that says only "no" meaningfully, there is only one possible outcome: increased hospital costs. With growing frequency, HSAs are being embroiled in local allocation decisions where they compromise by buying political peace by authorizing higher expenditures, such as the struggles over CAT scanners.

Since HSAs do not have to pay for their decisions, they are not accountable in the marketplace. Planning agencies are one step removed from operational experience and are more likely to plan future medical schemes on the basis of "what ought to be," rather than "what the public will support." The operational mode of this type is a further displacement of forces that insulate both providers and consumers from the marketplace. In essence, HSAs cool down the centralized heat in Washington and increase controversy at more diffuse local levels of government. It is a time-honored political ploy.

The coming tragedy of HSA failure is that the national conclusion that they do not work will not be reached. What will be concluded is that pluralistic financing and health care services have failed because of their high cost and unresponsiveness to regulation. The obvious solution will be to eliminate private administration and institute public administration. A careful review of PL 93–641 leads a person to think that its authors anticipated such an outcome.

AN UNLIMITED SUPPLY OF MONEY

Cost accountability is most frequently measured at the level of the individual entity or corporation. What is one person's price is another's cost. With today's system of multiple sources of financing health care, there is an ever-expanding source of money. Every resource allocation or operating decision is paid by someone else, since no one person is faced with a specifically defined sum of money. Hard choices are never made when people anticipate a lack of consequences for their choices.

Patients are not concerned about the corporate financial status of Blue Cross when they are hospitalized. Physicians and hospitals do not need to care about it either. Each is worried only about his or her own economic survival. Until attention is focused on individual financial matters, there will be no cost accountability for health care.

THE HOSPITAL AS A MONOPOLY

Historically, the hospital industry has possessed some of the economic characteristics of a monopoly. Its market forces are inelastic, and there is no reimbursement formula that properly balances the legitimate interests of government, patient, and institution. In a given community, two major forces tend to reinforce this concept of hospitals as a monopoly. The first is the physician. Most patients in hospitals today are attended by specialists, since 82 percent of all physicians restrict their practice to a specialty. When patients are older, have more than one disability, or are admitted for trauma, several physicians may be involved in their care.

Other physicians are chosen by the attending physician, based on his or her personal knowledge of their abilities, judgments, and skills. This knowledge of a colleague's abilities is acquired over time and is limited by earlier experiences. This is a reality of medical practice, reinforced by a public that selects and prefers to remain with one source of primary care. Economically, this practice supports a monopolistic hospital market condition, since a physician's knowledge of a colleague's competence is limited to those with whom he is in frequent contact.

Community attitudes are a second element reinforcing monopoly. Demographic studies repeatedly report patients' preferences for hospitalization near their residences. Most patients want their families nearby in time of severe stress. Until patients' problems are recognized as being clearly beyond the capability of locally available physicians, they will not be transferred elsewhere.

These two factors are sufficiently important to override difficulties caused by a difference in hospital charges. In addition, third party payers, such as government programs, insurance carriers, Blue Cross, and Blue Shield, provide coverage for more than 85 percent of hospitalizations. Consequently, price differentials mean little to a substantial number of patients. The public is more concerned with monthly insurance premiums than with the cost of a hospitalization.

In effect, hospital market behavior is what it is because physicians and patients make uneconomic decisions.

REIMBURSEMENT SYSTEMS

For some time, efforts to rethink reimbursement schemes have been going on because of an awareness of these realities of the marketplace. The goal of these efforts has been to separate the efficient hospitals from the inefficient and to reward efficient ones for superior performance. The difficulty is that external forces determine a large part of the cost of operating a hospital.

If a hospital is in a labor market where the minimum wage is $4 per hour and another hospital is in a $3 market, the higher cost hospital is not necessarily less efficient. Higher labor market rates would raise the overall costs of operations approximately 19 percent. Since between 52 percent and 58 percent of hospital costs are wrapped up in wage and fringe benefit costs, such differences have substantial impact. Older hospital plants usually have higher operating expenses than newer ones. Generally, an inner-city hospital is older and more expensive to operate, as well as to remodel, but it has lower depreciation costs.

The total effect of these factors is incompletely understood. Any reimbursement system that attempts to categorize hospitals according to these variables will produce inequality, because the cumulative magnitude of the effects is unknown. In addition, it is difficult to separate the efficient from the inefficient institutions. Furthermore, whenever a new payment system is introduced, hospitals will not all be equally situated. Any standardized approach will, therefore, fail to keep all hospitals fiscally sound, since efficiency in adversity will go unrecognized and some inefficient hospitals will have to be maintained because there is no reasonable alternative for the population they serve.

The problem of the efficient but unneeded hospital is a political dilemma. Realistically, the only acceptable decision is to allow it to continue to operate but to prevent its expansion. Over a long period of time, the establishment of more modern services in other hospitals will increase their attractiveness to physicians and patients and decrease that of the unneeded hospital.

In some minds, cost accountability for health care is best achieved by use of standardized hospital charges at the national, regional, or local levels. Such thinking is dreaming, because cost factors of production differ significantly among institutions. Rates charged for services must reflect the uniqueness of the particular set of problems with which an individual hospital copes. To pay the same rates to two hospitals in entirely different circumstances may cause the better one to fold. Equal rate structures imply equal community medical needs and support of hospitals; this is not the actual situation.

A successful reimbursement system that is accountable must be designed to consider individualized institutional programs and needs. Any modification that attempts categorization of hospitals will result in inequities. The initial effect will be the downgrading of medical quality in high cost efficient hospitals.

If cost accountability is to become reality in any new reimbursement system, the system must accommodate the realities of a pluralistic financing mechanism. The essential characteristics of such a system are:

- an established rate structure that has been reviewed by an outside authority and approved on the basis of acceptable standards of efficient operations, and that has used performance indicators and case mix as the fundamental inputs;

- the establishment of a reasonable relationship of the institution's size to total debt and annual capital expenditures, so that 1122 reviews are required less often for larger hospitals;

- a review of the results of hospital care by an external agency to assure that the quality of medical care meets minimally acceptable standards;

- no postaudit adjustments that eliminate cost factors or limit net surplus;

- a workable and equitable hospital payment system, based on an institution-by-institution decision-making process with each hospital responsible for the outcomes of its pricing decisions.

The goal of cost accountability must be the maintenance of fiscally healthy institutions that are needed to provide readily accessible care of a quality nature, at a desired level of service, and in a reasonably efficient manner.

At best, cost accountability for health care is a handle difficult to grasp, and at worst it is a will-of-the-wisp idea within a pluralistic financing mechanism. To be accountable there must be appropriately placed responsibilities. To continue to maintain the limited perspective of focusing control mechanisms on general hospitals without fixing specific responsibilities on consumers, physicians, and government is to assure their failure. It is in the interest of the public good that persistent efforts continue to devise workable schemes to maintain a constructive tension between accountability and responsibility.

NOTE

1. George Bernard Shaw, *The Doctor's Dilemma* (Baltimore: Penguin Books, 1913, 1941), p. 7.

Part III

Restraint and Regulation

Chapter 11

How Revolting Is
Regulation?

Since late 1966, the hospital industry has learned that a Washington paper blizzard has more meaning than a daily flyer from the Department of Health and Human Services (HHS).Regulation has grown from a paper tiger into a man-eating beast.

After an active period of new regulation pronouncements, it is easy to conclude that all regulation is bad. In quieter moments, most hospital administrators would concede that some regulation of the hospital industry is desirable.

WHAT AND HOW TO REGULATE

The basic issue is what should be regulated and how should it be done. The answer to this simple question is difficult.

All forms of regulation are based on a notion that solutions exist to the problems the new regulations are supposed to eliminate. In the societal arena, particularly health care, this viewpoint is a misunderstanding of the nature of the issues.

In recent times, Western civilization has come to accept instinctively the scientific method as the way of solving all problems. As long as a problem is of a scientific or engineering nature, this method is correct. A solution exists to a chess game or to a structural engineering problem; the game is won, or the bridge continues to stand in a hurricane. The result can be observed and is correct.

Social problems do not have these characteristics. They are not totally definable because each issue intermingles with a larger set of issues. Only under severe assumptions can difficulties of dealing with open systems be handled, and then the assumptions must be so restrictive that it is impossible to achieve optimal solutions.

113

The Nature of Open Systems

The traditional use of regulation has been to achieve greater efficiencies in one sense or another. Hospital licensure, for example, was first promoted nationally in 1946 to improve hospital care. If more hospitals met minimum standards of operation, a greater number of people would be discharged in healthier conditions. Was this goal achieved? Today the population of the United States lives longer; but was this due to hospital licensure, or better nutrition, education, or housing?

One open system interacts with other open systems so that it becomes impossible to isolate cause and effect. Whether or not, or to what extent, hospital licensure has promoted longer life remains unknown.

Concepts about regulation have an implicit assumption that the future can be whatever society wants it to be by the use of reason. Tomorrow will be perfect; it is malleable, reasons the regulator, and the wider price to be paid is not counted.

Experience with the upward spiral of health care regulation has demonstrated an institutional loss of equity and liberty. Medicare regulations have placed percentile caps on hospital costs, removed the program's participation in net operating surpluses and bad debts, and ignored the equity of private patients. Liberty has been lost by requiring Section 1122 reviews and certificates of need. In essence, regulation writers have said that liberty and equity are luxuries that society can no longer afford to maintain for American hospitals.

Goal Definition

Hospital regulation in the past decade has provided insufficient time to assess past and present modes of regulation. However, many hospital executives sense an inappropriateness in current federal regulation. Their uneasiness is expressed in a commonly asked question: "What should new regulations accomplish?" Too often in the past their concerns were focused on what new regulations required.

When hospital industry representatives testify before Congressional committees, or work with HHS officers, a first priority should be obtaining a definition of the good being sought by proposed regulations. Goal definition is crucial to accomplish good regulation. The greatest amount of Medicare and Medicaid regulation in the last five or six years has been aimed at reduction in costs for both programs.

The ultimate in cost reduction would be either the abolishment of the programs or the closing of all hospitals. Obviously these values are not held by the vast majority of the public, and they have little political meaning. Cost control regulations that have been promulgated fall somewhere short of these points.

In the past, the federal government adopted a procedure that required departments to prepare cost impact statements for new regulations. Federal departments preferred not to be bound by this requirement because of the difficulty of estimating cost effectiveness of proposed regulations operating in open systems.

Some time ago, the Food and Drug Administration initially estimated a cost savings of about $80,000,000 for the Maximum Allowable Cost (MAX) program for generic drugs for Medicare. After 18 months of negotiation and the threat to file a Freedom of Information request, this estimate was pared to $26,000,000.

The Medicare program may save this money by using generic rather than brand name drugs. However, the compliance cost to hospitals, physicians, and pharmacies may easily exceed two to three times this amount of dollars. Existing accounting systems will never reflect why additional operating costs were incurred or the impact on the quality of patient care when physicians' prescriptive practices are limited. Ultimately, the cost effectiveness of MAX drug regulations will be blurred by the interactions of different open systems, the difficulties of measurement, and the values held by its participants. No one will ever be totally certain of the net effect of this regulation.

Regulatory ideas that seek cost limitation on hospital care are perverse since lower inputs for health services are assumed to mean greater efficiency. If there is an unequivocally definable goal, a concept of efficiency is useful. In health care there is no clearly defined goal, because no rigid standard for measuring health exists. Efficiency means measurements of outputs. In open systems, outputs in one system are inputs in a related system.

Where there are networks of interconnected systems, regulatory interventions must be sure which system is the focus of a problem and how to intervene to achieve a desired goal.

Regulations of health care work from a model based on the scientific method. They believe in systematic procedures, identification of goals, forecasting techniques, devising alternative strategies, evaluating planned outcomes, statistical monitoring of the action, and feedback mechanisms. Hospital planning legislation, such as P.L. 92–603 and P.L. 93–641 are examples of this kind of thinking. Because several open systems are involved, it is questionable whether such a plan will succeed over time. Denials for CAT scanner units have upset many a hospital, with a result that neurosurgeons and neurologists have purchased scanners for their offices and avoided the regulatory mechanism.

Experience in regulatory interconnected open systems would have predicted this outcome. Their planning model did not work. Because of the basic technological advantage of scanning techniques, most hospitals will sooner or later acquire scanning capabilities. Efficiency in spending dollars was temporarily accomplished, but will be overturned by values about the quality of patient care.

Other planning issues will follow the same path. The current effort to define hospital service areas and program the number of hospitals and beds needed will never achieve optimal results. As long as population movements cannot be controlled, it is folly to believe that a new suburb of 80,000 people will not sooner or later have a hospital, despite a citywide 50 percent occupancy rate in hospitals.

Problem Definition

Problem definition is difficult in open systems. No tightly defined paradigm exists. There are conflicting sets of values that contend with differing objectives. Mandated planning can never solve these problems; they are elusive and ensnared in an arena of political judgments. The best that can be accomplished is a continual resolving of previous solutions. This is so for all public policy issues.

Regulatory control of open systems faces unique problems. In solving scientific problems the solution does not have to be visualized in a statement of the problem. In public policy matters a description of the problem must include a guess as to how the problem will be resolved.

Definition of a problem is the formulation of a proposed solution. For example, if deficient mental health services are a problem, then improvement in mental health services is a solution. To accomplish this goal, the next step is to expand the number of community mental health centers and the availability of staff, new therapies, and so on. The problem has been identified in terms of the solution, not in terms of its context.

How does a person know when the mental health problem has been solved? There is no endpoint because there can always be better mental health. Realistically the endpoint is reached when money runs out, or enough is enough; not because poor mental health has been eliminated.

On public policy issues there is no trial run for the new regulations. Even demonstration projects have a tail of never-ending consequences. The lives of individuals who participated are changed, money is spent, and its impact is irreversible. Then another round of solutions is initiated, other consequences occur, and new dilemmas need to be faced.

The history of Medicare regulation illustrates the problem. In the last decade, its regulations appear to have chased one problem after another, with the regulations becoming increasingly specific and restrictive, and no end is yet in sight. Officials at HHS must have a sense that hospitals are like balloons, they squeeze at one point, and a bulge appears elsewhere. Every problem seems to be a symptom of another problem. This is the nature of open systems.

Regulatory thinking is an effort to change the present state of affairs from what is to what it ought to be. Reasons are sought to explain the difference and resolutions suggested. However, a remedy at one level is a problem at a higher level. Solving the problem of medical cases overloading emergency rooms is an example of this chicken and egg thinking. To eliminate medical patients, the most common proposal is to educate the public to have a family physician. This recommendation then raises issues about who is to do the educating, how it is to be done, and whether it will be effective. The proposed solution has set off a series of issues at a higher level.

As solutions become broader, implementation becomes increasingly difficult. For this reason regulators attack their problems in small steps in the hope that a systematic approach will lead to overall improvement. However, when a problem is approached on too low a level, its elimination at one level may create more severe problems at a higher level. The regulator often fails to consider that marginal improvements do not necessarily guarantee overall improvement.

For example, the current proposals of HHS requiring uniform reporting of accounting forms as required by PL 93–641 may result in reduced Medicare costs or make audits easier, but they will straightjacket hospital organization structures and increase the costs of future change.

Regulators think about problems of regulation in terms of their own experiences. They tend to choose explanations that are plausible to them and conform to their understanding of the real world. Whether or not they accurately perceive reality is seldom questioned. The elimination of any net operating surplus from Medicare and Medicaid reimbursement formulas is an escape from the realities of hospital financing in an inflationary economy.

Regulators need to understand that they are liable for the consequences of their actions. The effects of what they do can matter a great deal to the people and institutions that are touched by those actions.

Part of the Political Process

Regulation is totally a part of the political process. Values held by a heterogeneous population affect regulation through politics. As the American scene becomes increasingly heterogeneous, there will be an increasing struggle over which set of values will be heeded. Physicians, trustees, hospital staff members, government employees, blacks, the poor, the wealthy, old, young, nonworkers, and workers each have priorities in hospital care that they want reflected in new regulations. The displeasure of ignored groups is then expressed in the political system.

The way to get regulators' attention is through a congressman or a governor. Administrators have a vague sense that mounting regulations are unnecessarily forcing hospitals into confrontations with one group or another at an increasing rate and into more and more interactions with the political process. Subpublics are learning to use the political system to regulate hospitals to serve their goals. HHS utilization review (UR) regulations are a good example of differing interests of groups and of failure to identify the appropriate system locus of controlling hospital lengths of stay.

Physicians admit and discharge patients. The burden for noncompliance, however, falls on the hospital. If a staff physician refuses to comply with a determination that a patient's continued stay is medically unnecessary, the hospital is denied reimbursement under Medicare.

Imposing this sanction on the hospital has little bearing on the actions of the physician, in whose hands the decision lies as to whether or not to admit or discharge a patient. The effect of placing the sanction for physician noncompliance on a hospital is to require a hospital to provide services without federal reimbursement, and thus to increase its charges to non-Medicare patients. A more appropriate regulation for an effective UR system would impose sanctions on a physician, rather than on a hospital.

This form of regulation has other consequences. Physician cooperation is essential for the effective operation of a hospital. By placing the hospital at the center of UR regulation, the medical staff/hospital relationship is damaged when hospitals are forced to oppose physicians.

STEPS TO IMPROVE REGULATION

Given the nature of open systems and a need for some regulation, what can be done to improve the regulator actions of government, particularly HHS?

In the first place, the regulatory process should be improved to ensure that HHS cannot act, as it has, without a full and open public debate. Two procedure changes would help to achieve this goal: (a) congressional review of major regulatory proposals; and (b) evidentiary hearings before HHS with a right of cross-examination. Taking these steps would make known the heterogeneous interests of different groups, rather than having them develop later at the institutional level.

Both procedures would help determine the appropriate level for interposing a new regulation. Advantages and disadvantages would be more sharply focused and the purpose would be made more explicit. The procedures would also provide a forum where questions can be raised, such as what standard is to be used to determine success and how it will be measured.

When the hospital field is surveyed, concerns about present and future regulation seem to be considerable. Past practices of waiting for the next spate of regulation and then struggling to comply are gradually waning as hospital administrators learn how to cope with a regulatory environment. However, a broad understanding of the constraints and methodologies of regulation will increase the influence of hospital administrators. They will learn that there are many issues to be faced to combat revolting regulation successfully.

Chapter 12

Alice in the Hospital Wonderland

In the story *Alice in Wonderland,* a little girl undergoes a series of disquieting experiences as she tries to find a way home. Ultimately, she succeeds, and a happy ending follows. This is the popular American dream, that misfortune will fail and goodwill will triumph.

Hospitals in the United States are like Alice in Wonderland; they are lost and trying to find their way. They are beset by problems they did not create, though public opinion convinces them to the contrary. What is occurring to this major industry in our country cannot lead to a conclusion that, like Alice, a happy ending will follow. There is much evidence that this will not occur, unless hospitals reassert some basic truths that are being ignored in favor of some popular myths.

A NEED TO CHALLENGE GOVERNMENT ACTIONS

For the past several years, hospitals have gone right along without challenging the basic thrust of the federal and state governments. While they have filed a spate of suits against government actions, they have chosen to fight on grounds that are irrelevant, in terms of bringing about change. Without challenging the basic assumption on which government acts, they have been a party to the present dilemma.

Government actions are based on an implicit assumption that hospitals are masters of their own ships. Until now, hospitals have gone along with the hoax. When PSROs were invented, and HSAs, prospective rates, and ceilings were proposed, hospitals participated without publicly informing

---

*Reprinted with permission from HOSPITAL PROGRESS, August 1978, © 1978 by The Catholic Health Association.

those who make laws that what was being enacted to control the rise in hospital expenditures was beyond hospitals' abilities to affect. Instead of explaining the total relationship between physicians and hospitals to bring about a full understanding, hospitals fell into a trap of responding to specific elements of proposed legislation rather than describing the milieu in which a general hospital operates.

As a primary premise, hospitals do not control admission of patients. Hospitals are only facilitating agents. They appoint members of the medical staff and establish minimum performance standards. The decision to admit a patient, the services to be ordered, and the decision to discharge are traditionally matters decided by a physician without interference from a hospital.

Yet, the efforts of third party payers of hospital bills have been focused on containing costs of hospital operations. On the patient side, UR and PSRO activities have attempted to control length of stays. On the administrative side, prior approval for the expenditure of capital funds has been required. Both efforts have been aimed at the wrong point in the health care delivery system, and not on the physician-patient relationship, where control must be effected. This is not to say that controls are not necessary; rather, they are secondary to the primary control point that revolves around the physician and patient.

There are three major reasons why controls on hospitals will never achieve the results desired by the federal government:

1. Hospitals, like any corporate entity, have an inherent drive for growth, fiscal viability, improvement in service, and prudent economic decisions; they pragmatically balance commitments against resources to permit the institution to survive.
2. Physicians, while part of an organized medical staff in a hospital, are primarily independent entrepreneurs and are regarded by the decision makers in hospitals as surrogate customers.
3. Physicians believe it is their prerogative to decide the mode of treating a patient without control by the hospital.

Controls now applied to hospitals are being used as guidelines by HSAs to evaluate certificate-of-need applications. This tends to force institutions to work against their own economic interests. Not only is the hospital expected to respond to the need for a requested service, but at the same time it is expected to seek support of the other hospitals in the same area for developing the proposed program. Stripped of idealism, this action calls for a hospital to use its creativity to make a marketing judgment and then to turn around and report to its competitors what is planned and expect them to support the program.

Government policies assume that hospitals are advocates of UR and PSRO activities. Both are aimed at shortening an average length of patient stay, and, in some cases, this can lead to an average occupancy rate that results in an unsatisfactory financial situation. Even when these programs work against the best economic interests of a hospital, it is expected that the hospital will pursue this approach with vigor. They may be desirable programs when a hospital has a high occupancy rate, but it becomes disastrous when a hospital has a marginal fiscal picture.

Another program of the federal government that works against a hospital's interests is to expect several hospitals in the same community to get together and seriously explore trading off clinical services, particularly emergency services, pediatrics, and obstetrics. Because of the ripple effect, a hospital that might be willing to give up an obstetrical service because of low volume finds that to do so it must also consider its gynecology admissions. The same holds true for an emergency room; admission of inpatients from this service must be considered. Treated separately, what may appear to be reasonable for a single service may turn out to be fiscally irresponsible when the ripple effect is taken into account.

The present trend of regulation is based on a naive belief that hospitals have not and cannot manage their affairs in the public's best interest without government agencies reviewing and approving all fiscal activities. This is a strikingly different position than a few years ago.

When the history of the relationship between hospitals and government is traced, the last 30 years have seen a remarkable transition. From the mid-1940s up to the mid-1950s, government was an advocate of hospitals, wanting to expand and increase their numbers. The Hill-Burton Program was directed to this end, but was focused on the lack of hospitals in rural areas. By the mid-1960s, advocacy changed to a position of partnership and was expressed through the passage of the Partnership for Health legislation. By the mid-1970s, partnership shifted to an adversary position with the intention of controlling activities of hospitals. This is the current situation.

Each new set of regulations issued brings forth a rash of suits contesting the positions of government on either substantive or procedural bases. In the period of three decades, the shift has been from advocacy to partnership to adversary relationships. To thoughtful observers it is clear that in the long run the present situation is not in the best interests of hospitals, government, or the general public. It is neither constructive nor positive.

Health systems in all of the developed countries have a similar history. Between 1870 and 1930, their major trait was one of expansion of the health care system. The United States went from a few hundred hospitals to over 4,500 in this period. Other countries experienced the same growth phenomenon. The period between 1930 and 1965 was characterized by putting financing mechanisms for health care in place. From 1965 on, all concerns were on controlling the rising costs of hospitals.

RESTRUCTURING THE HEALTH DELIVERY SYSTEM

Promotion of HMOs

Looking to the future, there appears to be two possible courses of action. One system receiving government support and encouragement is the widespread promotion of health maintenance organizations. From the standpoint of the third party payer, this arrangement appears attractive. The patient/subscriber deals with a prepayment system that in turn deals with both physicians and hospitals, and exerts pressure to balance the provision of hospital and physician services against premiums paid by subscribers. It is a closed loop system, where fiscal interests have primacy over other interests. This model envisions patient days per 1,000 population as absolutely no higher than 1,000 per 1,000 population, preferably around 500 to 600 patient days of care annually, rather than the existing 1,250 patient days now seen in many communities. It is doubtful that this model can successfully be applied to an entire population. HMOs are aimed at enrolling employee groups and do not address themselves to the aged, chronic, alcoholic, or mental patients who are not in the working population.

An HMO pattern, if widely applied, could serve the interests of third party payers at the expense of the total range of services needed by the public. It is understandable why government would support this model. Not only does it require fewer days of care to be paid for by Medicare and Medicaid, but it keeps government out of administration of the program. Rather than dealing with 350,000 practicing physicians and 7,000 hospitals, it need only be concerned with approximately 200 + HMOs.

Protection of Legitimate Hospital and Government Interests

The other system for hospitals is to move toward protecting the legitimate interests of both hospitals and government. Each role in this system needs clarification. Government has to stop placing unrealistic regulations on hospitals and expecting them to police the utilization of both hospital and medical services.

The present method of penalizing hospitals for all weaknesses in the health delivery system has reached a point where Blue Cross and the federal government have both been active in putting restraints on hospitals. In the process they have not looked hard at what they might do to control costs. For example, Blue Cross for many years has paid first dollar costs of its subscribers' hospital expenses when they entered hospitals. Clearly this action separates an episode of illness from its direct economic consequences.

To make matters worse, subscribers usually believe that during hospitalization they are entitled to have all services paid since they have paid a monthly premium for this protection and are now entitled to collect on this insurance. The fact that Blue Cross offers policies that encourage hospital use is justified from their viewpoint because of marketplace competition. The fact that hospitals act similarly is not considered appropriate institutional behavior by third party payers.

In a restructuring of the health care system a major priority should be given to forcing third party carriers to move away from paying for first dollar costs for their subscribers during hospitalization. Until this is accomplished, payments to hospitals will continue to rise.

This is no small task since both labor unions and employers have fought bruising battles over this issue for years. Both sides would probably be reluctant to reopen the issue, yet it is necessary if inpatient hospital use is to be affected.

One of the myths the public believes about health care is that the government and Blue Cross are upset by the rising hospital costs. Their expression "rising hospital costs" is merely a way of reflecting concerns about the rapidly increasing number of dollars paid to hospitals for services received by subscribers.

Payments to hospitals by Blue Cross and Medicare have two basic parts: (a) the days of care they pay for on behalf of subscribers; and (b) the average cost per patient day of care in the hospital. Even though there are two parts to this equation, both the government and Blue Cross have elected to focus on only the half that is safest from their point of view; cost per patient day. The other half, subscriber usage, goes unmentioned.

Since neither government nor Blue Cross has shown any serious interest in dealing with elements of usage that are under their control, it seems appropriate for hospitals to suggest strongly to both government and Blue Cross the need for doing so. Since economic leverages are usually required to get another group's attention, hospitals should work through their state hospital associations and adopt strong measures to force the Blue Cross and Blue Shield to undertake the necessary correction.

Focus on the Physician-Patient Relationship

Political peace by the mid-1980s can only be achieved if hospitals force attention of the third party payers on the physician/patient relationship, rather than on hospitals. Past negotiations with Blue Cross have usually been a debate over the adequacy of reimbursement, which casts hospitals in the role of being money hungry and unconcerned with public considerations.

If hospitals were to join together in a coordinated effort to insist that Blue Cross develop programs that move away from first dollar coverage for hospital stays, they would succeed. If Blue Cross resisted these efforts, hospitals should consider threatening to terminate employer contracts with Blue Cross, on the logic that the Blue Cross and Blue Shield are less interested than hospitals in the amount of monthly premiums paid by subscribers. Unless Blue Cross is put between a rock and a hard spot, it will probably not look seriously at moving away from first dollar coverage because of the countervailing pressures from labor unions and employer groups.

Malpractice Insurance

Another consideration that needs to be dealt with is the malpractice insurance situation. Given the legal climate that pervades society, physicians and hospitals need to be given protection against capricious lawsuits. If third party payers want physicians and hospitals to use ambulatory approaches for medical care as much as possible in order to reduce inpatient admissions, physicians and hospitals need assurance that they will be protected.

To expect physicians to exploit ambulatory care to the maximum feasible extent may be asking them to take unnecessary risks. In order to eliminate the risk, the federal government should consider the establishment of a federally-created insurance corporation, so that physicians and hospitals are protected in the exercise of reasonable clinical judgment. This kind of legislation needs support from the Social Security Administration in order to assure public and congressional representatives that this type of legislation is not motivated by vested interests, but by an agency concerned with appropriate use of health care resources. In this type of program, panels of experts would probably have to be developed to review pending cases and pass on the quality of professional judgment in each situation.

Fee-for-Service Concept

If the physician/patient relationship is to become a focal point for economic decision making, care must be taken to preserve the fee-for-service concept. To move away from the traditional fee structure is to invite physicians to find avenues around programs or not to participate at all. Concerns expressed about fee for service usually center around the amount of fees charged and the incomes generated by some physicians. This criticism has led to seeking alternative methods for reimbursing physicians for their services. To follow this line of reasoning is to assure failure of any proposed program, because a total alienation of the medical profession will occur. It would be far more productive to have medical representatives indicate a desire to retain fee for service. Having clarified this point, attention could then be turned to defining methods that provide patients and third party payers with recourse when they are dissatisfied with professional fees.

What has been lost sight of throughout the years is that fee for service is a system of payment in which patients pay only for services received. This system provides the maximum in flexibility and encourages a physician to spend optimal time on professional activities of direct patient care. When a physician opts to work fewer hours per day or per week, fewer patients will be seen, and there will be a lowering of physician payments. When a physician works harder and sees more patients, the reverse is likewise true. Incentives for working are automatic in such a system. When a physician stops work, is sued, takes a vacation, falls ill, or retires, no organization is responsible for the related costs. The system is highly efficient; there are no built-in inefficiencies. This must be kept in mind when dealing with proponents of closed loop systems who advocate salaries for physicians; they are pushing for a less productive system.

Because of its flexible nature, fee for service can be used to accomplish the objectives of the third party payers in limiting hospitalization. For example, the professional fee schedule for a cystoscopy might be higher when performed on an outpatient basis. The same could be true for ambulatory surgery; the fee schedule could make it in the surgeon's economic interest to perform it on an outpatient basis. The procedures to be included should be developed with the recognized specialty groups in organized medicine, and not simply be determined by HHS, the work of the intermediaries, or Blue Cross and Blue Shield plans. The key to workability lies in the cooperation and support of private practitioners and the organized medical group to which they relate. Rather than have the American Medical Association (AMA) as the only point of contact, the representation of physicians' interests should be broadened to include that of the specialty organizations.

Reimbursement

In the course of restructuring the health delivery system, the existing cost system of reimbursement must be abandoned. Economic forces at work must be allowed to become a major determinant of the use of hospital services. To pay a hospital its costs, no matter what the level, is not an incentive to sound management. Neither is it wise to substitute government regulation for all of the managerial and financial decisions of a hospital. Both practices lead to increases in costs and politicization of the decision-making process.

Little can be accomplished until the incentives and behavior of physicians, patients, hospital management, and governing boards are permitted to make rational economic decisions from their respective viewpoints. These must also be compatible with the self-interests of the payers of these services. Ways need to be found for increasing competition between health care providers. Physicians and patients have to have an incentive for selecting an institution on the basis of relative quality and known cost of service.

Patient Economic Responsibility

As part of restructuring the health delivery system, patients must be brought into the economic decision making. As things now stand, typical patients neither know nor can anticipate physicians' fees or hospital charges. They have no economic stake in paying for the costs of these services, except as the costs are ultimately reflected in the monthly premium that they pay. Since that cost is lumped together with thousands of other subscriber payments, there is no direct relationship between an episode of illness and a monthly premium. Neither are patients penalized if they do not follow their physician's directions for either improving health or staying out of a hospital.

There is a growing concern about the way to limit health care expenditures by concentrating on the issue of keeping persons healthy, rather than on the question of returning them to health after they have incurred an illness. Hospitals, by their very nature, are repair-oriented; they see the patient after a physiological change has occurred. There has not been a concerted effort among physicians to prevent illness either. Physicians are problem-solvers who are concerned with discovering disease and treating it. They, like hospitals, react to what is discovered and do not have a primary concern with human preventive maintenance.

A prepayment plan might offer a variety of premium rates. For persons who have had a heart attack or a stroke, there might be a surcharge on the basic premium rate unless the subscribers could present evidence that: (1) they are on a regular exercise program; (2) their weight is controlled; or (3) they have attended a course for victims of heart disease dealing with how to change life styles to live successfully with the disability.

An annual certification might be required in order to demonstrate continued adherence to the program. Upon receipt of an attesting statement, the premium would be lowered to a standard rate. In the event a subscriber is healthy, he might be given credit for proper diet, exercise, nonsmoking, and other positive indicators, thus having the benefit of a reduced premium. Where an employer now bears the full cost of premiums, the subscriber might instead be paid the difference between the regular premium and the reduced premium, or conversely, the subscriber might have to pay the difference between a regular premium and the surcharge that might be levied for poor health practices. Such a program would most likely be effective. The role of the hospital would be to provide training programs for each specific disease entity.

BEGINNING A NEW ROAD

For years, those in the health field have believed that no compromise in quality of care can be permitted. The public may no longer share this belief. The public may have undergone a permanent shift in attitude and may now be concerned more with cost than quality.

Future efforts should be directed toward the demand side of the equation and not on cost containment that cripples the health care industry. The hospitals of New York and Massachusetts are keenly aware of the disastrous effects of limited reimbursement. They know the importance of affecting the physician -patient relationship so that economics come into play at this point in the system.

With increasing frequency, public representatives are raising health care economic problems they want considered. They are questioning relentlessly capital costs of hospitals at HSA meetings. However, to hospital professionals, this seems to be a reaction to a set of beliefs they hold and not from a philosophical basis of what they expect in hospital care. The present status of the relationship between hospitals and government cannot continue indefinitely, but must be permitted to evolve into an era where programs, services, and controls square with the forces at work in a free marketplace.

As things now stand, hospitals and physicians are being caught up by arbritrarily imposed standards that require the knuckling under of the private health care sector to government dictates and edicts.

The government's game plan has three major thrusts: (a) programs designed to cope with physician activities; (b) programs aimed at reducing inpatient use of hospitals; and (c) control of the operating and capital funds of hospitals.

To date, the controls being applied to physicians have lagged behind those on hospitals, but a change can be anticipated. The federal government will impose controls on physicians through PSROs and by encouraging the development of HMOs so that increasing numbers of physicians will be forced out of private practice and into HMO medicine due to economic necessity.

The leverage needed for accomplishing the government's objectives for hospitals will be through HSAs and the reimbursement programs of Medicare and Medicaid. Since funding for HSAs is federal funding, requirements can and are being laid down that require an HSA to submit an acceptable plan to HHS if they are to receive annual funding. Their plans must follow the guidelines determined at the federal level.

At an institutional level, controls are exercised in the form of reimbursement, which is manipulated by HHS to force conformance with federal standards. Remaining largely outside the sphere of control is the physician-patient relationship. This is a crucial point in the entire health care delivery system. To be successful, patients and physicians must be so affected that, in acting in their own best economic interests, they are also acting in the best economic interests of the body politic.

As the problem now stands, government controls are based on taking financially protective measures solely against hospitals for matters having to do directly with patient care. At the institutional level, restrictions are twofold: control over capital expenditures above $150,000 and any substantial change in programs or services under the threat of losing depreciation and interest expense if not approved. This is cost control, not control of demand. The difference goes unrecognized.

No doubt Alice knew she was a long way from home when she was in Wonderland. Hospitals apparently don't attach enough significance to their own position since they let others continue to apply cost controls. Hospitals are unlikely to have the same success as Alice.

To those who read the *Federal Register,* who meet with staff members of congressional committees, who provide testimony at public hearings of Congress, and who are acquainted with the names, faces, and positions of persons in the executive branch dealing with health care, the distinction between the legislative and executive arms is striking. If hospitals are to move to a position of neutrality over the next decade, they would do well to remember the sage observation of H. L. Mencken, who said, "The urge to save humanity is almost always only a false face for the urge to rule."

To those who watch the main actors at HHS and read the increasing number of rules, regulations, guidelines, and standards, this pithy comment seems appropriate.

One of the major instruments available to hospitals in dealing with HSAs is a long-range plan that delineates not only what the hospital is now providing in programs and services, but looks to its role in the future. The more accurate the projections, the more defensible its methodologies, and the better the chance of establishing credibility in a review of projects by the HSA. In addition, hospitals are going to have to face a choice.

If they elect to continue to deal primarily with HHS and only casually with Congress, they will probably be caught in a unified system, dominated regionally by 200 HMOs and nationally by HHS.

On the other hand, if hospitals choose to expend most of the efforts and dollars at the congressional level and keep HHS as a secondary concern, then the chances of deliberately plotting a course of action that ultimately evolves into a neutral role for hospitals has some hope in the future.

Responsiveness at the federal level is far more apt to come from the Congress than from HHS. To be effective, though, representatives from Congress and the Senate need hard facts, solid analysis, and an understanding of the issues involved. With their own small staffs and far too many commitments, they are not in a position to do this for themselves, but must rely on HHS or else turn to agencies and persons outside of government circles who are affected by their decisions. Capitol Hill needs to hear not only from the AHA, but from constituents back home. More than casual thoughts are required. They need to see carefully reasoned positions presented in easily readable fashion.

Moving the health field to neutrality will not be an easy task. It will be opposed by persons within government as well as outside. Focusing on the right issues will be hard to do because of the previous practice of looking at the wrong policymakers. Working closely with Congress appears to be a route that will be most productive. The health field needs to be heard on a continuing basis at this key level of government.

What does all this mean for the individual hospital? Recognizing that the thrust of government is to reduce payments to hospitals through the application of more and more stringent fiscal controls and to make it harder for them to keep up with technological change, what can the hospital do in the hostile climate that now exists? At the national level, hospitals must become more involved politically with a Congress that will appreciate the limits hospitals can effectively control.

Today, a hospital response requires something more than a continuation of existing trends, but must be responsive to the guidelines as put forth by HHS. Priorities may have to be shifted, innovations developed, attitudes changed, the fact recognized that the ways of the past are gone forever and that the future belongs to those institutions who regard the years ahead as a challenge. Changes in the future are not something to be avoided or shunned because they break with tradition. This is not the end of the road, but the beginning of a new one.

Chapter 13

The Caterpillar and the Butterfly

In the past, I had thought that the coming decade would be characterized by the development of economic competition in the health field through the rapid expansion of capitation plans. In explaining why this is apt to be the case, I had concluded that the road down which the industry is now marching—of increasing regulation—would eventually reach the point of bringing the hospital field to a standstill. Thinking more from an emotional standpoint than anything else, I concluded that the piling on of more and more regulation would lead to this result.

On reflection, such a conclusion is unjustified. No matter how much bureaucratic tinkering is done to the health field and no matter how many unfair and inequitable regulations are laid on hospitals, the health care industry plays such a vital and integral part of daily living that it will survive. It will neither grind to a halt nor will trustees give the front door keys of hospitals to the federal government to operate. Battered and buffeted by the hail of regulation, the health care delivery system will continue to operate, but in a different configuration of services.

EMERGENCE OF THE HEALTH FIELD

Over the past 40 years, the health field has moved from an almost invisible part of any community to a position of prominence. Years ago a 200-bed hospital was considered by health professionals to be a substantial institution, even though it often occupied less area than a city block and blended unobtrusively into its neighborhood. Automobiles parked along the streets around the hospital were a minor irritant to the homeowners of adjacent property. Physician offices went unnoticed, since they were typically located over drugstores or in innocuous-looking office buildings scattered throughout the community. Hospital equipment rental stores were difficult to find unless someone had the exact address. The only large, visible facilities were state health insitutions, which were located on the town periphery at the end of streetcar lines or in rural areas.

Today the scene is visibly changed. The 200-bed hospital has grown into a complex covering six to eight square blocks that may include a 600-bed general hospital with an emergency room handling 30,000 to 50,000 visits annually, a skilled nursing home, a mental health center, an ambulatory surgical facility, one or two large professional office buildings, and a road network specifically designed to handle high volumes of traffic flowing on and off the health campus. Throughout the town, much evidence can be seen of other health related activities, for example, drugstores on busy corners and rows of one- and two-story small office buildings housing a wide array of specialists, clinical psychologists, holistic medical programs, comprehensive health screening programs, community blood banks, and individual offices for optometrists and podiatrists. Hospital equipment rental stores now look like large supermarkets. Taken together, the wide spectrum of health activities has now become a highly visible part of every city and town in this country. Thinking back to what it was like 40 years ago, health care has become a larger and more important part of the resources used by every family. The continuous and substantial demand by the public over the last four decades has changed the caterpillar into the butterfly as a result of the growing public interest in mending, fixing, and repairing the human body.

Shift in Public Attitudes

The demand for more health care has undergone a remarkable change. Citizens no longer are willing to accept their physical condition as something over which they can do nothing. Persons employed by public agencies do not accept a passive attitude toward social or health problems they encounter.

This drastic shift in attitude is highlighted in James Michener's book, *Chesapeake,* where he describes Timothy Turlock as a penniless man living off the land who has lost all of his teeth in later life and simply accepts it as inevitable.[1] Had Turlock been living today, he would be receiving a monthly welfare check, and arrangements would be made for him to receive a full set of dentures at the taxpayers expense.

Expenditures

This shift in public demand for health care services is apparent when the personal health care component of the gross national product (GNP) is examined. The results of the last 28 years contained in Table 13–1 show what has happened.

In this period, health care expenditures, as a percent of GNP, have slightly more than doubled, which means that the public is willing to spend directly, or to have spent on their behalf, twice as much of the portion of the pie than they did in 1950. For whatever reasons, they think health care is worth this share of the GNP. Physicians may have influenced the demand for health care services, but the public agrees with this increasing share being spent in this manner.

This shift has been aided and abetted by the news media, who appreciate the public interest in all things concerning health. *The Wall Street Journal* is a good example of the current level of interest in this subject. As a financial paper primarily concerned with business and finance, a reader would not expect to find many full-length articles devoted to the health field. Yet, two or three times a week there is a major piece detailing some aspect of the industry. The newspaper reflects the shift in public attitudes that has taken place.

This shift can be verified in another way. Since 1965, total health spending has grown an average of 12.2 percent per year, while the economy, as a whole, has averaged 9.0 percent per annum.[2] If this has been induced by government programs, the government's share of health care expenditures as a proportion of all health care would be rising each year, but such is not the case. In 1975 and 1976, government programs accounted for 42 percent of all health care dollars, but this dropped slightly in 1977 and 1978 to 41 percent.[3] The continued shift for a greater share of the GNP indicates that the demand for health care is strong and growing stronger each year. What may be an ugly caterpillar to the federal government may turn out to be a butterfly when viewed from the perspective of the public.

Table 13-1 Personal Health Care Expenditures as a Proportion of the Gross National Product

Year	Percent of GNP	Amount (Billions)
1950	4.5	12.7
1960	5.3	26.9
1965	6.2	43.0
1970	7.6	74.7
1975	8.6	131.5
1978	9.1	192.4

Source: *Health Care Financing Review* (Washington, D.C.: U.S. Department of HEW, Health Care Financing Administration, Summer 1979), p. 22.

Increase in Intensity Factors

When intensity factors are examined, they reveal the same trend. From 1970 to 1978, inpatient days increased 8 percent, while the population in that same period rose 6.9 percent, and the average length of stay declined from 8.2 to 7.6.[4,5,6]

Physicians also experienced the same phenomenon. Total physician visits from 1972 through 1977 stayed relatively constant, resulting in a per capita decrease from 5.0 to 4.8 visits per year.[7] During this period, however, emergency room visits increased from 60.1 million to 77.6 million, a 29.1 percent rise.[8] Meanwhile, hospital laboratory tests went from 850 tests per 1,000 physicians to 1,510, an increase of 77.6 percent.[9] Both the public and physicians are using more services; the public does so when a physician is not readily available, while the physician is using more of the backup services in order to obtain a more complete clinical picture. As is to be expected in today's world, the physician prefers to deal with as much quantitative information as can be reasonably secured before outlining a specific course of therapy for a patient.

The reasons behind the increase in the intensity factors need to be examined in greater detail. Several reasons have brought about this shift and are woven together. Though they can be separately identified, the proportionate weight of each cannot be measured.

First, public demand plays a part. When a new service becomes available in a community, such as the start of a renal dialysis program, this is often reported in the news media to inform the public. A family, on its own initiative, may call their physician and inquire about the new service if some member has a condition that might be aided by it, or they might call the center and secure the needed information.

Second, physicians in a town also have the same kind of interest as the public, but for different reasons. Knowning they are likely to be asked about the new service, they will chat with other physicians who they believe may know more about it. If satisfied, they will begin to make referrals to it in order to be able to make up their own minds about its usefulness to their patients. If this proves out, they will begin to refer appropriate patients routinely. As referring physicians, their motivation is not economic since they have nothing to gain by it. Rather, it stems from their desire to see that their patients benefit from an available resource. Whether or not patients take advantage of the referral and how they pay for it are questions that referring physicians consider outside their purview. In physicians' minds they have discharged their professional responsibility by making the appropriate referrals.

With the proliferation of specialists and health related services that has occurred, referrals are now an everyday occurrence in physicians' offices. Physicians draw on a wide range of available resources including specialist consultations, freestanding clinical laboratories, x-ray units, cardiopulmonary laboratories, ambulatory surgeries, mammography, CAT scans, and physical therapy. Practicing physicians are now at the hub of a large network that has grown and expanded as a result of their desire to see to it that their patients are properly treated.

Third, intensity has grown as a result of new medical knowledge becoming known to the practicing physician. This occurs in two ways. In medical schools, often with the financial assistance of a National Institute of Health (NIH) grant, experimental projects are undertaken. If the project is successful, such as a speech and hearing clinic sponsored by an otolarnygology service, the physicians heading the project will begin to train nonmedical personnel. If the informal training program works out, a formal course of instruction will begin, and soon graduates will be found in nonuniversity hospitals and otolaryngologists offices. As the number of therapists grows, a certification program will develop, and a formal career path will be established. Ultimately, these therapists may develop their own practices and establish freestanding speech and hearing clinics. In a decade, this full course may be run from an experimental project to certification.

In the same vein of development, a slightly different course may occur. Private practicing specialists may take the lead in splitting off these programs from universities after learning about the results being obtained through research papers appearing in their journals or through seminars they have attended.

If the demand for new services becomes strong and sufficient volumes develop to make them economically viable, the snowball effect takes place, and the armamentarium of medical resources grows. This has occurred time and again as can be seen in Table 13–2.

In addition to this list, another one could be compiled of physician specialists. In general certifications, 23 fields have been accepted by the American Board of Medical Specialties and an additional 28 in subspecialties.[10]

A fourth reason that has increased the intensity factor has been the malpractice situation. The rapid rise in premium costs for malpractice insurance in the mid-1970s brought home to physicians the need to practice defensive medicine. Not only do they ask themselves if they have enough clinical information about each patient, but they also give consideration to whether or not they would be able to demonstrate adequately the reasonableness of their thinking if they had to defend themselves in court.

Table 13-2 Examples of Specialty Trained Nonmedical
                Health Field Personnel

Bacteriologist	Medical laboratory technologist
Bio-medical engineers	Medical records librarian
Blood bank technologist	Medical secretary
Certified laboratory technician	Nurse anesthetist
Clinical psychologist	Nutritionist
Cystologist	Occupational therapist
Dental hygienist	Optometrist
Dentist	Operating room technician
Dietician	Pharmacist
Electrocardiogram (EKG) technologist	Physician assistant
Food Service manager	Physicist
Health educator	Podiatrist
Hospital administrator	Radiation therapy technician
Histotechnologist	Speech and hearing therapist
Licensed practical nurse	X-ray technician

Source: Health Education Commission, Board of Higher Education, *Health Education Information System And Program Directory*, (Springfield, Ill.: June 1972).

Lastly, physicians now have far less concern about patients getting into life-threatening situations than they had in the past. This narrowing results not only from the availability of more medical knowledge about the clinical problems they face in practice, but from their counting on and taking advantage of the widespread use of automobiles and telephones, and the availability of backup services in the community. As a result, they can rely on patients or their families getting in touch with them if a patient's condition changes markedly. In terms of time, they may be less than a minute away if they need to be reached by phone. If a person needs an examination, physicians typically think that the family can transport the patient to their offices or to a nearby emergency room in a matter of only a few minutes. In the past, neither the automobile nor the telephone were readily available to nearly all the population. Knowing that major physiological changes can take place within minutes or a few hours, physicians were reluctant to take chances, and they followed the course of making broad assumptions about what constituted life-threatening problems. With the widespread acceptance of telephones and cars, they can now narrow their definition with safety. In addition, physicians often see patients long before they are in life-threatening situations, and they take corrective action or refer them to the appropriate specialists or program so that risk is substantially reduced. The use of cars and telephones has reduced the physician's definition of life-threatening situations. House calls are just a memory because of these two developments.

For the five reasons listed, the physician enjoys greater freedom in treating his patients on an ambulatory basis. The trade-off has been an increase in intensity of the use of health services together with a rising demand on the part of the public.

Specialization and Decentralization

This push toward specialization of effort and decentralization of services is not unique to the health field. It has been going on in society for more than a century. The job shop has been replaced by the production line, and the large department store has felt the impact of the specialty shop. Medicine has been caught up in the same trend that sweeps through the general economy. The car and the telephone have simply speeded up the process.

With this perspective in mind, it is appropriate to relate these trends to the impact of increasing regulation. The following benchmarks should be remembered:

- Hospitals have become larger, technologically-oriented enterprises that are both labor and capital intensive.

- Hospitals have demonstrated a willingness to respond to the interest of the public and the medical profession in rapidly introducing new equipment, space, and trained personnel.

- Physicians utilize specialized resources not under their control when the results give them a more complete clinical picture of the patient.

- Physicians willingly refer to specialized resources when they come to appreciate that their patients benefit from their use.

- Patients and their families are unconcerned about the costs of providing service, particularly if shielded by a third party payer mechanism.

- Patients expect to utilize the full range of appropriate services available in the community at the time of the episode of illness.

- The federal government has placed its major emphasis on controlling the costs of the hospital and has largely avoided regulating the use of ambulatory services.

The result of the government's efforts is that it has concentrated its regulations on the inpatient, where nearly 47.9 percent of the health care dollar is spent. This is reflected in Table 13–3.

The 52.3 percent unregulated portion of the nation's health bill is going to physicians, dentists, optometrists, clinical psychologists, podiatrists, hospital rental firms, drugstores, and freestanding professional buildings. The controlled parts are general hospitals and long-term facilities.

PATTERN FOR THE FUTURE

The pattern for the future is clear under increased regulation. The growth and development of programs will occur in the uncontrolled sector as an effort to avoid regulation. As controls are compounded, those persons who are now providing services in the hospital will increasingly look toward moving their activities outside of that environment, from the controlled to the uncontrolled arena. This will be resisted by hospital administrators who will be concerned that this will reduce the volume of any given activity and lead to higher unit costs of operation, because the indirect expenses will be spread across a smaller base of direct costs. This shift will ultimately find the general hospital offering only those services required primarily for inpatient care. A harder look will be taken by physicians in an effort to do more on an ambulatory basis for patients. As long as such shifts lower the cost of providing these services and continue to be paid for by the third party payer, they will be applauded by government, carriers, and the public.

When this trend begins to take hold, the rate of increase in hospital outpatient activities will decline. The gap between actual patient days and

Table 13-3 Use of Health Care Dollars—1978

Type of Service	Percent of Total	Expenditures
Hospital care	39.5	
Physician services	18.3	
Nursing home care	8.2	
Drugs and drug sundries	7.9	
Dentist services	6.9	
Expenses for prepayment and administration	5.2	
Research and medical facilities	4.9	
Government public health	2.6	
Other personal health services	2.3	
Other professional services	2.2	
Eyeglasses and appliances	2.0	
Total	100.0	$167.9 billion

Source: Health Care Financing Review, (Washington, D.C.: U.S. Department of HEW, Health Care Financing Administration, Summer 1979), p. 24.

adjusted patient days annually reported to the AHA will then begin to narrow.

The growth of out-of-hospital health services will include freestanding programs, adjunct services offered by multispecialty group practices, or part of HMOs that will be growing extensively during the next decade. This will take place alongside increasing regulation and will add to the confusion. As HMOs expand enrollments, they are likely to discover that they can offer services to their members on an ambulatory basis at a lower cost than they can purchase the same services from the hospital. At the point they have sufficient volume to undertake such a service at a cost that is lower, they can be expected to commence it. As an HMO, they are exempt from the requirements of PL 93–641 and will not have to apply for a certificate of need. This is an advantage that they will use.

If an HMO foresees that it is unlikely to have sufficient volume for quite a while, it may, along with other HMOs in the same area, contract with a freestanding service, provided the price is cheaper than can be obtained from the hospital. In some cases, it may even encourage the establishment of a freestanding service if the price is favorable.

Under the recently enacted amendments to PL 93–641, HMOs are encouraged to follow this route if they have 50,000 or more enrollees. Hospitals, on the other hand, in order to qualify for certificate-of-need (CON) exemption, must have 75 percent of their admissions from capitation plans. Few hospitals will be able to meet this requirement in the foreseeable future with the exception of those, like the Kaiser-Permanente Hospitals, who have been part of a system for a number of years.

Candidates for moving substantial volumes of patients out from under the hospital umbrella include deep therapy, renal dialysis, physical therapy, diet instruction, and stress testing. Other services are likely to be split between hospital and freestanding programs and to include laboratories, pharmacies, and diagnostic x-ray. The greater the amount of regulation, the more quickly it can be expected to take place.

Behind this kind of movement stands the prevailing attitudes of the medical profession. Physicians in private practice are there because they enjoy that form of organization. They believe in fee for service and have demonstrated time and again their depth of feelings about its importance to them. Part B of Medicare recognizes this, as do all of the carriers that pay Usual, Customary, and Reasonable professional fees. This widespread feeling of independence and the fierce desire to maintain it suggests that physicians will act as they have in the past when threatened by external controls. Where they have clinical interests that can direct ambulatory patient volumes, they will move toward establishing them out of the hospital as part of their own operations, under their own control, and not subject to federal dictates. In many cases where separate programs are begun, they will unnecessarily duplicate that same service in the hospital, and there will be insufficient volumes to maintain both at reasonable degrees of efficiency. Because of physician biases, patients seen in the office will be referred to the ambulatory setting rather than to the hospital, even though it is for the same procedure.

As this course of events unfolds, the general hospital will become more inpatient oriented and will be caring for more acutely ill patients. Also, costs will rise even more sharply because of the intensity of the services that will be required. The trend to locating more related activities on the hospital campus will be reversed. Physicians developing competitive services and programs to those of the hospital will do so on offsite locations. The local health care delivery system will still be a cottage industry, but one that is highly visible and a substantial employer in town. It will function in a loosely coordinated manner, held together by physician referral patterns, the telephone, and the automobile.

The maintaining of controls on inpatient activities and leaving ambulatory care in a free marketplace leads to the reshaping of the system in the manner described. Those in government who are attempting to control personal health care expenditures are aware that the ambulatory side needs to be dealt with through an expansion of regulations over that segment of the industry. To date they have been reluctant to move directly into this arena because of the deeply entrenched viewpoints of the medical profession regarding their prerogatives in a free enterprise system. They know that the fee-for-service concept cannot be directly challenged without doing battle with all physicians. Rather than confront this issue, the government has taken an indirect approach aimed at restricting the amount of federal dollars used to support health manpower programs. For the fiscal year ending 1977, the Bureau Of Health Manpower awarded grants totaling $526.7 million. In 1978, this was reduced to $521.6 million, but if a 12 percent adjustment factor for inflation is applied, the effective amount turns out to be $458.4 million, a real difference of $68.3 million, a reduction of 13 percent.[11]

This trend will eventually dampen off the number of medical students and others enrolled in health professional schools. Even with this taking place, the number of physicians in practice and the number of physicians per 100,000 population will continue to rise through 1990. There will be 219,300 additional physicians practicing in 1990 over 1975, an increase of 58 percent. This suggests that the trend just outlined will be pushed along by physicians who will be looking for ways to enhance their income and will seek opportunities to establish those programs where they see the possibility of offering the same service as the hospital's, but at a lower price.

There are a number of services that can be incorporated into the office practice setting that will generate revenues. The potential list is shown in Table 13–4.

The competitive effect on hospitals will be substantial as illustrated by the changing sources of revenue. (See Table 13–5.)

During the 1970s, the hospital became increasingly dependent on ancillary services for its revenues. Where routine services used to provide the majority of its funds, this has slacked off to where it is less than half. As alternatives for hospitalization increase, physicians can take their practices out of the hospital and center them in their offices. This will be particularly true where HMOs become firmly established, as in Minnesota where this has happened. The results are already evident.

Table 13-4 Potential Outpatient Services in a Prepaid Multispecialty Group Practice

Preventive

Health education
Multiphasic screening
Industrial medicine
Alcoholism services

Curative (diagnostic and therapeutic)

Laboratory
  Clinical
  Anatomic
Radiology
  Nuclear medicine
  CAT scanning
  Ultrasound
  Radiation therapy
  Endoscopy under fluoroscopy
Cardiology
  Cath lab
  Noninvasive cardiology
Surgery
  Local anesthesia
  General anesthesia
Ophthalmology
  Laser assisted
Endoscopy
  Diagnostic
  Therapeutic

Curative (diagnostic and therapeutic) (cont'd)

Sick call
  Daytime
  After hours
Intravenous (IV) therapy
  Chemotherapy
  Hyperalimentation
Obstetrics
  Prenatal care
  Normal deliveries

Restorative (and terminal)

Physical medicine
Occupational therapy
Social services
Vocational evaluation
Cardiopulmonary rehabilitation
Kidney dialysis
Extended care
Life care
Home care
Hospice

Source: TriBrook Group, Inc.

Table 13-5 Shift in the Nature of Hospital Service as Indicated by Changing Sources of Revenue

	Percent of total		Percent increase (decrease)
	1969	1978	
Inpatient service			
Routine service*	60.2	43.7	(27.5)
Diagnostic service**	5.9	14.2	140.7
Other inpatient services	27.7	29.8	7.6
Subtotal	93.8	87.7	(6.5)
Outpatient service			
-Diagnostic service**	2.5	5.0	100.0
Other outpatient services***	3.7	7.3	97.0
Subtotal	6.2	12.3	98.4
Total services	100.0	100.0	—

*Room care
**Laboratory, x-ray
***Includes emergency room
Source: Reprinted, with permission, from *Hospitals,* published by the American Hospital Association, copyright February 1, 1979, Vol. 53, No. 5.

Table 13-6 Percentage Distribution of Expenditures of Minnesota Health Maintenance Organizations

	1975	1976	1977	1975–77 Percent Change
Hospital services	32.9	32.1	31.2	(5.2)
Ambulatory care	55.7	56.5	60.1	7.9
Administration	11.4	11.4	8.7	(23.7)
Total	100.0	100.0	100.0	

Source: "1978 Report to the Legislature on Development of Health Maintenance Organizations" (Minneapolis, Minn.: Minnesota Department of Health, December 18, 1978), p. 4.

The threat to the hospital from the uncontrolled sector of the health field has not yet been recognized. But, as regulation continues to increase, the application of lopsided controls in the industry will lead to a worsening of the existing situation. If bringing about economic competition in the health field is needed, it cannot be accomplished by resorting to free enterprise for part of it and a high degree of regulation for the other part. The amendments to P.L. 93–641 are intended to stimulate the now-missing economic competition by providing freedom to HMOs. This is an objective worthy of support, but it will not take place without providing an equal measure of freedom to hospitals.

The current position of the American Institute Of Certified Public Accounts (AICPA) on hospital financial reporting, which requires consolidations of related organizations onto the hospital balance sheet, also works to the detriment of the general hospital in the same manner as the federal regulations.[12] In the event a hospital causes the formation of a service organization, such as one to contract laboratory procedures, or a foundation where it is apt to benefit from its fund raising, these assets and liabilities could be required to be consolidated and would, therefore, fall under the regulations of the controlled sector of the industry. Not only do hospitals have to be concerned with the federal government, but with auditing firms as well.

Before all of the pieces of the puzzle just described fall into place and lock hospitals into a position that prevents them from having any discretionary revenues to utilize, they should take steps to protect their long-term financial outlooks. One of the major strategies a hospital can employ is to develop its own HMO and thereby be able to take advantage of the legislative loopholes and protect freestanding services they may have developed. If, because of medical staff attitudes, a hospital finds it cannot take the initiative in forming an HMO but must watch its creation under some other auspices, the consequences of this position need to be appreciated.

The health care industry, in all aspects, is unlikely to become totally regulated. The hospital component is equally unlikely to become totally deregulated. Successful institutions will be those that are able to keep a foot in each sector.

Regulation is going to be with hospitals for a long time to come. The problem today is to ensure that it is applied in a fair and equitable manner to all component parts of the industry. Given a choice beyond that, hospitals should move as rapidly as possible to become deeply involved in fostering economic competition and to establish a pivotal position in this emerging trend.

NOTES

1. James A. Michener, *Chesapeake* (New York, N.Y.: Fawcett Crest Books, 1978).
2. *Health Care Financing Review,* (Washington, D.C.: Department of Health, Education, and Welfare, Health Care Financing Administration, Summer 1979).
3. Ibid.
4. Ibid.
5. *Estimated and Projected Population By Age And Sex, 1950 to 2000,* (Washington, D.C.: U.S. Department of Commerce, Bureau of the Census, Population Reports, Series P–25, Nos. 210, 311, 519, 704, and 721.
6. *Hospital Statistics,* 1978 ed. (Chicago, Ill.: American Hospital Association, 1978).
7. *Health Care Financing Review.*
8. *Hospital Statistics,* 1972 ed., (Chicago, Ill.: American Hospital Association, 1972).
9. *Health Care Financing Review.*
10. *Annual Report,* (Evanston, Ill.: American Board of Medical Specialties, 1978). Table 1.
11. *Manpower, A Change In Course,* Annual Report (Washington, D.C.: Bureau of Health Manpower, 1978).
12. *Exposure Draft on Hospital Related Organizations* (AICPA,1979).

Chapter 14

Government, Politics, and Health

Government regulations are persistently nibbling away administrative independence and forcing hospitals to quit solving a variety of operating issues by preempting decision making. On the other hand, administrators are gradually making up their minds to quit trying to exercise independence and are wondering how long the candle is worth the game. Rather than quit a little each day, hospital leadership should strive to develop an attitude that each day they succeeded in squeezing the government back a little.

CHARACTERISTICS OF GOVERNMENT

To get into this position, some observations about government characteristics are useful. None are new; some are more important than others. There are four central driving forces in today's legislation and regulation.

First, legislators seek to maximize their chances of remaining in office. Politicians live from one election to the next election; consequently, their time perspective is limited to their current term of office. They are not disinterested or uneducated about health care problems; rather, they are limited by the attainable. In other words, they are restrained by the limits of public opinion. An individual legislator's actions seldom will affect a legislature of several hundred members who are swayed by their perception of the public will. Health care and its economics are not of public concern unless they are in clear, unmistakable terms.

Second, bureaucrats also express public opinion. During the past 40 years, pervasive government and collective control of all activities has been preferred to individualism and limited government. There has been a shift away from the rule of law toward a rule of officials. The future is for even more government imposition, with greater waste, rigidity, insensitivity to

147

individual concerns, authoritarianism, and a concomitant loss of efficiency. Because bureaucrats do not stand for election, they can afford to give greater weight to social concerns and ignore institutional needs and survival.

Third, program failures of government are most often not admitted, but are used to justify new interventions in society. The past fifteen years of Medicare and Medicaid show that if a regulation fails, it is followed by the issuance of a score of new regulations, all in greater detail and laying the base for even further interventions. It is futile to believe that program failures will be corrected if legislators and bureaucrats would only understand health care institutions, traditions, and financing. What they clearly perceive is public opinion, and what they clearly do not see is that government direction in some activities is beyond their abilities.

Fourth, fiscal accountability in the public domain is rigid, stifles initiative, and is regulated by strict rules. America has long pursued a course that government allocated dollars should be spent exactly as prescribed. Efficiency and effectiveness of programs are of small consequence when compared to expenditure authorization. This is a uniquely American fetish. The converse is found in the English system, where common sense is the rule, and government officials are given discretionary authority. In some United States complicated government activities, flexibility is accomplished through the use of private contractors, such as in the National Aeronautics and Space Administration (NASA). This accountability hangup is the result of the basic structure of the American government and a public belief that politicians and bureaucrats are second class citizens who need supervision in fiscal affairs. In England, civil servant status is an assurance like "sterling on silver." This is not an American viewpoint.

These four characteristics affect developing government health care programs. Fundamentally, they imply that standardization in many different ways will be attempted, whether it is in payment for hospital services to government program enrollees, PSROs, mandated planning, utilization review, MAX drug regulations, or any other current issue. This drive for standardization in a field of activity that has traditionally been individualistically oriented is just now beginning to unfold, but is inevitable. Institutional, patient, and physician concerns of equity will be swept away in the continuing torrent of regulation. Courts will not be a realistic source for fair play, (for example, the July 30th ruling of a District of Columbia federal district court sustaining the 80 percent cost reimbursement level against the pleadings of the American Association of Medical Colleges (AAMC).

From a government point of view, equity is achieved if everyone is treated alike, even though circumstances vary. It is similar to not saving either one of two swimmers, when one might be saved, because it is unfair to the other swimmer.

When PSROs begin to roll, physicians will understand the effects of efforts to standardize medical care. Treating all patients with the same disease alike isn't what physicians believe is their ideal role.

An effect of these four government characteristics is that reimbursement, or, as it is more appropriately labelled, payment for hospital services, is likely to remain less than true cost. Only sick people and health insurance program managers worry about medical care costs. This means that housing, foreign policy, energy, schools, and other issues that daily touch most people are of greater political concern. Likewise, in legislatures, the interests of the medical consumer in the political arena take priority. The public images of hospitals today are distorted by political words that promise greater benefits than their funding of inflated promises will permit. The whole ballgame of the unlamented Secretary of HEW, Casper Weinberger, was premised on cost shifting rather than cost saving.

ACCEPTED VIEWPOINTS IN WASHINGTON

There are three viewpoints that currently have widespread acceptance in Washington that influence thinking about medical care costs. They are that (a) hospital and medical costs are controllable; (b) fee for service of the private practice of medicine is inefficient; and (c) health care manpower can be redistributed to areas with unmet needs.

Each of these opinions flies in the face of worldwide experience. In most countries, the current rate of increase in health care costs exceeds that of the United States. A variety of schemes to contain costs have been tried, and all are notable for their failure. It is both amusing and sad to watch an alleged erudite Washingtonian take a statistic, such as the percent of GNP going for medical care, point out that it is increasing, and then extrapolate it to the point that it engulfs the whole economy. The sad part is that, whenever a ratio statistic is increasing, this is the theoretical result and, of course, never occurs.

Uncontrollable Costs

Costs are uncontrollable unless demand is controlled and the costs of resource input for hospital services are fixed. Despite these facts a constant, forceful effort must be maintained to contain costs within the limits of the possible.

Fee for Service Is Inefficient

The thinking about private practice versus group practice efficiency is true. However, a good manager with authority is necessary if any efficiencies are to be realized. Per capitation group medicine is still an idea that has not been generally accepted by the public. All the cost savings in the world will not bring it into universal use unless the public will accept it. To date, it is a useful concept only in special situations.

Redistribution of Health Care Personnel

The hope for redistribution of health care personnel into ghetto and rural areas is specious in a democracy. All of the monetary incentives and societal concerns in the world cannot overcome the cultural and personal deprivations that exist in these pockets of society. As long as this country remains a democracy, there will be a shortage of services.

PUBLIC OPINION

If elected officials and government bureaucracies have little leeway to defy public opinion, then its origins should be understood. Generally-held public opinions have great stability, but over long periods of time, they gradually change, and occasionally they revert to their earlier points. For example, before World War II, this country had an isolationist point of view. Isolationism was then discredited by the war, and internationalism became popular. Yet, once again this opinion has risen after a 30-year hiatus.

On most widely-held public opinion issues, there is also likely to be one or more countertides. If the shift of the opinion is to be reinforced, then the countercurrents must be sought out and encouraged. How can this be done?

In most fields, new ideas and theories are proposed by researchers and scholars. These are then disseminated by intellectuals such as teachers, commentators, and writers, who cull this material and pass pieces of it on to a wider public. If the material has passed professional muster and has been replicated, a new understanding gradually evolves to replace earlier opinions.

However, health care opinion making does not follow this general pattern. Meaningful research on the organization and delivery of health care services is rare. There are HHS grants for this purpose, but, for a variety of reasons, hard, useful data is seldom delivered. This means that the traditional base of new knowledge is missing and that the intellectuals are not restrained by facts but are free to propose and sell any idea that appeals to them.

The effect of this lack of a knowledge base is frequently seen in Washington. Most often, in discussions about a particular new regulation or legislation, an article from one of the health field journals will be brought out to support a line of argument. Generally, the article will only have limited application because of its scope or inadequate methodology. This fact, however, is ignored, and unjustified generalizations are drawn.

If the basic responsibility of hospital administration is organization and delivery, then university faculty people in hospital administration and their allied researchers in sociology, medical economics, and organization should be doing meaningful research on these problems. Unfortunately, in most instances, they are not working on significant and burning issues. The present situation in health care research is similar to building a fire with the fire department standing around discussing how much air should be in the tires of the pumpers.

When it is recognized that the state of public opinion is the root problem and that legislators have a different priority system than the health field, administrators will be in a position to develop plans for shifting public opinion with new facts. However, this will have to be done without the help of university researchers. This means that administrators are going to have to do the job.

Is this possible? Administrators must define needed research areas and come up with the staff members and money to do the job. Also, once the data is developed, administrators need to be the spear carriers, or the intellectuals to disseminate their work.

The American Hospital Association (AHA) and the state associations are doing this work, particularly the Research and Education Trust of the AHA. However, the work that the authors have seen from these sources only occasionally centers on the issues that are important in terms of changing public opinion, and the work is not expressed in popular language.

Much of the public information is misinformation. Some of the speeches that are made year after year in health association meetings are overstated or misstated. Yet, administrators sit through them without challenging and do so because they cannot quickly and easily cite a refuting reference.

However, administrators often have a feeling that what is being said does not square with their experience. When this occurs, they should remember that they are the ones in touch with reality, and research data is only an abstraction of their reality.

The approach outlined here does not suggest a public relations program in the traditional sense. It does suggest an organized research effort with subsequent publications to report findings. It means discussing infant mortality in terms of socioeconomic classes, access to medical care, and effects of illegitimacy. Or it means finding out the excess number of cobalt units in the United States, as well as where communities should have them.

This kind of approach requires administrators to stay on top of the literature. If this order is too tall for most administrators, then they had better set up a permanent task force to monitor new findings continually and to be able to focus attention on them.

There is another current myth. Practically every person in health insurance activities agrees that cost-based reimbursement is no panacea for cost containment efforts. Therefore, prospective reimbursement is the only way out of the maze. But what is meant by this cliché?

When a person digs hard enough, he will find that prospective reimbursement must also mean postaudit adjustments and a formula approach to establishing rates. In reality, this is nothing but rate setting with cost caps. Yet, who has heard the counterargument in loud and unmistakable terms from hospital administrators? Rather administrators nod their heads that, yes, prospective reimbursement is the answer.

Too often people feel that a response is someone else's responsibility. This is not so! If it is more appropriate for an association to respond, then administrators must insist that their associations go about the work at hand.

If Medicare and Medicaid were trial marriages, then national health insurance will be a permanent one. The probability of this being a happy marriage should be carefully measured.

In 1966, administrators began the Medicare trial marriage believing that what was promised was so and that it was unthinkable that a system so large would be used to undermine the financial stability of hospitals. Yet, this is exactly what has happened. If it had not been for the broadminded view of Indiana Blue Cross in covering uncovered government program costs, most hospitals today would be in serious financial difficulty.

On national health insurance, the federal government will again need administrators' signatures on the dotted line. Administrators should not easily sign a participating contract. Eight years of struggle should have taught administrators that reasonable cost is looked on by bureaucrats as unreasonable and as a pillaging of the public purse.

Next time, administrators should talk to government contractors to find out what cost-plus contracting means and how it works. Also, they should find out what the government's definition of perspective reimbursement really is and not how they plan to make it work. Also, where do loopholes exist for achieving equity and for formal appeals on a low-cost basis from bureaucratic irresponsibility?

Government decision makers at the state level must understand that a hospital can only be successful medically if it is first successful financially. Medical care accomplishments must be financed adequately, and to be underfinanced limits both the quality and scope of hospital medical care.

Hospital financing has become a densely intertwined structure of regulations that overlaps, contradicts, and leaves gaps. The current government trend to proliferate rules to overcome specific problems has created an accounting maze in which no one person remains an expert on all financing issues. Its ultimate end will be caused by a realization that an unworkable financing system has evolved and patient care has markedly deteriorated.

Much more could be expressed on the foibles that interlock hospitals and government.

A quotation from President Franklin Roosevelt's Jackson Day dinner address in 1940 summarizes the present dilemma. He said "But the future lies with those wise political leaders who realize the great public is interested more in government than in politics."[1]

Roosevelt was correct. Administrators need to work persistently to remove political sham and shortsightedness from forming health care programs and to help lead public opinion into an understanding of what is possible in the hospital world.

If administrators do not try, they will drop deeper into the abyss of lowering quality medicine and its availability. Perhaps problems with government are the result of playing the role of health care politician rather than insisting on the imperatives necessary for success.

Administrators must take large risks and speak clearly, thoughtfully, and forcefully on the areas within their expertise.

NOTE

1. The Public Papers and Addresses of Franklin D. Roosevelt (New York: MacMillan, 1940) p. 28.

Part IV

Administrative Roles and Thinking

Chapter 15

Putting Humpty-Dumpty Together Again

In the days of yesteryear, a hospital administrator could sit on a wall in his pink polka-dot bow tie and survey his world with composure and aplomb. With the cascade of federal and state regulations, he rolled off the wall, with the same consequence as Humpty-Dumpty: his perspective has been splintered, and he is groping to put himself back together again.

If the nature of hospitals has changed, then the hospital executives' role has been altered and become increasingly stressful. No one needs to look far to see the effects of this stress. In an unscientific, purely random fashion, early coronaries, bleeding ulcers, and nervous tics are increasingly manifested by administrators. These conditions are apparently the battle scars of sustained conflict with trustees, physicians, hospital staff, the community, and the government.

In the last quarter of a century, the level of complexity in hospitals has gradually and steadily increased. Hospital executives have reached a level of daily frustration, with constant worry about decreasing medical quality and money, and fear that there is a lack of ability to control the organization. Uncertainty, rashness, impulsiveness, and a lack of predictability in the health care field are causing a loss of focus in administrative activities.

How can Humpty-Dumpty get a fresh view? One of the keys to the future is to look at the administrative staff of a hospital and seek ways to coalesce their efforts. In times of stress, differences in management philosophy, priorities, and organizational tactics, which under usual circumstances are minimal, are often exacerbated and become major obstacles to a united administrative effort.

STAFF MANAGEMENT

There are no magic formulas to produce desired performance. If a chief executive officer believes that the administrative staff of a hospital is a reservoir of talent and experience—and the vast majority do—then he ordinarily does not adopt a "yes man" point of view. Rather, he works to encourage an expression of differing viewpoints among his associates. This habit improves solutions to both policy and procedural issues. Yet, in tough times, this practice can be carried too far, and urgent decision making can be postponed interminably as the problem is debated. Because the final choice of an alternative may carry serious consequences, individual administrative staff members may hold to their positions unreasonably long; conversely, the chief executive, knowing the seriousness of the situation, may delay and even encourage debate beyond a sensible point.

There are several management techniques that may be helpful in focusing administrative priorities and interests. Probably the most useful practice is keeping the management process open, that is, no hidden agendas, no secret meetings, and no special deals. This also means keeping trustee meetings, committees, and all activities of the medical staff open to all members of the administrative staff. The priorities and problems of the decision makers are then clear to the decision proposers. A corollary practice is an open office of the chief executive officer to the total adminstrative staff.

To prevent organizational chaos, administrative responsibilities cannot be parceled out on a restricted basis, such as an assignment to lead the professional departments or the service departments as a total responsibility. Every administrative person needs some responsibilities that are corporatewide, such as staffing board and medical staff committees or clinical divisions, and being accountable for their performance. A unified administrative perspective is a difficult goal.

A persistent concern of all chief executive officers is the achievement of optimal performance by the administrative staff and the use of appropriate incentives to stimulate them to strive for maximum results. Typically, the greatest failure of chief executive officers is too much concern over administrative style and too little attention to final results.

In essence, an administrative staff member should have clearly defined responsibilities and then be left alone to achieve these goals. This means management by objective, budget accountability, and quality measurement and assessment. Without annual performance budgeting, adequate criteria for evaluation of administrative performance will be inadequate.

One of the major roadblocks to outstanding administrative performance is the human trait of not wanting to extend one's scope of responsibility. Too often, assistant administrators see or know about an inadequacy in some other part of the organization and willingly ignore it because it is not their responsibility. This goes all the way from burned-out light bulbs, to failures in adequate patient care, to sensing a new avenue for hospital programming. A sense of security must be felt by all staff members if they are to be responsive.

While the business world has spent several decades playing with stock options, bonuses, and profit sharing, little has been done along these lines in the nonprofit corporation. The best incentives appear to be opportunities for innovation, considerate personal relationships, additional education, and participation in the larger health care world. Successful managers create their own positions. Unfortunately, some administrative staffs are bottlenecked by chief executive officers who are driven by insecurity, on ego trips, or believe that the fewer the administrative risk-taking ventures the better.

Every chief executive officer owes a responsibility to his associates to discuss their performance periodically, commend success, identify weakness, and lay out the path ahead. It is helpful also to have a sufficient level of respect and trust so that he will be used by his associates as a consultant, on a privileged basis, for both organizational and personal problems. Associates should feel that the chief executive is sufficiently concerned about them and will always go an extra mile to help them.

TIME MANAGEMENT

Because a hospital has thousands of procedures and must be sensitive to the needs of patients, community, and physicians, every chief executive officer sooner or later struggles with the issue of where to direct his personal attention and to know when he is bogged down in detail. Too often the human response to an increasing workload is working faster and longer. Under time pressures, taking even more time to reflect on the process and decide what should be done to manage things is most dificult. What needs to be done is the exact opposite of what people feel they must do.

Obviously, the first step is to decide which decisions are most important to the organization and which ones can be reassigned to other competent people on the staff. In other words, is the chief executive shoring up weak assistants by doing some of their work? If so, then the problem is slowly compounding.

Delegating

After the decision-making process has been analyzed and the workload is still too large, adding an administrative assistant to help analyze projects in detail should be considered. The assistant can investigate issues so the important elements of a decision are pinned down before the chief executive must consider the problem and make a decision. Fundamentally, administrators manage from a few people up to hundreds of thousands. By reallocating decision making and establishing a sufficient number of positions, accommodations from one size level to another level are made.

Much of the problem of maintaining an appropriate equilibrium is tied into the psychological aspects of the executive. All delegation of decision making involves risk taking. The more the administrative staff is in the act, the greater the potential for failure, while the accountability of the chief executive officer remains the same. Since the top person is probably the most competent, he is apt to see how he can improve the work of an assistant. The crucial issue, though, is to figure out whether or not the improvement is worth the extra effort.

An often overlooked aspect of organizing the chief executive's job is personal behavior related to workflow through the office. How often has an executive with appointments early in the day visited for 45 minutes or so before getting down to business and then wonder why he is running· behind all day. Paperflow, scheduling, interview techniques, report reviewing, relations with assistants and medical staff, and telephone conversations are all areas that are subject to analysis for improved efficiency. There is also the need to know when judgment should be used to work fast or slow. At times, going slowly and deliberately may save time in the long run. People have their own theories and their own personalities to integrate into how best to get the job done. But, they should think about how they are running their offices and where they are wasting time and effort.

Responding to External Affairs

Parallel to the problem of the organization controlling the administrator rather than the administrator controlling the organization is the issue of an appropriate response to demands to get involved in outside activities.

In most communities, it is easy to get involved with a dozen or more local activities. Without restraint, an administrator can be invited to participate in everything from pancake breakfasts to sunset receptions.

At the same time, local health and hospital affairs and health systems agencies are additional areas of effort. On top of this, regional and state level hospital activities and work at the national level add to the workload.

These activities can be full time if not controlled. How does an administrator know where to concentrate his interest? Obviously, the primary issues are the worth of this work to the hospital and whether there is a hospital goal that necessitates influencing a wide sphere of health affairs.

The chief executive officer's posture should be determined by what the trustees of the hospital think is appropriate as a total scope of concern.

Unfortunately, many trustees have not caught up with the facts of modern administration. With new government regulations pouring out from the state and federal levels, an administrator must be involved. If recent state and federal hospital regulations are reviewed, the message is clear: a chief executive may control daily hospital operations and save several thousand dollars, while national regulations cost the hospital several hundreds of thousands of dollars annually.

This means that time is better spent on external affairs than on internal operations. Administrators need to convince trustees of the value of this work and then restructure the organization to allow enough freedom to engage in a larger scope of activity. It is passé to believe that the administrator's only responsibility is that of daily operations.

Complexity of regulation and the increasing interrelationship of health care institutions with programs like PSROs mandates outside concern and participation.

One peculiarity of hospital operation compared to any other industry is worth noting. In almost all other American industries, 15 or 20 large, major corporations dominate the industry. In the hospital industry, there are almost 7,000 independent corporations, with no dominant companies. Because there are government, investor-owned, religious, rural and urban, specialty and general, and university and community hospitals, there is fragmentation of primary interest.

When government is approached with such a diverse constituency, legislatures do not differentiate the hospital industry from the typical industrial situation, and they become confused. Likewise, the AHA, the lobbying arm of the hospital field, has difficulties developing a consensus with this kind of diversity. The moss-covered strategy of divide and conquer works well against the hospital field.

ROLE MANAGEMENT

When the hospital field is in a period of instability, of rising expectations for hospital performance, and of inadequate financing, administrators increasingly look like Humpty-Dumpty. Frequently, the question is asked about who worries about the welfare of the chief executive officer. At least Humpty-Dumpty had all the king's horses and all the king's men trying to put him together again.

Irrational and irrepressible pressures are now at work that make all hospital administrators worry about whether or not they possess the stamina and talent to keep the hospital corporation functioning effectively and with a sense of humanity. Historically, boards of trustees are responsible for appointing, directing, protecting, and evaluating their chief executive officers.

The problem with the traditional role is that most trustees, at best, only see a part of the iceberg with which the administrator must daily deal. In fact, trustees, medical staff members, hospital staff, city hall, the state board of health, and HHS all have different standards and perspectives for judging adequate administrative performance. In many areas of administrative responsibility, these groups are in direct conflict. How then does an administrator find anyone who is concerned about him?

Obviously, trustees cannot abrogate their responsibility; however, administrators need to be persistent and articulate in explaining and defining today's real world to them. It is the height of folly to accept the old view that a board of trustees will exercise, initiate, and have a comprehensive understanding of the role of the administrator.

Competent, experienced administrators are a scarce resource and are not easily replaced. Recently, one major medical center in the United States began a search for this type of executive. They considered about a dozen executives, redefined the executive's role, and raised the salary to almost six figures. They are still looking.

Because trustees have some comprehension of current complexities in hospital operation, the status of effective administrators has gradually increased. With improved status has come greater concern for preserving and protecting able executives. Trustees realize that the penalties for poor executive judgment have increased for the hospital. Even though trustees may not know the daily risks, they have become aware of the trend.

For a board to worry about the welfare of the administrator, the executive must let trustees know that he is concerned about his own interests and the hospital's well-being. If he continues to accept increasing responsibilities without proposing a broadening of the administrative staff, he has no one to blame but himself. If trustees turn down such a recommendation, the administrator has an obligation to explain how it will retard or prevent the accomplishment of hospital objectives and he has a duty to be as persuasive as possible. Similarly, the administrator must be responsive enough to inform trustees that there are limits to the amount of pressure he can personally absorb.

A parallel problem to an administrator's welfare is that of the difficulties faced by experienced administrators who have problems adjusting to an increasing rate of change. What was sound thinking in hospital operation a decade ago is now illogical and irrational in making appropriate decisions.

Times have passed him by, and daily he wonders and worries about how he and the hospital fit into the current state of affairs.

Too often trustees do not realize that administrative *rigor mortis* is due to their lack of foresight. The shortsighted and popular view is that an executive is hired to run the hospital, and, at the time a new person is appointed, trustees make a determined effort to find the best qualified individual for the position. Twenty years later, having foregone many vacations and inadequate time off for rest and advanced education, the board suddenly realizes the executive is no longer the competent individual they selected earlier. Often, the administrator has contributed to the situation by not working to keep skills up, by always putting the immediate demands of the hospital ahead of personal needs, and by failing to point out what is happening to him.

Thoughtful boards are gradually learning to correct this situation by providing opportunities for time off for prolonged study and travel. It is both cruel and poor management judgment to have high initial employment standards, and then fail to provide opportunities during a person's career· to improve his knowledge that cannot be learned on the job but is needed to remain competent.

A person who fails to adjust to change in middle age is partially the victim of an American education. American school systems and universities are mostly vocationally-oriented and do too little to develop a liberally educated person, particularly in the graduate administration curriculum. The pursuit of excellence requires an understanding of societal forces in its many different manifestations. The older a person becomes and the higher he rises in responsibility, the less the need for technical skills and the greater the need for a liberal education. Unfortunately, at the entry point to administrative work, craft skills are valued most highly, so that broad understanding about a society comes only through personal motivation and informal education pursuits at a later time in life.

When Humpty-Dumpty is put together again, there is always the possibility of a second fall from the administrative wall. It can be avoided by learning to cope with continual change in the future.

How anyone learns to cope with change has been an endless topic of discussion for psychiatrists, educators, political scientists, as well as the corner saloon crowd. The excitement and stimulation of hospital administration comes through new experiences. Change should be welcomed as a challenge to do better, to rise to meet the demands of a new situation, and to stretch, and stretch again, intellectually.

Coping with change is a state of mind. Continual change is a normal state of affairs. Problems of adjustment are difficult when the rate of change rises quickly and unexpectedly. One comforting thought in times of high-speed change is that everybody else is having the same set of difficulties.

If a person learns to accept change, then there is no need to worry about being a Humpty-Dumpty administrator.

Chapter 16

Men of Iron

Standing in the eye of the storm now blowing through medical care and hospitals throughout the country are career hospital administrators. As they strive to cope with disparate demands on their institutions by trustees, medical staff, employees, the community, and the government, they are paying a serious psychological price.

The consequences of job stress caused by working in public situations over which they have little control are producing strains that affect their mental and physical health. The present stressful situation has occurred because hospital administrators are responsible for organizational responses without having sufficient managerial authority to enact these changes.

They are ensnared in a web of mixed accountabilities that reflect past organizational practices, where medical staffs still believe in independence within the institution, where communities expect more services at lower costs in an inflationary economy, and where governments purchase hospital services at less than full-cost reimbursement.

STRESS FACTORS

As hospital administrators struggle to achieve adequate institutional responses to these forces, their psychological well-being has been ignored. Apparently, it is widely assumed that administrators are men of iron capable of maintaining their emotional balance no matter how severe the organizational pressures and how inadequate the institutional response.

The stress factors that affect the administration of a hospital need to be examined. It may be helpful to describe them in the context of what is now occurring in hospitals.

In the past, administrative education, experience, and training contributed to the administrator's ability to handle conceptual problems, to understand statistical information, and to be knowledgeable about operations, but these are now only part of the backdrop for the daily activities of an administrator.

Trying to survive in the organizational jungle of a large governing board, a suspicious medical staff, restrictive third party reimbursement, and inappropriate decisions from the local HSA requires the hide of a rhinoceros and the single-minded determination of a bulldog. Intellectual skills need to be blended with emotional maturity.

Working in an environment filled with uncertainty, increasingly unreasonable demands from a variety of sources, bureaucratic double talk, arbitrarily imposed rules and regulations from outside agencies, and a growing list of unresolved problems and issues requires a level of internal stability not previously needed. Analytical abilities are now superseded in importance by a sense of humor, a state of optimism, an ability to absorb unwarranted criticism, an understanding of group dynamics, stubbornness and perseverance in the face of unreasonable odds, and an ability to anticipate questions and answer them before they are even asked. Obviously, this is a set of performance requirements difficult to fulfill.

For chief executive officers (CEOs) who used to spend most of their work day having individual conferences with department directors, reviewing progress on assigned projects, mapping out changes in detailed procedures, and reviewing reports, their day is now often a steady round of conferences and committee meetings, disrupted by frequent full-day absences from the hospital to participate in meetings with those external forces that affect the operation of the hospital. The loss of control of their own time may well be the single most important change for hospital executives in the last two decades and one that prevents them from following the kind of advice that psychologists and physicians offer.

They are caught up in a daily web of meetings that demand substantial chunks of available time. When these meetings are not important, executives become particularly upset because they know that phone messages are piling up; reports, memoranda, and letters are doing the same; and the list of people wanting to see them for conversations continues to grow. When they return to their offices at the end of such a day of meetings, they find that the list of things to do has grown substantially, even though they have been at work all day.

Their feelings are reinforced when they look at their calendar for the next day and see a day similar to the one they just experienced. This is particularly annoying because it does not square with the work habits they have developed over the years. In the course of their careers, they have internalized a sense of urgency about what they do. They are always anxious to get finished with whatever they are doing so that they can tackle the next problem. They become impatient if meetings with subordinates take too long; they want to get to the bottom line and skip the details. This drive to resolve the unresolved makes an executive a restless person, a skimmer of information, and a person who concentrates not on what has been accomplished, but on those matters to be dealt with as soon as possible.

Eventually, this pattern leads to problems on three levels that chief executives must face: (a) their role in the institution; (b) their feelings about themselves in this role; and (c) the growing imbalance between their corporate and personal lives.

Chief executives need to understand that their role is in transition and is now different than what it was in the past. Their immediate office staff often recognizes this before they do, and the executives set up barriers that make it difficult for anyone but an immediate subordinate to penetrate the organizational wall. This brings isolation and leads to the need for an associate to head up the internal operations of the hospital. This is a double-edged sword since, on one hand, it is a way to reduce the number of troublesome problems, but on the other hand, it leads to a greater feeling of being alone. No longer do executives have the opportunity of wrestling with a clear-cut problem in a one-on-one relationship. These are now the province of their associates. Instead, chief executives are left with the indecisiveness of group meetings, timetables that keep slipping, an inability to exercise accustomed authority, and a feeling of being responsible for matters over which they no longer have control. They find themselves as participants in this setting where their thoughts and opinions are received with less warmth and appreciation than was the case when they were dealing with department directors.

This shift in the way chief executives now spend their days is particularly difficult because it affects their own set of values that have evolved over the years. Even though they may have been in the same position for two decades or more, the performance requirements are no longer the same. Over the years, their work habits led them to reduce organizational uncertainty and to seek to ensure predictability in every phase of the operation. Organizational uncertainty is to an executive what a missed diagnosis is to a physician. This is now accomplished at the secondary level of the organization. But at the top, the chief executives are still left with more to do than time available. Without having been planned, they find their workdays growing longer. More often than not, their days commence at 7:00 a.m. with a meeting of the medical staff, proceed to a mid-morning administrative staff meeting, followed by a noon luncheon meeting, are succeeded by mid- and late-afternoon appointments with key subordinates, and culminate with a dinner meeting that may not adjourn until 9:00 p.m. Such a schedule requires the stamina of a bull. If they tend to overeat and shun regular exercise, this kind of routine leads to excess weight, slack muscles, and a loss of mental agility. This is a brutal schedule when kept up month after month, year after year.

Too much pressure, constantly applied, from too many directions leads to a decreasing ability to cope with the demands of the organization. If uncorrected, the pressure may affect chief executives' personal lives and their feelings about themselves; may reach the point where they lose their sense of humor, become preoccupied, lack enthusiasm, suffer anxiety, have feelings of depression, seek relief in alcohol, and lose their sense of personal worth; or, in extreme situations, may undergo a personality shift. These are the dangers of living with too much stress for too long a period of time. In addition, even though they may be aware that they are under continual pressure, others in the organization not knowing the full extent may be less than charitable about behavior traits they see exhibited in their dealings with them.

Chief executives in such settings may discover that their feelings about their work and their role in the organization have shifted to where they feel trapped by their work environment. They may find themselves climbing out of the car in the parking lot wishing they didn't have to go into the hospital and their office; and they may recall with a startling thought, that it wasn't so long ago that they just couldn't wait to get into the hospital and go to work. They appreciate the fact that a continuation of their negative feelings about going to work may lead to a slowdown of organizational momentum, and a lack of enthusiasm will act as a brake on the emergence of new ideas within the organization. These negative feelings are reinforced as they repeatedly rediscover that nothing is clear, accomplishments require disproportionate investments of time, and accomplishments are minimal. They find themselves on a treadmill they didn't create, and they are running faster and faster. Problems continue to grow faster than solutions. This is particularly burdensome because the ability to perform effectively in a managerial role requires concentration on matters that need to be resolved.

Chief executives of hospitals live with a great deal of organizational uncertainty because of the peculiar organizational relationship of the medical staff. They may find themselves in a dilemma; the governing board expects vigilance about the quality of patient care, but, at the same time, expects cooperation with the medical staff. If administrative steps need to be taken that affect physicians, the hospital CEOs accept the fact that they are creating a stressful situation for themselves.

It is not an unreasonable rationalization to suggest that chief executives of hospitals are subject to unusual conditions. They cannot exercise direct control over a medical staff, the governing board, or the external factors that operate on the hospital; however, in the board's mind, they remain fully accountable for the total hospital. This level of accountability severely restricts their ability to adjust, even if they are competent, secure executives. Their frustration arises out of their awareness that they see the need to respond to changing conditions, recognize the organizational steps needed to be taken, but can't get persons who need to agree to the changes to see the necessity of doing so. This is compounded by demands on their time.

At the core of the stresses that now affect them are three factors:

1. Their organizational relationship to the medical staff is clouded in ambiguity.
2. They are accountable to a governing board that cannot meaningfully measure their organizational performance.
3. They function at the apex of an organizational structure that requires participation in many activities that cannot be delegated to others in the administrative structure. Stated another way, their ability to manage their own time is severely restricted because of the expectations of those they cannot control about what they should be doing.

Collectively, these three factors severely limit CEOs' abilities to exercise a full range of coping mechanisms. Even though they have the ability and willingness to put themselves in other people's shoes—be it board member, physician, agency official, or consumer—they cannot effectively respond to all of them. Their time is too limited because of the perceptions of others about their role and others' demands on their personal participation .The fact that the others may be unrealistic goes unrecognized. The problem is not that hospital executives fail to see these pressures, but rather in knowing how to extricate themselves from these constraints.

PSYCHOLOGICAL TRAUMA

These unrelenting day-to-day pressures on hospital executives are gradually debilitating hospital administrative staffs. One effect is a decrease in administrative effectiveness, as the cumulative effects of frustration and anxiety are felt.

The psychological price paid by hospital administration is now escalating at an unrecognized rapid rate and will continue to do so until the traditional corporate structure of hospitals is recognized as unsuited to current institutional leadership needs.

The extent of the pyschological trauma now being experienced by hospital administrators has not been systematically studied or reported. When aberrant behavior of administrators is recognized in an institution, it is usually handled privately by a member of the medical staff or a concerned trustee. In either instance,there is a lack of awareness that trustees and physicians in other hospitals may be handling similar situations.

Symptoms of too much stress on administrative staffs abound. Its manifestations vary according to the personalities of individuals and the characteristics of the institution. Overstress in an individual is difficult to identify because any one act is not usually sufficient to cause concern; rather, a set of behavior manifestations collectively become significant.

Hospital administrators live in two worlds, one private and personal, the other institutional and personal. The linkage between the two worlds is personal, hidden, and typically known only to the administrator. However, the pressures of one world spill over into the other world, unknown to the people in either world.

As the number of unmanageable institutional problems increase, their effects are observable in both the private and organizational behaviors of hospital administrators. As anxiety and frustrations increase in the hospital, administrators' private behavior may reflect the inability to cope with the institutional demands on them. They may appear preoccupied with institutional problems, and they may demonstrate a lack of tolerance toward urgent family affairs that interrupt their train of thought. Their children may quickly learn that their parent has a short "mental fuse," while the spouse may notice frequent periods of depression and listen to comments that reflect periods of depression, along with comments that reflect disillusionment with choice of career or position.

As problems continue unresolved, sleepless nights often follow. Subsequently, risk-taking behavior may begin with an increased use of alcohol and tranquilizers, and reduced physical activities. At a later stage, there may be frequent private discussion of either early retirement or a career shift to another field.

Underlying these behavioral changes is a sense of loss of personal worth and a weakening ego. Both feelings are serious losses in hospital administrators because their organizational role requires them to provide continuously a sense of accomplishment and worthwhileness to the hospital and medical staff.

Personal losses in family relationships may occur because of administrators' anxiety and frustration and their desire to avoid private responsibilities. As working hours lengthen and weekend days in the office become commonplace, their weekly participation in school and church activities, trips to the beach, or movies with the family are ignored. Later, planned vacations are cut to a few days in an effort to find additional time for solving institutional problems. In some cases, private losses may result in divorce, serious illness, or a prolonged period with a psychiatrist.

Because of the personal connection between private and institutional life, the behavior changes noticed in the family situation will also appear in organizational behavior, but in different ways. These behavior changes are usually quickly noticed by the hospital staff because of their daily interactions with the administrative staff. When reimbursement restrictions increase from third party payers, and as a medical staff simultaneously pressures the administration to increase the quality or number of hospital staff members, while trustees are insisting on a reduction in a contemplated rate increase, administrative organizational behavior may change.

Change occurs because the key element of predictability in administrative leadership has been substantially lost. When withdrawal or indifferent administrative behavior is manifested, hospital staff members can no longer rely on past administrative behavior as a guide for determining what decisions are desired or acceptable in the current situation.

Withdrawal from decision making is a commonly used behavior adjustment to cope with unmanageable situations. An administrator may begin to find reasons for being away from the hospital in order to avoid being asked to grapple with current management problems. A variation of withdrawal behavior is to remain at the hospital, but, when a management problem is discussed, to either ask the person presenting it to suggest an answer that is immediately accepted or to project an attitude that any suggestion is acceptable since the larger institutional problems are unmanageable anyway.

Another withdrawal coping behavior is to increase the delegation of authority to associates at lower levels in the organization to avoid requests for direction. At times, this kind of behavior is often preceded by an effort to increase centralization of decision-making authority. When this fails, the administrator may suddenly and unpredictably shift authority for decision making to lower levels in the organization.

A similar type of behavior may occur with the board of trustees and the medical staff. An administrator may either initiate increased use of the committees in the organization, in order to let them make decisions rather than have to make a decision, or reduce the number of committee meetings to avoid facing problems and pressures and, instead, ask the hospital administrative staff to make the necessary decisions without his or her participation.

In order either to avoid confrontation with the medical staff or to buy their support, administrative efforts to control clinical activities may be reduced or stopped. In addition, administrative supervision of the hospital staff may be tightened beyond a reasonable level to meet the demands of the medical staff for improved performance of hospital personnel, even when these demands are unreasonable.

Essentially, the administrative response to a limited authority and increased accountability is to stop leading the institution and to make decisions only when consensus from institutional power groups has been achieved, which is basically riskless decision making.

Along with these changes in administrative leader behavior, personal behavior in the institution may also shift. Interpersonal relationships may be altered from an even-handed tolerance and good humor to behavior that is abrupt and abrasive.

The overall effect of these changes may have serious organizational consequences. Decision making will be slower than usual, and lower management levels will soon express reluctance to assume the same or greater degree of responsibilities as they perceive that their administrative risk taking has been increased. As new events unfold, the total organizational response will be different than what people had previously learned to anticipate.

The morale of the institution will also be lowered because of attempts to shift blame for apparent administrative inadequacies to other personnel. Prolonged pressures that are not relieved will ultimately decrease management levels of performance, and the institutional quality of care to patients will slowly deteriorate.

Administrators experiencing psychological trauma are in a poor situation to look for outside help. Their organizational position and the behavior expectations of those around them often preclude the use of the therapy resources that would typically be sought for assistance. If used, the stigma that might be attached to their use may further deteriorate administrative performance.

People in organizations want to believe in the myth that their leaders are invincible and capable of coping with any event. The secret drink, the surreptitious taking of a pill, or a private feeling of dispair are unthinkable in the mind of the organization man. To the extent that the leader is found to be mortal and human, insecurity is increased by this amount for all members of the organization.

Such prejudicial attitudes heighten an administrators' fears, as well as their awareness, that their behavior is being scrutinized in many ways by the people around them. Under these conditions, it is easy to conclude that the only way to make adjustments must be totally private.

As the national and local environment of hospital administration is surveyed, institutional pressures are going to increase indefinitely in the future. As they increase, the psychological price of being a hospital administrator will also continue to go up. This means that more and more administrators will experience psychological difficulties. If new ways of helping administrators are not developed, there will be an increasing scarcity of experienced people to fill these positions and a decrease in attractiveness for young people to enter this field.

In troubled times hospital administrators have almost no place to turn for help. They know that the medical and health care professions keep few secrets from each other and that a move in their direction for help will be quickly known. Even in a large metropolitan area, they know that the monthly gathering of specialty societies is a place for exchanging gossip, and this knowledge will forestall their looking for professional help outside the institution.

A sense of isolation and lonesomeness aggravates administrators' deteriorating mental health status. They feel increasingly trapped as institutional pressures rise, and there is no place to turn to for help without telegraphing the message that they are no longer invincible.

HELPING THE CAREER ADMINISTRATOR

In the foreseeable future, it is unlikely that boards of trustees will understand the complex realities of today and expand the institutional authorities of hospital administrators to allow them to cope better with today's demands. The psychological price of being a hospital administrator will continue to increase.

Because of the damage already done and the anticipated damage in the future, the field of hospital administration needs to recognize what is occurring and to plan ways to help moderate these effects upon career administrators.

There is one major way the situation can be eased. It is to define and develop a program for hospital trustees to help them understand the modern role of hospital administrators and the existing limitations of management authority for dealing with external pressures now applied to hospitals.

Achieving this goal is clearly beyond the capability of educational programs aimed at hospital governance. In the last decade, there has been a plethora of such programs with little meaningful impact. This is reflected in an organization structure that is designed to provide sufficient administrative authority to control the total hospital organization.

When trustees have had to come to grips with a medical staff or tilt with community power groups, they have often been unwilling to modify the hospital organization to structure the administrative role properly. Usually, it has been easier and more acceptable to rationalize the authority needs of the hospital administrator, continue an unworkable arrangement, and wind up with a frustrated administrator.

To begin to develop a new level of understanding in hospital governance and insight into the current organizational role of the administrative staff, it will be necessary to find out in an organized way the extent to which administrative authority is too limited to meet today's institutional needs.

External demands by regulatory bodies on hospitals have created a complex, intricate management environment that is difficult even for full-time administrators to understand. How then can voluntary boards of trustees understand the current administrative milieu?

Recently national and state hospital associations have started to document the excessive regulation of hospitals and the variety of contradictions found between regulatory agency demands. Likewise, traditional hospital organization structure contradicts regulatory assumptions that hospital administration can control medical staffs and medical practice.

As the next step, beyond the identification of contradictory and excessive institutional regulation, it would be valuable to undertake a comprehensive organizational study in order to identify the limits of hospital administrative authority and accountability, of a medical staff, and of a board of trustees, in terms of meeting external regulatory demands. This kind of study would identify the shifts in authority, accountability, and organizational responsibility needed for a hospital to respond effectively to the present and future administrative demands on a hospital.

A realignment of authorities among governance, medical staff, and hospital administration that reflects current institutional needs would significantly reduce the psychological pressures currently experienced in hospital administration.

Unfortunately, the present no-win situation of hospital administration often blocks reasonable adjustments to relieve institutional pressures. No professional administrator wants to be perceived as a "cry baby," but impossible demands need to be pointed out for what they are, and a realistic appraisal needs to be made about expectations for hospital administration.

Probably the first step for administrators trying to avoid mental health problems is to learn to maintain a sense of humor about their present dilemma. They must also recognize that the pressures of the here-and-now in the health field are unrealistic and that an administrator's ability to change institutions is limited. Finally, they should try to do only those things that are achievable. Until administrators stop trying to meet every demand—reasonable and unreasonable—the psychological price paid will continue to rise and make hospital administration a perilous career.

Chapter 17

The Power Broker—
Prototype of the Hospital
Chief Executive?

MACHIAVELLI'S CONTRIBUTION TO MANAGEMENT

In the hospital environment, a thorough grounding in the way people are apt to behave is of primary importance to the hospital chief executive. Machiavelli in *The Prince* described behavior in this way: "Men are of three different capacities; one understands intuitively, another only understands so far as it is explained, and a third understands neither of himself, nor by explanation: the first is excellent, the second commendable, and the third altogether useless."[1] Because of an imbalance between the responsibilities and the constraints on administrative authority, an understanding of people's behavior is crucial.

The gap between responsibility and authority may lead hospital executives into an administrative style that becomes a life of leverages and of using tonal qualities, facial expressions, and body language to buttress their skills in carefully controlling information, agendas, and timing. They need skills of persuasion in one-on-one situations, but they also need to appreciate how such conversations fit into an overall plan to solve multifaceted, complex problems. This is a unique set of skills that can be acquired only by repeated exposure and frequent mistakes. It is an organization game designed for risk takers and experienced hospital executives, not for the uninitiated.

The hospital is an ideal organizational structure for a power broker because of the multiplicity of hospital departments and clinical services. It

---

* Reprinted, with changes, from the Power Broker—Prototype of the Hospital Executive by Richard L. Johnson from *Health Care Management Review* with permission of Aspen Systems Corporation, copyright 1978.

is difficult to trace the ill-defined decision-making process accurately. Chief executives may be the only common thread among the hospital's committees and governing board. This provides them with an opportunity to wield real power by reporting information to the various groups in a manner most advantageous to the course of action they desire. While they should not deliberately misrepresent information, they may emphasize certain aspects to one group and other sides of the problem to another. Both groups will receive the facts, but they will act on them from slightly different perspectives.

CHARACTERISTICS OF A POWER BROKER

Probing for New Information

Power brokers demonstrate observable behavior characteristics. First, because they possess long and sensitive organizational antennae, they are constantly probing for new information and listening to informal channels of conversation. Not only do they want to know what is being said in various circles, but who is saying it.

This goes on in almost every contact that is made. Although concealed by a smile, a joke, an arm around the shoulder, or a verbal pat on the back, the intent is the same: to disarm other people so they will say whatever is on their minds. In effect, the other person is dealing with a warm, friendly, information-processing system that has its radar screen in use constantly, sweeping the organizational structure.

Anticipating Behavior

A second characteristic is the ability to anticipate the individual behavior of those involved in the decision-making ladder. Because of their understanding of behavior patterns, chief executives may read a situation as the prelude to a gale, while all others may see the unfolding events as a whispering breeze. Recognizing where the problem is headed may lead them into vigorous action and a flurry of telephone calls.

Younger executives and associates, who lack these understandings and sensitivities, may wonder why the chief executive is so upset. They fail to appreciate that the chief executive is trying to get a jump on a potential problem in an effort to steer it into an organizationally safe channel.

By concentrating their efforts at the onset of the problem, chief executives avoid spending large chunks of their time later in committee meetings. In addition, they stand the best chance of working out a solution to their liking because opposition has not had an opportunity to organize.

Focusing Attention on the Problem

A third characteristic of power brokers is their ability to keep their attention riveted on the problem. Once they know their preferred solution and have it clearly in mind, they will devote their time to planning how to overcome any potential objections. Being single-minded, power brokers are not distracted by how well people dress, how much wealth they may possess, or how charming they are as conversationalists; their eyes see all the decision-making participants as parts of a jigsaw puzzle that must be fitted together to bring about the desired results. Because their own time must be rationed among competing priorities, power brokers single out those elements they consider most likely to interfere with their decision and devote their time and talents to those aspects.

Controlling Information

A fourth characteristic of power brokers is that they have access to more information than the other participants and are in a position to control how and when it is dispensed. Although they cannot hold the information to themselves for prolonged periods of time, they can withhold it for limited periods. The degree of urgency of action determines how long it can be sheltered. Depending on circumstances, this may vary from a few hours to several weeks.

The ability to withhold information permits the stage to be set for its reception. For example, chief executives may walk through the emergency room suite, glance into the cast room as they go by, and observe a technician casting a patient with no physician in attendance. Not only have they observed a poor medical practice, but they have gleaned a useful piece of information that can be tucked away in their minds until they decide to use it at an appropriate time.

UNDERSTANDING THE ORGANIZATIONAL PROCESS

If a given issue involves a two- or three-step process, power brokers may opt not to divulge all the relevant information at once, but to withhold parts of it until near the end of the normal channel for such decisions. Chief executives may do this for a variety of reasons. If the problem is disciplinary in nature, they may conclude that enough information already exists for the committee to reach a proper decision without disclosing anything further in order to limit additional embarrassment. If the course of events goes as planned, they were right; if not, they can still bring out the information at the next step in the process.

In another situation, information may be withheld because one or two committee members might misuse it if they have personal animosities toward the person who is the problem. By keeping back part of the information, unnecessary personality clashes might be avoided.

Where one of the committee members is known to be a gossip, power brokers may carefully screen the information they divulge, knowing that they can provide a more detailed account at the next level.

Crucial to the credibility of power brokers is the intent behind their decision to withhold information. If they intend to protect an individual from unfair or harsh treatment, or to ensure objectivity and evenhanded organizational justice, they are usually on safe ground. If the information is withheld for punitive reasons, their decision will ultimately breed mistrust of all their administrative actions.

When power brokers recognize that an issue may lead to heated discussions in committee meetings, they can use another tactic. From their vantage point as chief executives, they usually control the scheduling of meetings. If they feel it is warranted, they may delay the call of a meeting in order to provide a cooling-off period.

Finally, they still have an ace in the hole: their ability to control the preparation of agendas for such meetings. This gives them the opportunity to determine the sequence of activities at a meeting. By carefully reviewing the discussion that is likely to occur, they can determine the order of items placed on the agenda.

As part of this thinking-through process, chief executives also should try to determine which persons involved in the decision-making ladder will or will not be present at the scheduled meetings. Those persons who are likely to support their course of action should be present. Executives often have ambivalent feelings about the absence of those who are likely to oppose their recommendations. Although the opposition's absence makes the meeting easier, it might be wiser to delay holding a meeting until the opposition can be present to avoid efforts to overturn a committee decision.

Power brokers are interested in ferreting out any strong viewpoints prior to a meeting to discuss a sensitive matter. Instinctively, they will take a head count. If they determine the group is likely to reach a stalemate or not be able to cope with the issue, they will search for an alternative route to follow to give themselves the widest possible room for maneuvering or negotiating at other points in the decision-making process.

TWO POWER BROKERS

Occasionally, a hospital finds itself with not one but two power brokers. In addition to the chief executive the other is apt to be the chairman of the board. With two power brokers, the others in this organization get conflicting clues and become confused. They do not know whether to relate to the chief executive or the chairman of the board. Subordinates who typically would support the chief executive become unsure of organizational channels and may keep both chiefs equally informed, hoping that this will give maximum protection.

Differences

Two power brokers may share common ground with respect to institutional goals, but it is unlikely that they agree on the ways to achieve them. Because of differences in personalities, styles will vary even though the organizational structure has been set up and is unlikely to change. Each will emphasize different points, timing will vary, the cast of characters involved will surely be modified, and the information provided will not be identical. There is bound to be confusion as each power broker maneuvers to offset the impact of the other.

A Test of Strength

Once a power broker recognizes that someone else is trying to play the same role, the manipulative process takes on a more serious aspect. Each gives top priority to getting rid of the competition. A problem is no longer something to be solved, but becomes a test of strength and guile between the two champions.

When problem solving has become secondary, it is usually well known by everyone except the two combatants. If they are equally matched, the institution gradually loses its forward momentum. Ultimately some third party, such as a trustee who is tired of watching the contest, may break the deadlock by seeing that one or both leave the organization.

If they are unequally matched, the stronger will create a set of circumstances that will lead to the organizational neutralization of the opponent. A two-power-broker contest usually begins when the second power broker is new to the organization. He operates on premises about the scope of his responsibilities and authorities that are out of keeping with the thoughts of the other power broker. Number one then tries to outmaneuver number two and to reduce number two's role in the organization until it is obvious to all that number one is still number one. In some hospitals, this same process may occur over and over again.

THE CORPORATION PRESIDENT MODEL

In the mind's eye of many hospital administrators, the corporation president is the preferred organizational model. Surrounded by problems over which they have limited direct authority, chief executives see the corporate model as a way of more effectively coping with those problems. They see corporation presidents as aggressive, no-nonsense, let's-get-it-done executives who are concerned primarily with, and have their performance judged by, the results on the bottom line. The appeal of such a model is strong and growing among administrators, as external agencies increase their insistence on hospital accountability to the public's interests. Although it is not totally applicable, the corporate model will be widely emulated and will result in modifications suited to the peculiar nature of the hospital organizations. The result will always be a combination of corporate president and power broker.

Increasingly, the hospital administrator is being renamed president and is serving on the governing board as a full-fledged member. However, there are basic differences between the corporation executive and the hospital administrator. In the industrial setting, the chief executive's performance can be measured with a far greater degree of accuracy than can that of their counterparts in the hospital. Although each corporation has its share of board problems and inadequate directors, both the president and the directors know that the year's results are quantifiable in terms of return on investment, net profit, and earnings per share of stock. No such weapon is available to chief executives of nonprofit hospitals to defend their position.

INFORMATION AS THE BASIS OF POWER

The core of a power broker's influence rests in having an information base that is wider and deeper than that of any other organizational participant. Power brokers' success with this administrative style depends on being psychologically sensitive and having a set of values respected by the people with whom they have contacts. They can be tough and shrewd, but not devious or divisive. In terms of technical knowledge, the greater their depth and breadth, the more consummate they can become in their role. The ability to deal adroitly with finance, nursing, personnel, organization, medical care, radiology, materiel management, reimbursement, fire codes, and building maintenance leads to substantial respect up and down the organizational chain.

Effective power brokers may use their authority as chief executives to grant exceptions to institutional policies or reward cooperation by providing needed equipment or space. They may use horse-trading ability to achieve institutional goals by using *quid pro quos*. For example, they may push a two-person ophthalmology group to add a third member and occupy space in the hospital's professional office building in return for which the hospital will purchase a ceiling microscope for an operating room. This kind of bargaining is understood by most physicians in private practice so long as the trade-offs are recognized as conforming with the goals of the institution.

As government intervention in hospital affairs has increased, the number of regulations and bulletins has rapidly multiplied. This is a ready-made situation for power brokers. Being the first to read and cite those bulletins enhances the poor broker's role as the major source of important information. First knowledge of a new regulation or a change in a government formula increases the dependency of others on chief executives for guidance. The wider the gap they can create, the more effective they can become as power brokers.

DEALING WITH THE GOVERNING AUTHORITY

In dealing with the governing authority, hospital chief executives cannot resort to letting the facts speak for themselves to the same extent that this is possible in a for-profit setting for two reasons. First, they lack clear-cut authority over the medical staff, and, second, their own performance cannot be reasonably appraised using quantitative measures. For these reasons, they are pushed toward the power broker style of management if they are to be effective in their relationships with the board and medical staff.

Trustees do not expect a hospital to be the same financial success as a business. Most expect administrators to see that the hospital runs a modest surplus after depreciation; at the other extreme, they would probably consider a surplus of ten percent after depreciation too high, even though this would be quite satisfactory in their own business. Should administrators turn in a year-end surplus of ten percent, board members might regard their motives with considerable suspicion and question their social consciousness.

Governing boards also lack knowledge about medical care and tend to listen more carefully to medical staff recommendations about diagnostic and treatment needs than they do to administrative recommendations on the same subject. Lacking some credibility in this area, administrators often feel compelled to resort to power broker techniques.

When hospital administrators state that they see no advantage in being a formal member of the governing authority, what they may really mean is that they have so adapted to the role of power broker that they are satisfied with their influence on board decisions. By not becoming board members, they may believe their actions are less observable to others. They can also tell themselves that their style is warranted since they are not part of the governing structure.

RELATIONSHIP TO THE MEDICAL STAFF

Inductive Versus Deductive Reasoning

Medical staff members are an organizational aspect unique to hospitals. They are both part of the hospital and apart from its functioning. They are surrogate customers on behalf of their patients. They do not view the hospital as organization people do. They solve their professional problems along lines that are unfamiliar to those schooled in the ways of management.

From their earliest days in medical school, physicians are taught to use inductive reasoning in solving clinical problems. Physicians collect a set of facts about patients—x-rays, laboratory reports, symptoms, and sounds—and arrange them in their minds to arrive at a diagnosis. In effect, they use logic: facts A plus B plus C equal diagnosis D. This reasoning process, which was so difficult to master in the early days of medical school, ultimately becomes automatic and tends to be used to think through any problem associated with physicians' work, including those of the hospital organization.

In contrast, hospital executives apply a deductive reasoning process to solve their professional problems. They decide on what they want to happen and then look for ways to bring it about; they start with a general premise and look for specifics, while physicians start with specifics and then look for the general premise. Power brokers decide where they want to go, and then move people and information around in a pattern that will produce the desired result.

Handling Information

Much of the need for power brokers is due to the positioning of the medical staff in the organizational structure of a typical hospital. New administrators quickly learn that physicians may talk quite openly in the privacy of the chief executive's office, but that this is no indication of their willingness to say the same things in an open forum, even if the group is composed entirely of physicians. Usually private talks center on the issues of quality of care and the exercise of professional judgment. These are matters of considerable importance to the institution, but they are also of a personal nature because they involve the reputation of the physician under discussion.

Experienced professional administrators appreciate that this kind of knowledge gained in confidence cannot be divulged in a straightforward manner, but that the stage must be carefully set and the matter engineered with sensitivity and caution.

This requires that they carefully think through a scenario that permits enough information to be reported to appropriate persons without labeling the source. They may seek out the same information from others so that this primary source does not stand alone. They may delay the reporting process until this can be accomplished. They then must present it in a manner that protects themselves. This is often done by invoking their responsibilities to the hospital and by saying that they personally find it regrettable. At the heart of their methods of reporting is their certainty that those with whom they are communicating do not interpret their motives as personal or subjective. To maintain future effectiveness, they can never, under any circumstances, give the impression they are vindictive, even when they might have justification in their minds for such a tough stance.

These factors usually preclude "telling it like it is." Chief executives must concern themselves with who to tell, how much of what they know to tell, under what circumstances to tell, how to tell it to achieve the result required, and, finally, how to sequence the decision-making process from committee to committee to governing authority. In thinking through these steps, they must continually balance the need to know against the development of an inappropriate solution because they failed to anticipate the reactions of all the people on the organizational ladder properly. This skill requires political judgment that can only be acquired through long exposure to the process.

How Others See It

The power broker method of dealing with physicians does not go unnoticed. Trustees appreciate it because it minimizes the risk of confrontation between the governing board and medical staff. They are anxious to avoid quality of care problems in which they might have to make decisions on their intuitive judgment, and they would much prefer the problem reach the boardroom table with a proposed solution that has the backing of the leadership of the medical staff.

On the other hand, individual medical staff members may view power brokers in an entirely different light. They may regard their approach as manipulative or underhanded. Many tend to be suspicious and may ascribe personal ambition or a hunger for power as the power broker's motivating force, rather than the pursuit of worthy institutional goals.

Not all physicians react in this manner. Those who have served on local school boards or have been active in community organizations have learned the limitations of applying inductive reasoning to all types of problems and are less likely to be critical of those who use the power broker's process. These physicians often become the confidants of administrators because they provide a communications bridge between the two thought processes.

LIMITS ON THE ROLE

Information Channels

Exercising the role of power broker in a hospital is relatively easy because of the multiplicity of information channels that converge at the door of the administrator. In addition to the financial statements and operating statistics, administrators are often alerted to sensitive problems through conversations with people in and out of the organization. These can include nursing personnel, pharmacists, pathologists, leaders of the medical staff, orderlies, nurse's aides, trustees, police chiefs, reporters, federal agents, as well as friends and neighbors. In nearly all cases, the information transmitted will be verbal and in confidence, and no written records are available. The subjects usually covered are drug addiction, unexpected pregnancies, alcoholism, discovery of terminal diseases, conflicts of interest, rapes, acute psychotic episodes, and involvements with local police. Administrators find out about such problems as criminal activity, serious social maladjustments, or other potentially embarrassing situations.

A Reservoir of Support

By virtue of their role in the hospital, chief executives become the recipients of a great deal of such information. Over the period of a decade, it enhances their position as power brokers in a way that might not be expected. Early in their administrative careers they come to understand their role as being helpful and sensitive when confronted with these events, and they learn to forget the events as quickly as possible after they have been resolved. Physicians, trustees, and community leaders who experience serious personal or family problems come to appreciate that executives can be trusted to be discreet and to never use such knowledge for their own benefit. This tends to build a strong reservoir of support and goodwill for their administrative decisions. Although they use a manipulative process, they do not abuse it. Many of those with whom they deal see them as persons of integrity.

Organizational Explosions

From time to time, chief executives will conclude that they cannot use a politically sensitive approach to solving a problem. They may ruefully conclude that no matter how carefully they orchestrate the reporting-out process, the result will be an organizational explosion. Under such circumstances, they must weigh the need to get on with the task immediately against the disadvantages of delaying it until a more favorable climate has been achieved. This is a judgmental decision that rests solely with chief executives and makes their position a lonely one.

When organizational explosions occur, there are two primary reasons. The chief executive either misread the situation or could not conceptualize a way to avoid it and accepted it as a last resort.

Overusing the Power Broker Style

One of the dangers of using the power broker style is that it may be used when it is not needed. Similar to physicians who use inductive reasoning on all types of problems, power brokers are susceptible to the same conditioning. Without meaning to, they apply this technique to all their managerial problems. Instead of using a direct, straightforward approach in their relationships with hospital department directors and assistant administrators, they continue to use the tools of manipulation.

This can be disconcerting to the directors and assistant administrators who see no need for the power broker approach. Until they become totally familiar with the motives, value systems, and adherence to solid performance of the chief executive, the directors and assistant administrators may remain wary of him and uncomfortable with this style of management. Working relationships with subordinates are more quickly achieved and maintained if chief executives operate in a manner that is familiar to them and appropriate to the organizational relationship that exists.

A REMINDER

The real world to an administrator may appear to be something else to others. The administrator needs to be reminded from time to time of the pertinent comment of Daniel J. Boorstin, who wrote: "We Americans suffer primarily not from our vices or our weaknesses, but from our illusions. We are haunted not by reality, but by those images we have put in place of reality."[2] All people use images to one degree or another to accomplish goals. Those who become hospital power brokers must not be tempted to use this administrative style for games. This style is a necessity for survival, but it must be used cautiously and judiciously.

To some people, power brokers are manipulators who use this approach because they lack a solid grounding in management. To those who have tried to cope with a considerable gap between responsibility and authority, it represents the difference between failure and success. Power brokering is not an equation of manipulation or management; rather it is the application of solid management techniques combined with a deep understanding of how people behave as human beings.

NOTES

1. J. P. Bradley, L. F. Daniels, and T. C. Jones, eds. *The International Directory of Thoughts* (Chicago, Ill: J. G. Ferguson Publishing Co., 1975), p. 735.
2. Ibid.

Chapter 18

Alligators and Hospital Administrators

STRESS

Coping with stress has become an increasingly popular subject. The theme is the same; the world is growing in complexity at an alarming rate, and this is putting people under constant pressures. People are being told that their survival depends on maintaining a sound body, practicing habits of good mental health, and taking charge of their environment.

To ignore these programs and to let life continue its present pattern is to run a risk of being swamped by events of the day's activities. People are warned that the best protection against losing humor, becoming preoccupied, exhibiting a lack of enthusiasm, suffering anxiety, and feelings of depression, seeking relief in alcohol, losing a sense of personal worth, or in extreme situations, undergoing a personality shift is to take the necessary steps before these symptoms occur.

Physical Remedies

On the physical side there are ten million people now jogging or running. Blue Cross is advocating exercise programs in its advertising, and bookracks are filled with a wide variety of exercise programs. The public is being encouraged to see physicians, receive clearance, commence an appropriate physical hardening program, and revamp dietary habits to complement their exercise activities.

In general, people are encouraged to have medical advice about how far to go in undertaking this kind of conditioning before embarking on a different life style. Stress tests, dietary counseling, and an outline of appropriate exercises are all part of the program used to determine how far is far enough.

Psychological Remedies

While physicians are offering medical assistance, psychologists suggest that stress is best controlled by people taking charge of their environment, establishing priorities, learning to say no, providing intervals during the workday for brief relaxation, avoiding work weekends, and balancing work, play, and physical exercise. Physical stress can be measured and persons advised about the limits to which they can go wtihout endangering their health. People can be put on regimens that build strength and provide conditioning that will improve ability to handle increased physical activity.

Psychologists are more limited in their ability to help a person cope with stress. Unlike the physician, a clinical psychologist does not put people through stress tests to determine their ability to handle emotional stress.

When executives change positions, they usually give little thought to seeing a psychologist to determine how much stress they can handle. Instead, they move into the new position, encounter emotional stress, and then seek professional assistance. At this point they may find themselves in a "Catch-22" situation, where testing and advice is helpful, but is akin to the physician telling a mother of three young children to stay off her feet for six weeks. It is sensible, but not very practical. This is particularly true for the chief executive of a hospital. He knows what he should do, but he operates in an environment that severely restricts his ability to cope. Because of the pressure cooker in which the administrator operates, he cannot take advantage of conventional wisdom on avoiding stress.

Even though stress factors exist for all people, they differ in intensity, in some cases because of the makeup of the person or due to organizational pressures and constraints.

COPING PROBLEMS OF THE ADMINISTRATOR

In the past, administrative education, experience, and training contributed to an ability to handle conceptual problems, to understand statistical information, and to be knowledgeable about operations; however, these are now only part of the daily activities of an administrator. Trying to survive in an organizational jungle of a large governing board, a suspicious medical staff, restrictive third party reimbursement, and inappropriate decisions from the local HSA now requires single-mindedness and discipline.

To Leave or Not to Leave

Continuing job-related frustration may lead an executive to consider taking his talents and applying them in some other industry. He may go so far as to have confidential interviews with corporate executives in his own community. However, he will probably conclude that the transferability of executive skills from one industry to another is really not a reasonable alternative, even though his executive skills may be held in high esteem. Lack of experience in an industry can be an insurmountable barrier in job moves.

Executives may then consider establishing their own business. However, since chief executives are usually 40 years of age or older, they realize that, if the business is unsuccessful, their life's savings will evaporate. Private business ventures usually turn out to be too risky.

The only option left is continuing the existing career in the hospital industry. While this is not what had been hoped for when alternatives were considered, the chief executive comes to appreciate that the only true course to follow leads back to hospital administration. He can then begin to assess realistically what he faces in trying to lead an institution through the transition period now in progress.

Disparate Elements in the Hospital

A major concern will be a continuing ability to cope with the disparate elements of the medical staff as the chief executives face increased control over all hospital functions. If some physicians suspect their abilities, executives can anticipate a search of the hospital for evidence that the facility is not administered properly or that some departments are not operating satisfactorily. As any executive knows, there are always examples that can be found. As the list of dirty linen is compiled, the administrator may become boxed in without any way out, because he has no end-product measurements that reflect the overall results of his organizational performance. He may be tempted to believe that a medical staff is vindictive, or that the board of trustees is indifferent. If the CEO comes to accept this view, he may begin to see all hospital problems from this perspective, which in the long run will be disruptive to the hospital.

Quality of Care Issues

Because hospitals lack clear-cut end-product measurements, there tends to be a lack of agreement when questions arise over quality of care issues. Hospital executives, who are aware of this problem, know internal conflict is heightened when these problems surface because they involve members of the medical staff. Tackling inadequacies of clinical performance frequently sets up a no-win situation for the administrator. After a few rounds in this arena, chief executives may conclude that they should get along by going along. In the past, they would only wrestle with their own ethical and moral set of values.

Dichotomy of Role Perception

As the hospital representative to outside groups, a chief executive is a key trustee without portfolio or title. It is a role that only the administrator can perform because it requires an in-depth knowledge of operations, as well as knowing the general attitudes of those involved in governance and the prevailing climate among the medical staff. A gnawing problem to many hospital chief executives is a recognition that their role has changed, but is neither understood nor accepted by either members of the governing board or medical staff. A dichotomy of role perception leads to increasing tension in professional relationships with both groups, which can spill over into personal lives, because they are unable to bring about the change in attitudes they believe is needed.

Administrators are always on stage, responding to the needs, desires, and demands of groups to whom they are accountable, both formally and informally. Because of a lack of an end-product measurement, they instinctively recognize that governing boards are going to judge their performance on how they go about work, paying more attention to form than to substance.

As he surveys the list of unresolved matters needing his attention, he may yearn for the good old days when he had little difficulty keeping his corporate and personal lives separate and neatly compartmentalized by adhering to a daily schedule that allocated time between the two roles. In general, he could predict his schedule one week, one month or six months in the future with a fair degree of accuracy. But then his world began to change and his organizational role shifted as he found both the institution and his own professional role in transition. Uncertainty and continued stress are now his lot in life.

THE CHALLENGE

A hospital chief executive lives in an organizational climate that has both stabilizing and upsetting factors, and his challenge is to find a bridge between the two. In his personal world he also has the same factors at work, but on the organizational side he can develop, modify, or change the formal organization and vary the use of resources. This cannot be done in personal lives. Stresses encountered in a corporate role are usually satisfactorily reduced by manipulating organization mechanisms into different patterns.

When organizational adjustment is possible, stress may not affect the CEO's private life or affect the CEO personally. Whatever happens is accommodated in a reasonably short period of time, and things settle back into a normal routine. Upsetting organizational factors can be stabilized as quickly as possible by objective methods, for example, by carefully reviewing information obtained from the various management information systems, conducting onsite evaluations, analyzing a problem, rearranging priorities, shifting resources, changing procedures, or modifying policies.

Though administrators can partially manipulate resources and rearrange structures in the organizational side of their lives, a different set of tools is used for their personal lives. Family members and their needs cannot be moved about in the same way as an organization.

An ability to manipulate resources on one side, but not on the other leads to imbalances that must be accommodated. The following outline shows the upsetting and stabilizing factors for the organizational side of an administrator's life.

Hospital Organizational Factors

Upsetting Factors

- inadequate operating revenues
- lack of adequate capital funds
- inability to keep up with technological innovation
- lack of adequate authority
- inexperienced subordinates
- conflicts among governing board members
- ill-defined end result measurements of hospital performance
- loss of organizational momentum
- anti-administrator attitudes by medical staff
- hostile public climate toward hospital
- governing board members more concerned with procedures than substantive issues
- lack of sufficient knowledge of hospital operations by governing board members

- having to learn to live with decisions made by outside groups that have no accountability for the results of the hospital operation

Stabilizing Factors

- setting and following schedules
- financially sound bottom line
- competent subordinates
- predictability in the operations of the hospital
- adherence to valid precedents
- institutional goals clearly articulated and followed
- annual growth in units of services
- acknowledged value of hospital to the life of the community
- up-to-date physical plant and equipment
- well-developed management information systems
- efficient internal operations
- continuity of governing board membership
- governing board leadership that is responsive and sensitive to competent management

Personal Factors

There are also upsetting and stabilizing factors in a chief executive's personal life as is shown in the following outline.

Upsetting Factors

- poor health
- compulsiveness
- poor work habits
- too low a salary
- inadequate fringe benefits
- social snubs

- intense preoccupation with job
- unbalanced work-to-play relationship
- feeling of job insecurity
- emotional problems with other family members
- sustained criticism from family members
- lack of appreciation of pressure of job

Stabilizing Factors

- self-discipline
- stamina
- realism
- strong survival instincts
- discretionary income
- satisfaction with position
- good family relationships
- job security (employment contract)
- good health
- adequate time for nonjob-related activities
- on schedule with career growth plan

Options for Maintaining Personal Stability

To keep a hospital administrator functioning and performing well under pressure while at the same time living within the organizational constraints that now exist, the activities in the following lists are available.

Personal Options

- sustained and adequate exercise program
- an avocation that has a potential for a second career
- outside income

- breadth of perspective

- sense of self-worth

Organizational Options

- well-developed budgeting process

- an employment contract

- sophisticated management information systems

- strong, competent key executives

- performance-oriented review of personnel at all levels

- an entrepreneurial view of responsibilities

In essence, an administrator's organizational load can be lightened by rearranging responsibilities, strengthening management systems, increasing security, and developing a physique that can meet a rigorous schedule. In addition, they have to develop an attitude that Harry S. Truman had in mind when he said, "Any man who has had the job I've had and didn't have a sense of humor wouldn't still be here."

The heart of the problem is clear. Stress on all chief executives is here, is growing, and is not going to go away, no matter what techniques are employed. His role is going to continue to evolve. If he is married to a saint, has angels for children, and the good luck to have inherited a fortune, the changing nature of his professional role will not throw him into a tailspin. The less fortunate, however, would do well to bear in mind the findings of Hans Selye, who, after years of study of human stress, summed it up as follows, "Don't be afraid to enjoy the stress of a full life nor too naive to think you can do so without some intelligent thinking and planning. Man should not try to avoid stress any more than he would shun food, love or exercise."[1]

Because of his unique role in a complex organizational setting in society, the modern hospital administrator has to appreciate that, in spite of all he may do to use sound managerial tools and techniques, he is still going to have to meet the challenges of working in an environment that is relatively unconcerned about the stresses of the chief executive. This is the price of admission if he is to survive. He would do well to recall the old adage: "It is difficult to remember your objective is to drain the swamp when you are up to your elbows in alligators."

NOTE

1. *The International Directory of Thoughts* (J. G. Ferguson Publishing Co., 1975), p. 692.

Chapter 19

The Lessons of a Profession

When prospective students for graduate programs in hospital administration ask questions to find out about the life and work involved, they want to know what work is done and what the quality of life will be in this profession. Too often, unasked questions on the students' minds are about happiness, contentment, fulfillment, and service. Answers are difficult, because they are personal.

THE ADMINISTRATOR PERSONALITY

Students first need to understand that a person's world is his own; its agonies and ecstasies are totally private. Also, personality is unique, singular, and beyond the complete understanding of another; an individual can be both silent and public; motivated and apathetic; and straightforward and unpredictable.

As administrators, individuals are decision makers, risk takers, intellectualizers about the good of society; people of love, concerns, and tenderness; and pragmatists who mold, move and decide other people's futures.

Beyond the quality of the person, an administrator is a mixture of competence and incompetence, of great ability and skill, and of maddening blind spots and insensitivities. As chief executive, he knows much and yet little. He is a generalist among a mass of specialists. He is seen by some as an earth-shaker and by others as a definer of goals or as a busybody without accomplishments. He can be both devil and saint simultaneously.

---

* Reprinted from "Lessons of a Profession" by Everett A. Johnson from *Hospital Administration*, 1972 (retitled *Hospital & Health Services Administration* 1976) Journal of the American College of Hospital Administrators.

197

THE HOSPITAL PERSONALITY

A society is a potpourri of expectations. Organizations function as vehicles of expression for personal worth; for identification purposes; for masking of hidden failures with accolades of public success; and as a *raison d'être* for making life worth living.

A hospital serves many expectations. The young twentyish nurse who has not found her own niche in life, privately working out her scheme of usefulness, differs from the mature nurse's aide who is complete in her family life and reaching for greater goals by serving people. The newly-certified medical specialist, sure of his skills and sense of the world, provides a contrast to the experienced senior physician, aware of the limits of the science of medicine, concerned about the future of medicine and its overall usefulness.

LESSONS FOR THE FLEDGLING ADMINISTRATOR

Trustees

Since an administrator directly serves the expectations of hospital trustees, the trustees' desires must be measured. He finds pressure abounding, pushing and demanding new programs and conveniences from the hospital. He finds administrative life is one change after another, and the only predictable element.

On the other hand, the administrator will find most trustees do not really desire change. Their position typically is, if the money can be found, persuade all key parties that it is a worthwhile improvement, and keep all dissonant voices to a murmer; then proceed. If the stakes begin to rise—particularly if the change appears to be generating active opposition from the medical staff—then adjust, delay, modify, or postpone to a more appropriate time. The new administrator will learn later that most of the needed improvements in patient care have floundered on this particular shoal.

It has always been an article of faith in hospital administration that boards of trustees are necessary and highly useful. When he sees local government hospitals with patronage and other political problems, he will know this is worse. When he looks at the rigidities of operation that exist in state and federal hospitals, he will also be disenchanted. Finally, when he sees many private hospitals with trustees continually involved in daily operations, he will also be aghast. He will wonder about the notion of trusteeship. As student life fades into active administrative work, he will need to believe that hospital trustees are motivated by good intentions and seriousness of purpose. He will learn to suffer privately the understanding that dedication and intelligence are no substitute for experience, specific knowledge, and appropriate behavior.

When the new administrator experiences the hospital boardrooms becoming a center ring for local power struggles, he will see how rarely patient care comes out ahead. When the local physicians mass together and lay it on the line, he will generally watch the local elite quickly ride off into the hills. Too often he will watch another administrator be left at the pass to cover the retreat and finally lose the battle.

Medical Staff

The fledgling administrator must learn the rationality and irrationality of an organized medical staff and its constituent parts, the physicians of the community. He will learn that whenever change occurs in a hospital, physicians will usually be slow to accept it, need personal attention to ensure their understanding, and offer comments about how to better spend hospital funds. He will also learn that medical staff members rarely believe that new boilers are a necessity, that administrative offices are mostly personal aggrandizement, that too much space goes into storage areas, and that home ranges ought to be satisfactory in the main kitchen.

The frustrations of unreasonable opinions need to be counterbalanced with an understanding that physicians' lives and interests spin around clinical concerns, their great sense of assurance and independence, their lack of awareness that medical care is now a process involving many people, and their unwillingness to accept the expertise of administrators. Such things will block an easy accommodation to change.

The Organizational Triad

When administrative innovations that are aimed at improving medical affairs in hospitals are tried, the rigidities of attitude and behavior of trustees and physicians are joined. Yet, the administrator's future will be filled with one pressure after another to use the hospital to force adjustments in the traditional practices of medicine.

Past administration-watching has shown that only foolish or independently wealthy chief executive officers have seriously believed that they could direct and administer medical staff. Even though most administrators have been seriously concerned all of their professional lives with medical administrative practices that abuse patients, they have been unable to do more than skirmish on its fringes.

Conformity and endless continuation of these existing practices have been part of past administrative life. The unvarnished lesson is that the organizational triad—trustee, medical staff, and administration—as the best way to run a hospital, is a myth.

When trustees hire and set conditions of employment for administrators and when physicians direct the financial future of a hospital by controlling admissions and dismissals of patients, only the starry-eyed neophyte believes all three parts are equal. In a major hospital crisis when stakes are high and both physicians and trustees make a hospital momentarily their primary concern, administrative leverage is lost.

In situations where physicians squeeze a board of trustees, the administrator will learn that trustees usually accede to this pressure because they do not have the daily administrative experiences that lead to understanding nuances of hospital issues. Trustees also do not know how much of a gamble to take and the importance of alternative outcomes. When one administrator must try to hold a board of trustees in line against an assault of 50 or 250 physicians, it is understandable for trustees to opt for the prestige and goodwill of medicine and to ignore the reasoned judgment of their employee.

Control for the Quality of Medicine

A young hospital administrator will probably learn another lesson. Only in rare circumstances does a board of trustees exercise control for the quality of medicine practiced in the hospital. He will early on find that this is a joint operation between medical staff and hospital administration, and this state of affairs bothers physicians. Not that trustees don't understand or aren't part of the picture; rather, administrative types have a nasty habit of recognizing medical problems being swept under the rug or remembering which closets hold which skeletons.

The Specialist

In the medical staff, the hospital-based, fulltime specialist requires special advice for an inexperienced administrator. For example, when a specialist is quite competent but has a personality like a friendly local car salesman, this is almost a guaranteed administrative dilemma. Older heads know that if it comes to a take it or leave it situation, the medical staff will choose to support one of their own, and the patient be damned. While trustees may get indigestion over these problems, they typically fold their tents and accede to the wishes of the medical staff rather than taking the bull by the horns. A bum steer is what is left to an administrator.

The Art of Delegation

Probably the most difficult of administrative skills to acquire is the art of delegation. Habits, psychological needs, self-discipline, ability to work with others, and individual analytical abilities are some of the personal factors that affect one's ability to use this mode of administration. As size of organization and complexity of operation increase, the time span of an administrator is outgrown as he attempts to expand his efforts to control centrally all important, and sometimes unimportant, decision making in the hospital.

Delegation involves accepting responsibility for other people's judgment and abilities. It means accepting a quality of work that may be somewhat less than superiors' abilities would be to achieve the same result, if he were free to handle a particular matter. A lack of flexibility and difference in thought processes of others also causes an instinctive rejection of another's work.

In the world-at-large, adequate administrative delegation of work seems to be the rarest of skills. It is discussed in graduate programs in management, but largely left unpracticed. Yet, its essence is to be able to use it in situations of much stress and confusion. Probably the only way delegation can be mastered is in the hustle and bustle of daily administrative events.

Combining Emotion and Control

Sympathy

In many administrative activities, demands of the situation seem to contraindicate a successful assimilation of emotion and control. Unfortunately most nonadministrative people experience a hospital organization emotionally. They become irked when housekeeping is asked to move furniture or when maintenance is asked to replace a light bulb, and it is not done immediately. When a nurse errs on a medication, physicians often react angrily, rather than trying to help figure out what went wrong, and how it can be avoided tomorrow.

Too often, physicians, department directors, or other persons arrive at the administrator's office door in a state of agitation, because they are reacting to some activity in the organization. They express a sense of justice, righteousness, and an impeccable logic on their side and a ready-made conclusion that hospital operation is stupid, inept, and poorly-run.

To be rational and logical at this time is to create even stronger feelings. An administrator has the dilemma of figuring out the cause of a problem, yet respecting a person's feelings, regardless of how irrational or unwarranted. He must react to another person's feelings, without losing control of his emotions, and still find a way to explain and regain support of the organization. To have feelings and sympathy, without losing emotional control, is a never-ending administrative struggle.

Respecting Others

At some point in an administrative career the skill of knowing how to conceal administrative skills and to maintain rapport with other people in the organization must be acquired. It is not an easily developed habit.

In the tumult of daily administrative-medical interaction, a fundamental perspective can easily be lost. The administrator always needs to remember and respect physicians as individuals who are delightful, well-meaning, hard-working people, who carry some of the toughest loads in society.

Security

Too often today, progress toward improving patient welfare depends on an unusually competent chief executive officer. When he leaves an administrative post, the drive for improvement and the skills and acceptance necessary for its accomplishment are lost. Because of the subtleties in medical staff and trustee relationships, the succeeding administrator will spend several years developing a position strong enough to win the respect accorded his predecessor.

Frustration

Frustration is the handmaiden of hospital administrators. The daily grist of hospital operation is often shackled by stodginess and the mediocrity of its institutional setting and structure. However, their status reflects the practices of the times and the restraints all organizations tolerate as part of a society with multiple interrelationships.

The prospective student for hospital administration at some point will need to sort out and develop an understanding of the basic relation between emotion and intellectual understanding and conceptualization.

REASONABLE EXPECTATIONS IN ADMINISTRATION

What then is an answer to the potential administrator's unspoken question: what are reasonable expectations in hospital administration for happiness, contentment, fulfillment, and service? The answer lies within another question: what kind of life does the potential administrator need to be happy at 40 years of age?

If individuals seek fame or fortune, hospital administration is a poor choice. If they need a strong sense of security, a well-structured work situation, and some spare time to contemplate the world-at-large, they should look elsewhere.

In hospital administration, happiness is having more work than time; greater demands than ability to respond completely; and a sense of continually helping other people. Happiness is enjoying painting a wall at home for immediate satisfaction, because instant accomplishments are almost never experienced at work. Fulfillment is knowing that at the end of a career the administrator will have lived and served as he would have wished throughout a lifetime of work.

The lessons of this profession are never found in textbooks. To experienced hospital administrators, these caveats have been lived at one or another place and time. To trustees, physicians, and friendly psychiatrists, these lessons will appear as one person's effort to rationalize and work out totally personal struggles. It is, however, a message of realism for the coming generation of hospital administrators and an invitation to join the fray, doing so with eyes open and minds informed about the real world in which a great profession works. This profession faces major problems, coping with some, failing with others, but sure of a demanding, exciting time ahead.

MOVING INTO TOMORROW

The issue is to move from being operators of support systems for medical care into becoming managers of medical care systems. No other health profession is more central to society's developing notions about the total medical care process than today's hospital administration.

To move from today into tomorrow, hospital administrators must now accept the responsibilities and perils of leading a medical staff, trustees, hospital staff, and community that must be led before tomorrow arrives, and administrators now face a time to stand up while the house is counted. They have passed the day when boards of trustees could be looked to for total leadership and administrators could gracefully pass the buck. Today, the buck is in the hands of hospital administration, and because it is there, sufficient leverage exists for major accomplishments.

If today's administrative milieu appears foreboding, frustrating, and turbulent, it should be remembered that the Hellespont could only be crossed by vigorous swimming.

The sense of well-being and happiness that hospital administrators can find in the tumult of today was well described in Kahlil Gibran's *The Prophet* when he wrote about work:

> Then a ploughman said, Speak to us of Work. And he answered saying: You work that you may keep pace with the earth and the soul of the earth. Work is love made visible. And if you cannot work with love but only with distaste, it is better that you should leave your work and sit at the gate of the temple and take alms of those who work with job.
>
> For if you bake bread with indifference, you bake a bitter bread that feeds but half man's hunger.
>
> And if you grudge the crushing of the grapes, your grudge distills a poison in the wine.
>
> And if you sing though as angels, and love not the singing, you muffle man's ears to the voices of the day and the voices of the night.[1]

Talent, commitment, and ability are needed in hospital administration. If young people believe that it is important in life to be stretched to their toes, to strive to touch the untouchable, then join up for the days ahead. Do it with the point of view once expressed by the German adage "Rustich, so rost ich" ["If I rest, I rust."]

NOTE

1. Kahlil Gibran, *The Prophet* (New York: Alfred A. Knopf 1923, 1951), pp. 25, 28.

Chapter 20

Health Care Executives and Specialists: Team Members or Competitors?

The title of this chapter reflects the sense of rivalry that exists among people working in hospitals. It is not a new feeling, but it has persistently broadened and deepened in the health professions. Professional antagonisms exist, however, not from a grand design or personal inadequacies, but from a congruence of a variety of societal forces that have steadily pushed past traditions into the untenable reality of today.

A ZIG-ZAG PROCESS OF DEVELOPMENT

One way to explain why this is happening is to describe the shifting emphasis on access problems in health care, the issues concerning quality of care, and the difficulties of financing medical care, and then gradually trace these issues back to their origins. This approach would probably lead to a conclusion that the present circumstances are a logical outcome of decisions that were made to solve problems 30 to 40 years ago.

The ramifications of these earlier steps were only dimly perceived at the time, if at all. From this kind of analysis it could probably be concluded that the present state of affairs came about through a zig-zag process of development through a series of periodic minor adjustments to unanticipated new problems every few years.

By looking widely at the essence of society and then gradually narrowing the focus, an understanding can be reached of how these forces have influenced the professions and institutions of medical services.

Social Philosophy

A society does not begin *de novo*. All new societies are an amalgam of elements of older societies that have come together at a particular time

205

and place, and give rise to a newly accepted order of values. This process is not entirely rational in a free society; consequently, there will be unresolved conflicts in social philosophy. These conflicts are not sufficiently serious, however, to disrupt a new social order, but are accepted because a sufficient number of people adopt them, and a new set of values is established that will indefinitely persist.

Traditionalist Philosophy

The current existing state of social philosophies have three roots. The oldest has been named the traditionalist philosophy. Its main thrust is the goal of developing intelligent people. Its basic belief is that the world is fixed and relationships are unchanging. Consequently, people are not trained in technologies, but are given an appreciation of the "good life." This is the basis of the academic argument about whether to teach the humanities or to encourage the development of newer university departments, such as a school of business or engineering.

Practical Philosophy

The next wave of importance was an outgrowth of the industrial and scientific revolutions. It was an empirical philosophy and gave rise to the "practical" man.

In the past several centuries, it has proved to be an efficient and effective way of looking at the world. A physician's education is a prime example of this school of thought. Specialization into narrow areas of knowledge is the end result.

Pragmatic Philosophy

The current era began in the twentieth century and is known as a "pragmatic philosophy." John Dewey was the innovator for this school of thinking, a blend of theory and practice, or, as Dewey showed, a mixture of education and experience.

This philosophy is problem-oriented, but aims at developing broad specialists who are able to see relationships among disciplines. This is an integrating point of view and is exemplified by the education for hospital administration. This philosophy encourages the acceptance of an ultimate goal that all professional education in the twentieth century should be the acquiring of an outlook that learning is a continuous process to accommodate never-ending change in the environment and society. This means that a professional curriculum should have a goal of preparing a person to function effectively in a career 20 years after graduation, rather than focusing only on training him to function in first assignments.

PRODUCTS OF EDUCATION SYSTEMS

Too often, university graduates become technique oriented and thereby quickly turn into organizational competitors, rather than team members. People educated in the traditional philosophic orientation find out during their careers that they may be charming, cultured, and imaginative, but they are handicapped by insufficient knowledge of technology to come to grips with modern enterprises. Likewise, people educated through a curriculum based on an empirical philosophy have serious difficulties rising to top organizational levels because they become total specialists rather than generalists.

The Dewey philosophy reflects a reality that people can remain in an educational setting for only a limited part of their life. A graduate program must be aware that its curriculum cannot provide students with all of the skills and knowledge needed through a career. The goal is to create a capacity for life-long learning.

Graduate education is the base on which life-long personal expectations and goals are developed. Competitors and team players are therefore both created by universities at an early age. It is unfortunate that many professional schools do not recognize that in all organizations, immediately above entry levels, there are no purists; that all higher organizational levels are a blend of both management and professional orientations. Forgotten is the view that management is a state of mind and something any reasonably bright and energetic person can grow into. If a person believes that doing a job is achieved only through technical competence and no organization competence is needed, then the educational process has failed, and it has failed because its orientation is out-of-date with current reality.

Organizational Competitors

An organizational competitor is a person who has not matched his expectations with his abilities. The empirical approach has indoctrinated an attitude that technical competence alone is sufficient for a lifetime of success. Real world experience then diminishes this viewpoint, as he finds an increasing need to approach organizational work with a gradually broadening perspective. This happens when he begins to have to act like a manager. He experiences the reality that he is blamed for someone else's errors, or that he is responsible for more things than he can do alone, or that he is left alone and everything that happens is his responsibility.

Team Members

A technically educated professional who becomes a team member has acquired some mid-career insights that escaped his colleagues, "the competitors." He is recognizable because he has adopted an acceptance of risk taking on his own initiative. The competitor type is knowingly not a risk-taker to protect his personal security in an organization, but he encourages the organization to take risks that will never directly bounce back as his personal responsibility. A team player has learned to take graduated risks as he expands his initiative and innovation over time. He is also characterized by an ability to create situations around which he challenges his subordinates to succeed and to find ways to teach them organizational decision making.

Organization Misfits

If by mid-career a professional does not recognize his part in a larger coherent structure, that he is involved in a pluralistic appraisal system, and that leadership is an integrative function, then the last part of his career will be one of growing frustration, anger, and small-mindedness. Such a person is an organization misfit.

Democracy and Participation in Organizations

With the roots of the organization misfit defined, some thoughts about democracy and participation in organizations are useful. In an academic environment, as well as in medicine, there exists a nonsensical idea that democracy should be practiced in an organization. This is equivalent to believing that large committees always have greater wisdom than individuals or small groups. By extension, the largest possible committee is the wisest. Not many people believe that statement.

The unvarnished fact is that organizations exist to control. Many writers have expressed ideas about the limits of control and the best ways to direct large aggregations of people, but there is no birthright of freedom once a person joins an organization. Leaders may decide to free certain decision-making areas for group input, but no rational administrator allows total freedom to a committee or individual, even when parameters of control are not explicitly defined.

Organization Theory

While organization theory has many definitions, jargon, principles, and acceptable practices, it has as yet to develop a coherent general theory of management and organization. It does not seem likely that such a theory will develop until the theories of behavior and learning are accepted as useful tools for directing and controlling organizations. The whole methodology of organizations must reflect the reality that they affect the people participating in them, and people in organizations affect the ultimate forms, processes, and objectives.

Learning and Behavior Theory

Applied learning and behavior theory are basics for developing strong, competent organizations. How people learn and how they act is controlled by interaction of individuals and institutions. What they know and what they believe is not static, but moves as society changes. One of the reasons that "knowledge people" exist in large numbers in organizations today is the shift in economic resources and educational capabilities of society in the past 100 years. An organization in 1880 had to be substantially different than its 1980 counterpart because of the shift in people's capabilities. Today, many more skills are acquired prior to employment than in any previous era.

Concurrent with this change, other developments such as increasing certification practices, selective professional societies, and professional recognition techniques, have been tied to job requirements in the medical world and have thereby significantly expanded job monopolies. The only other worlds with similar restraints are churches and schools, and neither are noted for administrative brilliance.

THE SKILLS OF TODAY'S HOSPITAL ADMINISTRATORS

Developing a Meaningful Program

The most essential skill of a hospital administrator is his ability to take the desired goals of a society or an organization and group their elements into a meaningful program. As hospitals move through the next decade, an administrator will be able to reduce some of the existing professional roadblocks. When this occurs, feedback to universities will take place, and faculties will increasingly adopt a pragmatic philosophy. They will gradually recognize that all health care professions must be practiced within an institutional mileu.

Dealing with Multiple Sources of Direction

Unencumbered private practice, with its values about noncontrol and free enterprise concepts that are widespread in today's medical sphere, will soon be seen as real world myths. In the past decade, a growing awareness of institutional imperatives has diminished the relative proportion of competitor types who populate the health care scene. More and more younger professionals understand the distinction between freedom to exercise independent judgment and administrative restrictions. Many no longer resent multiple sources of direction and control.

Administratively, there is an urgent need to lay to rest the old chestnut that every person in an organization should have only one boss. The modern, complex, interrelated technology of hospitals and other industries cannot function with such a simplistic notion. Project, team, and functional organizational models require multiple sources of direction and reporting if the use of current knowledge is to be maximized.

Reducing Professional Rivalries

Because the process of decision making has become increasingly complex in hospitals, the need to reduce professional rivalries is of growing importance to administrators. Even though a chief executive understands why these persons act as they do, he must also develop two skills if the organization is to function at an optimal level. One skill is to practice administrative techniques that work to minimize the competitor attitude. The other skill is to have the ability to handle the stress they create for the organization.

THE SPECIALIST ISSUE

The world of hospitals is different today than it was yesterday. In the past, a fledgling administrator knew in detail most of the activities for each hospital position and the decision making expected from it. At one time or another, an administrator had to fire boilers, hold retractors, wash dishes, take blood pressures, and do a multitude of other operating duties.

This sounds ridiculous in today's setting. Now an administrator reviews memorandums, attends a variety of committee meetings, and has a staff of assistants to negotiate positions and make decisions. An administrator is now a decision reviewer and an advisor to operations.

Today an administrator must recognize the authority of knowledge of the specialist. He knows only in a superficial way what is involved in day-to-day operations; in fact, he has little or no direct control or authority over a vast number of specialists' decision making. The complexity of interrelated factors that affects major policy decisions as well as a host of procedural issues can be met only by bringing together all of the people affected so that no elements are missed in making a decision. No longer is there one person with sufficient knowledge to make an intelligent decision.

The specialist issue permeates all levels of hospital operations. To outsiders it is a bewildering chain of authority, and there are no magic formulas to achieving desired performance.

COALESCING TEAM PLAYERS AND COMPETITORS

How then do hospital administrators and organizations join the new world? How should, and should not, they behave as leaders to coalesce an organization into one unit when there is a mixture of team players and competitors?

To know what to do and how to do it, they must put into practice some of the theories about behavior and learning. Several different aspects of organizational life can be guided by these theories.

Understanding Characteristics of Organizations

The first is to understand the essential characteristics of an institution and how they affect the behavior and attitudes of individuals in the organization, from the nurses aide to the chief pathologist. There are organizational characteristics that influence individuals.

Institutions Have Purposes

The most basic one is that institutions have major purposes; they are established to carry out certain ends. All people who work in an organization must accept its goals. If a person believes it is immoral to kill other people, he should not join the army. If he believes in the importance of life, he may wish to work in a hospital. The goals of an organization and an individual must point in the same general direction. If an administrator faces a protracted situation in which an employee's goals are clearly different than those of the hospital, the employment should promptly be terminated. Otherwise, the personal adjustments required would be so deep that a prolonged period with a psychiatrist would be the only hope of bringing them into agreement.

Institutions Are Peopled

Another organizational fact is that institutions are peopled; that is, they require a number of persons to carry on their activities. If people dislike a variety of human interactions, then they ought to consider becoming forest rangers in Yellowstone National Park.

Institutions Require Structure

The third characteristic of an organization is that the achievement of its objectives requires a structuring of tasks, and these must be interrelated with other tasks. Typically, tasks are defined and interrelated before the selection of people to fill these tasks or jobs. This means that there must be a clear understanding of the demands, interrelationships, freedoms, and restrictions by a person considering working in an organization. It is far better to undersell a job applicant than to create future difficulties by a hard sell.

Institutions Are Normative

An often obscured facet of organizational life is that institutions are normative. That is, there are role expectations for all employees, and these are obligatory. To say it differently, there is a value system in the organization that forces compliance in most instances. Interestingly, there are variances in norms by hospital position. It is more acceptable for a physician to be less courteous than a nurse's aide.

Institutions Have Sanctions

Finally, institutions are sanction bearing. They have positive and negative sanctions for ensuring compliance with their values. Good people are promoted.

Controlling Behavior

The essential characteristics of an organization impinge on individual persons. Their job behaviors are on a continuum from required to prohibited. In between there lie other behaviors that are recommended or mildly disapproved. This flexibility feature of a job is what makes it possible for people with different personalities to fulfill the same role and give it the stamp of their individual styles of behavior.

The "competitor" types take advantage of the looseness between the poles of the continuum of behavior. Since organization values are rigidly enforced only at extremes, they ignore or are insensitive to the informal cues and signals used to control behavior between its poles.

This behavior probably occurs with specialists because they are aware of an organizational need to use their knowledge. They are likewise unaware that all positions in an organization derive their meaning and usefulness only in relationship to other roles. For instance, a licensed practical nurse cannot be defined without also defining a registered nurse and a nurse's aide.

To control behavior other than that which is absolutely required or prohibited requires at least *three* understandings.

People Live up to Expectations

People tend to live up to what is expected. The application of this principle can be used to make people grow and mature in organizational behavior. It is not only the behavior of the leader, but his disciplining and reinforcing of other people's behavior that communicates the standards that are expected as a norm. Too often the more prestigious hospital employees are not confronted by administrators when their behavior is undesirable. Confrontation of specialists who are few in number in the organization, such as a nuclear medicine specialist or a computer programmer, can be dangerous for the hospital administrator and can have serious consequences to the hospital if unsuccessful. Often, reasonableness for achieving overall objectives prevents needed discipline.

However, if an administrator can make specialists feel that their superiors and peers disapprove of their behavior, the behavior can be altered. In general, subordinates copy techniques, because all adults are skilled mimics.

A useful variation of this fact that will help to create a desirable organizational environment is to insist that all management levels reflect to their subordinates the norms or standards of behavior and performance of the chief executive officer. If this is not done, the values of the administrator will permeate only one level in the hierarchy.

For example, the chief executive must not place his psychic needs ahead of others in the organization. Since actions speak louder than words, he must behave in a way that maintains respect for individual rights and dignity. He cannot tell a department director that he exercises excellent management judgment and then not allow the director the freedom to make departmental decisions.

Organization objectives must constantly be clearly defined and be referred to for guidance at all management levels. Job descriptions should be changed when functions are shifted in the organization structure. The relationship of a position to the organization must be clearly perceived in an employee's job description.

Penalties and Rewards

Another useful administrative tool is to improve the use of penalties and rewards within the organization. Too often hospitals rely totally upon the salary structure as their only technique. A penalty and reward system should be defined in as great detail as possible, with definitions of desirable and undesirable behavior.

Together with this system should be a careful use of organizational status symbols. There is a psychic income for each person in an organization. Manipulation of these symbols can reinforce the informal norms desired by the hospital. The style of office, attractiveness of uniforms, the appearance of the environment, and communicating material all deliver unspoken messages.

Role Perception

The key to desirable job performance lies in the perception of role for everyone in the hospital. To accomplish this goal is difficult because all elements of organizational life must consistently reflect and reinforce its standards. This means that all organizational signals must be so clear that they can properly be interpreted. Also, the administrator must remain predictable in his behavior. This is the ultimate administrative technique for moving an organization toward its goals.

THE HUMAN ELEMENT

In the present age of computers and functional programming, the importance of the human element can be lost in the shuffle. Despite automation and computers, which require the programming of people up to a point, the human element is still crucial. People are important whenever there are unknown situations that cannot be accurately forecast. People, for the most part, are not programmed and are the most flexible part of an organization. Machines are used to replace personnel to increase both productivity and predictability. Machines, likewise, do not file grievances or go on strike.

Conversely, an organization does not exist to make workers happy, but to accomplish its objectives. There is a loss of efficiency when employee welfare is placed ahead of the patient's or hospitals welfare. That is the difficulty with the old human relations approach to management.

In the eyes of the competitor, the organization has increased in complexity beyond its ability to cope. The organizational imperatives today require human behavior adjustments beyond the ability of the specialist to change, particularly for the long-term employee.

How an organization can be effective in the midst of today's forces, caught in the bind of needed adjustment, is a dilemma. However, in the day-to-day operation of a hospital a set of criteria has gradually evolved to evaluate and thereby to enforce norms for the work of department directors and knowledge of specialists. The following criteria are used in one form or another to apply to management judgments about performance and behavior:

- supporting the department director and professionals because they respect job performance and abilities; conversely, criticizing inadequate performance and behavior

- knowing when and to what extent to compromise goals of the organization to meet the needs of an individual by recommending exceptions to usual practices

- knowing when to stop lobbying activities for a particular program after a decision has been reached; accepting the idea that appropriate behavior is to enter into discussions before the final decision and then to support the decision, right or wrong, once it is made

- having an ability to discriminate between facts and hearsay, and knowing how to use appropriate methods to ascertain the true facts in particular situations

- having the ability to remain silent when the necessary timing for the release of information to the hospital organization is crucial if predictability is to be maintained

- following through on tasks and decisions when assigned by administration or when an issue arises through interdepartmental activities

- demonstrating self-reliance and assurance in decision making

These factors are used both subconsciously and consciously by administrators. How they are used will be varied by the competence of the hospital staff, the economic condition of the community, and the size of the institution.

There is no magic wand that can be waved to make the competitor into an organization man. Severe limits of time and knowledge exist to changing individual behavior in organizations. It is both trite and true to observe that the final test of an organizational leader is to insist consistently on everyone respecting the dignity and worth of all persons in the hospital.

How anyone learns to cope with the peculiar demands of the knowledge specialist is an endless topic of discussion, as well as the subject of dozens of articles by human behaviorists and political scientists. The integration of competitors into the organization is a problem often recognized and seldom solved.

The need to think about the unthinkable is apparent. Just remember, in necessity the unthinkable becomes thinkable.

Coping with change is a state of mind. Continual change is a normal state of affairs. Problems of change are difficult only when the rate of change rises unexpectedly and quickly. A comforting thought in times of high speed change is that everyone else is having the same set of difficulties.

Part V
Managing Physicians

Chapter 21

The Managers and the Medical Staff

One of the first surprises encountered by a neophyte in hospital administration is the attitude of the medical staff toward management. Like the public, the beginner believes that since both are striving toward the same goals, they are partners. It comes as a shock to learn that physicians see it differently. Some administrators never overcome the hostilities that develop and spend a career making sure that physicians lose as many organizational battles as possible. Others learn to cope with this frame of mind and can keep it in perspective, even though they appreciate the necessity for never taking the medical staff for granted. The mistrust that exists between medical staffs and hospital executives is so widespread there has to be underlying causes for it. Why physicians and administrators often fail to see eye to eye is important to understand.

DIFFERENCES BETWEEN PHYSICIANS AND ADMINISTRATORS

Inductive vs. Deductive Reasoning

When students enter medical school, they are confronted with an enormous amount of factual information to be assimilated, as well as a whole new technological vocabulary. They become immersed in the scientific method and quickly learn that a conclusion reached about a patient's condition must be based on amassing as much readily available quantitative information as possible in order to justify their tentative diagnosis. They are repeatedly reminded that $A + B + C + D$ is the route by which a determination is made. Inductive reasoning becomes a way of life in medical school. By the time residency training is completed, it often has become a way of approaching all of life's problems.

In contrast to physician career training, the hospital administrator has never become imbued with quantification or the scientific method. His undergraduate days may have been largely devoted to nonquantifiable subjects with only a passing acquaintance with the other approach. At the graduate level he is exposed to quantification, but is taught that these are only part of the skills he needs in his career. Of more importance is philosophical grounding in social and ethical considerations and in business management. Between graduate education and early years in the field observing senior executives, he comes to appreciate that the way major problems are solved is to decide first where the hospital should go and then figure out what steps are needed to get it to that point.

Successful hospital executives most often use deductive reasoning in making their decisions. This approach to problem solving is alien to physicians, who tend to view it with suspicion because it seems to be illogical. On the other hand, administrators have difficulty relating to clinicians who put every subject through the filter of inductive reasoning. Hospital executives tend to get close to those physicians who have an appreciation of the deductive reasoning process. These medical staff members become the informal bridges between management and medical staff because they can easily relate between these two different schools of thought.

Entrepreneur vs. Organization Person

From another perspective, the administrator is the organization man and the physician is the entrepreneur. This difference has been recognized in terms of the organizational structure of the medical staff since early in this century. The Hospital Standardization Program established by the American College of Surgeons (ACS) had model medical staff bylaws that referred to the medical staff as self-governing and stated that the hospital administrator was expected to cooperate with that body. These bylaws were distributed to hospitals, and, by the end of World War II, a verbatim version was found in nearly all hospitals. When this activity was taken over and expanded by the Joint Commission on the Accreditation of Hospitals (JCAH), this element was retained.

Whenever hospital disputes arise involving individual members of the medical staff, these key points are usually invoked as reasons why physicians cannot be treated administratively as part of the operating departmental structure of the institution. The phrase, "the medical staff shall be self-governing," is still found in bylaw language in many hospitals. Even where this phrase is no longer contained, most medical staffs behave as if it is still there. Chester I. Barnard, writing in his classic text on organization structure, *Functions of the Executive*, deftly put his finger on the problem.

He pointed out that an executive's authority can be exercised only to the extent that those over whom he is exercising it accept his right to do so.[1]

Medical staff members usually deny that this right exists for chief executives of hospitals. In fact, in many hospitals, they deny it exists for another physician who may be in an administrative position, such as a medical director.

CONFLICTING VIEWS

Medical Staff Membership

The meaning of membership on a medical staff is seen differently by the two parties. Physicians see it as a process of presenting their clinical abilities to a peer group to determine if they meet the minimum eligibility requirements of the hospital. They accept, though sometimes grudgingly, that in the hospital they are part of a larger system of medical care, requiring them to abide by adopted professional standards.

In their office practice they view themselves as individual entrepreneurs, solely responsible to themselves for the diagnosis and treatment of patients. They are aware that through the education and training they have acquired, there must be a continuing concern about a level of competence that must be adhered to in the office as well as the hospital. They believe the same degree of skill should be applied in either setting. Thus, when seeing patients in the hospital, they believe they should be left alone to do as they see fit, as long as their personal standards of performance exceed those required by the institution.

The Hospital

Physicians do not view the hospital as a control mechanism that decides for them their hours, work schedule, income, or professional direction. Any steps taken by the hospital that they interpret as being even remotely in this direction are usually met with sharp reminders about their independence.

These attitudes have been in place for many years and have remained relatively unchanged. Yet the hospital has undergone a profound change, from a charitable, limited diagnostic and treatment capability, primarily oriented to nursing care, to a large, heavily capitalized, technological enterprise operating in an increasingly complex social setting. Many physicians think of the hospital as a support system for their own decision making. With the amount of long-term debt being carried by many hospitals to finance the facilities and equipment needed to support a wide range of specialists, the hospital executive has more and more difficulty reconciling these physician attitudes with the imperatives of meeting his debt service requirements, of coordinating a wide range of diverse talents, and of responding to a variety of external community pressures, while at the same time providing a future course for the institution.

The Chief Executive Officer

Problems are not alleviated by the other caveat in the bylaws that the chief executive is expected to cooperate with the medical staff. As a result, the chief executive of a hospital lives with a great deal of organizational uncertainty because of the peculiar relationship of the medical staff in the organizational structure. He may find himself in a dilemma; the governing board expects him to be vigilant about the quality of patient care, but at the same time expect him to cooperate with the medical staff. If administrative steps need to be taken that affect physicians, the hospital CEO accepts the fact that he is creating a stressful situation for himself. He is aware that physicians regard his lack of clinical training as preventing him from reaching valid conclusions about quality of care. Even though he does what senior executives in other industries do, operating on the basis of second- and third-hand information and statistical reports, these sources are often not regarded as valid by physicians. Because the hospital CEO can claim neither clinical competence nor direct authority over the medical staff, he is forced to undertake a series of maneuvers to bring about the needed results.

Quality of Care Issues

Because a hospital lacks clear-cut end-product measurements, there tends to be a lack of agreement when questions arise over quality of care issues. Hospital CEOs are aware of this and know that internal conflict is heightened when they surface problems of this type that involve members of the medical staff. To tackle inadequacies of clinical performance is all too frequently a way of setting up a no-win situation for themselves. A few rounds in this arena may lead chief executives to conclude that they should get along by going along. In the past they could do this knowing that they need only wrestle with their own set of values. But even here, the option to ignore these problems may be foreclosed because the internal information reporting system now documents the work of the utilization committee and the findings of PSRO activities.

The Governing Board

Because of both education and experience, a hospital chief executive often views the medical staff in a different light than do trustees. From long exposure he knows he has to deal with physicians with caution and great sensitivity, even though he may see the medical staff as part of the management responsibility. Although he would like to deal with it in the same manner with which he handles all of the other operating departments, he recognizes he has to treat physicians differently from how he deals with other management people. The chief executive may fail to understand why this is so, even though he appreciates it must be.

A governing board usually sees the medical staff as an anomaly not found in other forms of enterprises. Board members acknowledge that physicians have to meet certain standards for admission to the medical staff, but once having been met, they see physicians as surrogate customers who must be treated in a manner reflecting this kind of relationship. Consequently, when physicians express displeasure with administrators, governing boards listen carefully and are inclined to be responsive. In many cases the board accepts the medical staff's recommendation without carefully and critically examining the issue. This happens for several reasons, all intertwined in the thought process of trustees.

Trustees recognize a hospital as a medical care institution; as a community activity; as a place where minimum standards for professional performance are enforced; where physicians make free choice of whether or not to use the facilities; and where the operating departments headed by the administrator provide the support systems that permit these other activities to occur. They do not see the hospital chief executive as the person who leads and inspires the medical staff in addition to other employed personnel.

CONFLICTING ROLES

Hospital chief executives head a system that is expected to do its job efficiently and responsively to medical care interests. Their role is to see that the adopted professional standards are enforced. They are not expected or permitted to raise these standards; they can only encourage this being accomplished. They are free to consult with the medical staff and receive their advice, but not to make a decision affecting them without their involvement and often concurrence.

The chief executive cannot get out too far in front of the medical staff. If he acquires too much influence in the community, if he controls the medical staff too directly, if he achieves too large a surplus on the bottom line, if, in other words, he behaves as an aggressive, brilliant, hard-working executive, he runs the strong risk of courting organizational disaster for himself.

If the medical staff feels threatened by the CEOs' performance, it often originates from their belief that CEOs are not in charge of the entire hospital itself and that their role of dispensing medical care needs to be protected. Physicians will act on this belief when threatened. Individually, this may take the form of informing either board members or administrators that they, the physicians, are free to take their patients to other hospitals and may well do so if matters are not righted to their satisfaction. Administrators often view this as a threat akin to blackmail, while physicians see it quite differently. To them it represents the exercise of a right they have maintained as a customer. To physicians, their role in the hospital and in the organizational relationship of the medical staff to the governing board and administration is sacrosanct and must remain in the future as it has in the past. Even though the government is forcing the hospital to become the control point of the health delivery system, typical physicians, finding themselves increasingly threatened, determine not to let it happen in the hospital where they view their role as being of considerable economic importance, thus providing them with the leverage to protect their interests and attitudes.

THE FUTURE OF THE PHYSICIAN/ADMINISTRATOR
RELATIONSHIP

Given the disparity between the changing societal role for the hospital and the inflexibility of physician attitudes, tensions between administration and medical staff members will mount over the next decade. This will not be ameliorated by converting to the corporate structure with increased authority for CEOs, even though this would enhance their ability to deal with the external pressures.

While patient care has come to dominate the hospital, coordination of administration, medical staff, and governance is now a necessity. There is no neat and tidy organizational structure that will satisfactorily serve the interests of the three legs of the stool. Physicians can be expected to be increasingly demanding of the institution. Governing boards will continue to listen carefully to physicians, and administrators will be subject to increasing demands as they attempt to bridge diverse interests that subject them to heightened organizational pressures. As many experienced hospital executives view their roles, they are aptly describing their situation when they say that the fun has been taken out of their profession. They are caught in a pressure cooker where the heat keeps getting hotter and hotter.

The Revamping of Hospital Structure

The revamping of the hospital organizational structure is not going to be accepted by physicians if it requires them to be accountable to the chief executive, even if through a medical director or chief of staff. The concept of a single, unified structure—given the prevailing attitudes of the medical profession—is a workable idea only as long as the decisions reached by the hospital do not trample over strongly held concerns of the more vocal members of the staff. In order to minimize this risk, policy development needs to involve appropriate physicians along the way from the first steps up to final approval by the governing board. The result may be no better and might not be as sound as if the administrative staff decided what to do, but by meaningfully including physicians in policy development, acceptance among the medical staff will be greater, and the chance of successful implementation will be enhanced. This is of particular importance for the near future until physicians come to realize that the additional constraints being placed on them have come from external factors. Until that time, internal tensions will increase, and as they grow, the decision-making process dealing with shifts in programs, services, and organizational structure will have to be slowed down to the speed with which medical staff acquiescence can be gained. This will require the hospital to go in two directions at the same time. In response to these outside influences, the hospital should be streamlining its decision-making apparatus so that it can rapidly respond to changing conditions, yet it must develop a more elaborate and cumbersome one in order to involve all of the internal parties that are demanding a seat at the policy-making table.

Parity of Authority

This kind of dilemma is being faced by many institutions. The need is not for increased authority for either the CEO or the leadership of the medical staff, but rather for a position of parity between them. An imbalance now exists in most hospitals that favors the physician. It is not in the best interests of anyone to further this imbalance. To run through a series of chief executives or to emasculate their role in order to assuage a discontented staff leads only to a loss of organizational momentum and an inability of the institution to respond to swiftly changing conditions.

This kind of loss is not easily recognizable in the short run. Solving immediate problems and dealing with internal crises often results in a blurring of vision of long-term consequences. The need to win a battle, or to avoid one, usually has precedence. Under such circumstances it is difficult to remember that there is always a tomorrow that will have to be faced, and that tomorrow is likely to be more difficult and complex than what is being met today.

Parity of authority between the two requires living with an uneasy organizational balance that will tilt from one side to the other from time to time. The governing board's role becomes crucial. It will need the best information and analysis of hospital problems that it can obtain. This can be provided if the following two conditions, which are not usually found in today's hospital are met:

1. an administrative staff that is knowledgeable, experienced, and not overextended in terms of workload;
2. a medical staff that has continuity and stability of leadership.

Both are necessities but need to be reinforced by a governing board that deals in an evenhanded way with all parties. This is, however, a pious hope that has little likelihood of coming about; it is an organizational appeal of the same kind as motherhood. Yet much can be accomplished if governing boards are exposed to measuring performance. New hospital trustees quickly learn that the ground rules of business do not directly apply to institutions because of the complexities of reimbursement, professionalism, nonprofit status, and external requirements. Existing trustee programs do not help much either, because they usually paint with a broad brush the concerns of the total health care field.

Free Market Conditions

If the hospital field is successful during the next decade in bringing about economic competition between institutions, the role of the administrator will become pivotal since survival will be dependent upon managerial acumen. Under existing conditions, his role is that of manipulator and power broker, but when it becomes important that they have a real and sustained interest in productivity, then he will be viewed in a different light by both trustees and physicians.

The development of free market conditions is an essential ingredient in maintaining the excellence that has been achieved over the last half century in the health delivery system. By striving to bring this about, the many issues that have been identified that now separate managers and medical staffs will fall into place. Parity of authority, accountability for quality of care, self-governance, and trustee education will lose their importance in an inverse ratio to the development of economic competition. When the dominant themes become market share, pricing policies, marginal costs, and performance, and when seminars and conferences highlight these subjects, hospitals will have completed the journey from social and religious agencies and will have joined the mainstream of American industry. The decade just ahead should be exciting.

NOTE

1. Chester Irving Barnard. *The Functions of the Executive* (Cambridge, Mass: Harvard University, 1938).

Chapter 22

Point of View: Medical Staff Liability

More than a quarter of a century ago, each member of the medical staff was a kingdom unto himself. To believe that the medical staff had a collective responsibility for the acts of an individual member was unthinkable, although the hospital accreditation program of the American College of Surgeons held such a viewpoint.

That was not to say that individual physicians and surgeons did not take responsibility for the acts and decisions of colleagues. They did, but in an informal way that was quiet, kindly, and in the patient's best interest. Implicit in their actions was an awareness that if physicians and surgeons did not exercise leadership and control, the hospital administration might do so.

Two decades later, the former HEW sponsored a medical malpractice commission, a specter of what was to arise. Since then, the malpractice issue has become daily fare in the press, television, and popular magazines.

As hospital administrators watch the number of medical malpractice claims steadily increase and bear the brunt of malpractice insurance premiums that jar their financial nerves, there is considerable soul searching about the effectiveness of medical staff organization for controlling the acts of individual staff members.

When contemplating a program to reduce the number of patient injuries caused by ignorance or neglect on the part of hospital or medical staff, a hospital organization faces two issues: control of the hospital staff and control of the medical staff. Most administrators would prefer to deal solely with the hospital staff through better inservice education, recruitment of

Reprinted from "Point of View: Medical Staff Liability," *Health Care Management Review* by Everett A. Johnson with permission of Aspen Systems Corporation, © 1978.

more competent personnel, and better supervisory techniques. However, with the current state of medical malpractice affairs, the hospital as a corporate entity must carefully examine the relationship between individual medical staff members and the hospital corporation, as well as the relationship between individual medical staff members and the medical staff as a whole.

CHANGING ATTITUDES ALTER ORGANIZATIONAL CONTROL

In today's world of medical care, changing attitudes about who is responsible for what have confounded and exacerbated the issue of organizational control between physicians and an organized medical staff, and between medical staffs and hospital administration. Overlaying this issue are two other factors: (a) the increasing complexity and medical specialization required by the newer aspects of medical technology and instrumentation; and (b) the increasing sophistication, knowledge, and competence of hospital personnel.

The modern hospital is now staffed with personnel who recognize the limits of an individual physician's knowledge and skills. This awareness has created a relatively new institutional milieu for the physician, increased accountability for individual acts.

In the past few years, hospital medical staffs have struggled to come to terms with this new accountability. Often underlying factors are unrecognized or not verbalized at the medical executive meeting, where an attempt is being made to cope with irresponsible or incompetent acts of individual medical staff members.

Because of the nature of current medical practice, a chief of a service is often not available when a hospital staff member has identified a potentially harmful practice of a member of the medical staff. Such a situation is the institutional beginning of a malpractice problem, and it often gives rise to a conflict of organizational authorities, which has a potential for wrecking medical staff/hospital administration rapport.

Conflict of Authority—Two Examples

Two such situations that typify the daily warp and woof of the interrelationships of medical and hospital staff illustrate the point.

The first situation developed when a patient was delivered to the operating suite with a signed consent form in which the patient crossed out all specific consents except the right to medical photographs. The chief of surgery was unavailable; the first surgeon, who was told about the restrictive consent, ordered pre-op medications and performed surgery. After discussing the situation with the surgeon, the operating room supervisor noted this in the medical record and later discussed it with the chief of surgery.

The second situation involved surgical privileges. A general surgeon advised the operating room office that he was scheduling a dilatation and curettage (D&C) for a follow-up case, for which he did not have surgical privileges. After a discussion with the surgeon, the supervisor of the operating room notified both the chief of surgery and the chief of obstetrics and gynecology of the surgeon's behavior. Each chief advised the supervisor to handle the situation herself, which she did by not bringing the patient to surgery. She was scolded by an irate surgeon who claimed she had no authority to interfere with his decision.

Both events were later reported to the professional standards committee of the medical staff through the hospital administration for disciplinary action.

It is highly probable that similar confrontations with organized authority and control occur in most hospitals in one form or another. As malpractice claims and insurance premiums continue to increase at recordkeeping rates, the need and desire to come to grips with control issues institutionally will increase.

Lack of Response to Changing Attitudes

Unfortunately, most medical staffs and hospital administrations will not come to grips with the demand for increased accountability until an institutional crisis has been precipitated by a half million dollar malpractice judgment, cancellation of the hospital's malpractice insurance, or a journalistic exposé concerning physician or institutional neglect.

Why is a crisis needed to reassess the functioning of a medical staff? The roots of inertia go deep. Fundamentally, most physicians, at least subconsciously, resent being controlled by persons outside the medical profession, even when, from a societal perspective, those physicians admit the need for control. Their reluctance is understandable.

MEDICAL/HOSPITAL ENVIRONMENTS

Medical and hospital environments are unique—fascinating, demanding, and all-consuming. They are filled with values that have been hammered out in a crucible that tolerates few myths, and serious errors in judgment in these environments can mean an irreversible finality or a prolonged period of pain and suffering for patients.

In this kind of setting, ignorance and incompetence of nonphysician opinions are not tolerated well. There is also reinforcement for physicians who flaunt their egos because of their organizational status and freedoms, and fail to strive constantly for excellence in performance. Yet the current push for increased accountability holds an organized medical staff and hospital corporation culpable for failing to control judgments and acts of individual staff members.

Freedom to practice is not unlimited; it is prescribed by licensing laws, an expanding body of common law judicial decisions, and a rapidly growing body of governmental regulation. The limits of freedom in the practice of medicine have been significantly reduced in the past decade.

Practicing physicians are busy with daily hospital activities, diagnosing and treating patients, and completing insurance reports and medical records, as well as dealing with daily life outside the medical or hospital environment. It is little wonder that these individuals ignore or fail to notice the larger affairs of medicine.

THE CHANGING PHYSICIAN/HOSPITAL RELATIONSHIP

In the past, physicians viewed the hospital as similar to the church. Like the church, the hospital was always there, was generally responsive to the individual's needs, and demanded adherence to its principles without penalizing the individual for unconscionable behavior. While physicians viewed their local hospital in this light, they respected the opinions and judgments of medical colleagues regarding their behavior.

The recent medical malpractice turmoil has changed this perspective. With the enactment of Medicare and Medicaid, the American government decided to channel their efforts through 7,000 hospitals, rather than 300,000+ private physicians. Thus, the local hospital has become the vehicle for mandating change in existing behavior and performance of medical staff. It has become the messenger of bad news and the chosen control mechanism. As the most immediate impediment to medical freedom, the hospital is often the cause of much resentment.

THE QUESTION OF LIMITING RIGHTS

With the rise of serious medical malpractice issues also came the question of the rights of a group to limit the rights of an individual. The concept of organization connotes direction, control, and limits of authority or freedom. Once physicians have applied for appointment to a hospital medical staff, they have implicitly and explicitly agreed to limit their medical practice freedoms to those allowed by the institution. They have accepted a higher authority and control. As they move toward greater participation in the hospital, the meaning and reality of this choice become clearer.

In a fundamental sense, physician members of the medical staff have assigned certain of their medical freedoms away for that part of their professional activities that occurs within institutional walls. They have become part of a larger organization and agree to abide by its standards. Policymaking in all organizations, if it is to operate as a coordinated entity, occurs from the top down. When physicians insist they have a right to abrogate institutional policy unilaterally, they are in effect arguing that the hospital and its formal medical staff are nonentities and that policymaking should be decentralized and uncoordinated. This is anarchy, not organization.

This is not to say that members of an organization should not be consulted before new policy decisions are made; good management practices understand that internalization through member participation increases the possibility of establishing workable and acceptable new policies.

LIABILITY

The word liability can be viewed in two ways: in a legal sense involving the concept of torts and in an organizational sense implying responsibility.

Legal Aspect

The legal aspect often arises within the specific facts and useful precedents that attorneys consider when drawing up a plaintiff's petition for redress. Lawyers are now including more and more physicians in subpoenas, along with hospitals, as defendants. This probably represents their growing knowledge about medical care and its practices, and their recognition that an array of physician specialists and hospital staff are now involved in rendering modern medical services. The older concept of suing just an attending physician and a hospital has fallen with the American Bar Association's rising awareness that complex medical care problems often mean the involvement of eight, nine, or ten physicians.

One of the more interesting legal aspects of a medical staff's liability is an increase in the number of lawsuits individual physicians have filed against hospitals and organized medical staffs, when an effort was made to reduce clinical privileges or remove medical staff membership. When a medical staff tries to exercise controls to ensure adequate performance of individual members in the interest of reducing malpractice claim possibilities, it moves from one type of legal confrontation to another.

If a medical staff is to exercise responsible leadership and is exposed to paying legal fees and being responsible for any personal judgments, it will not accept such exposure beyond the first lawsuit. It is mandatory that a hospital be prepared to pay defense and judgment costs when a medical staff is acting responsibly and is sued.

Responsibility Aspect

Liability, in a broader sense, generally means organizational responsibility and is the heart of the matter for developing better controls to prevent patient injuries caused by a physician's action or inaction. The responsibility aspect has many elusive qualities that are not easily identified or approached.

Many observers of the medical malpractice scene have stated that the patient-physician relationship is the most critical aspect in determining the frequency of medical malpractice claims. Yet a medical staff has great difficulty attempting to cope with an individual physician's behavior toward patients and staff when he or she is irascible and insensitive to the feelings of others.

PROBLEMS OF CONTROL

Lack of Rules and Regulations

The rewards and penalties most frequently used in organizations for monitoring medical staff behavior are phased along a continuum. They go from mandated to prohibited behavior. For example, physicians must complete their patients' medical record, and they are prohibited from being drunk in the hospital. In between the two extremes, there is a large range of acceptable or undesirable behavior for which there are no organizational rules, merely approbation or dislike. This is the area of greatest difficulty to control.

For example, some physicians make hospital rounds late in the evening, after a full day in the office. They arrive at the hospital tired and worn out, and treat their patients brusquely and inconsiderately. What can a medical staff organization do about these physicians? Some of these physicians do not have active practices for long, but this is not always the case. Can a professional standards committee order physicians to adopt a pleasant attitude? About the best that can be done is to have respected members of the medical staff talk with the physicians and discuss the implications of their behavior.

Chiefs of Service Conflict

Another area of medical staff operation fraught with difficulties is the annual election of chiefs of service by the members of their clinical departments. This organizational practice may be seen as democratic by physicians, but it frequently leads to uncommitted chiefs of service and an uncontrolled medical staff. For example, elected chiefs of service seldom are accepted by their colleagues if they insist on quality performance and are willing to battle for its achievement. At best, their tenure as chiefs of service will be short.

The economics of private medical practice likewise influence control of medical staff. Unpaid chiefs of service usually must rely on other physicians' referrals for their livelihood. If they stir up a lot of animosity, their bank accounts may soon look like they took a three-month, around-the-world cruise. This means that control actions are limited to the most flagrant instances of poor medical judgment that have existed for a prolonged period. In such cases, the members of the chief of service's department are supportive of such action.

On the other hand, if chiefs of service try to control the medical care standards of practice when physicians generate a lot of referrals and practice a level of medicine that does not overtly injure patients, but who wander around the medical countryside diagnosing and treating patients, they will stir up trouble in their departments.

Because chiefs of service are typically well established physicians, they often have a relaxed attitude toward patient problems. They are likely to react to chief-of-service responsibilities with a similar lack of commitment. For example, if the hospital is shortly expecting a visit from the JCAH, there will probably be a drive to complete medical records. Outside of cajoling and issuing memorandums to get the job done, there will be a stepped up suspension of medical staff privileges of physicians with delinquent charts.

For the chief of surgery this can be a troublesome time, because the younger surgeons, who burn the midnight oil for nonpaying gunshot wounds and stabbings, may have their admitting privilege suspended. This means that the chief of surgery is back in the salt mine at 2:00 A.M. because they voted to complete the medical records, and no other surgeons are available who will accept the responsibility for completing them. A few nights of these chores and they, too, begin to bend the rules.

Organizationally, a medical staff has a difficult time meeting its responsibilities because its decision making is handled largely through a committee structure, and its actions depend on the goodwill and unpaid time of individual physicians. If medical staff leaders are conscientious in their personal medical practice and somewhat idealistic in their professional viewpoints, they generally expect their colleagues to meet the same standards. When that does not happen or there is active opposition, their frustrations may lead to their resignation, either in fact or in spirit.

ASSESSMENT OF MEDICAL STAFF ORGANIZATION

The present day medical malpractice control issue in a medical staff cannot be ameliorated without a hard-nosed analysis of its current level of functioning. The scorecard of results is now easily kept by merely looking at the annual malpractice insurance premium of the hospital.

It is in the subtleties of medical staff organization that the roots of malpractice issues are found. There is a medical staff liability for acts of individual physicians. Hospital boards of trustees have typically delegated hospital medical care responsibilities to the medical staff. They may not, however, delegate their accountabilities for patients and the public. Sooner or later malpractice matters, PSROs, and utilization review activities will force improved management practices on a medical staff if the staff does not face the issues for itself.

Organizational control of a medical staff is not a will-of-the-wisp activity full of ambiguity. It is an area of knowledge where techniques are known and can be usefully applied to medical staff affairs. These may sound like fighting words to a physician of an independent persuasion, but they are realistic if the number of medical malpractice claims is to be decreased.

DEVELOPING MALPRACTICE PREVENTION PROGRAMS

Many technical decisions are needed from a medical staff before medical malpractice incidence is reduced. These include a detailed working out of such issues as informed patient consent (what constitutes it, and how can it be accomplished), acceptance of a standard definition of death, protection of physicians who respond to "code blue" calls, protection of the confidentiality and safety of medical records, protection of patients, safe operation of electro-mechanical devices, infection control, and measurement of the clinical competence of physicians.

None of these topics can be satisfactorily dealt with through the traditional committee structure of the medical staff. Detailed study, rational thought, and concern for patient care, without organizational overtones, are needed if reasonable policies and procedures are to be developed. A committee that meets monthly for 90 minutes, is interrupted by coffee and sweet rolls, and gives no thought to the issues between meetings is not the vehicle of choice for developing adequate malpractice prevention programs.

This is not said to denigrate the good motives of the vast majority of physicians. It is simply that the complexities of modern day medical practice have outgrown the control structure of the traditional medical staff organization. Until that is recognized and faced, medical malpractice claims will remain a matter of constant concern.

Policy Versus Procedure

How can a medical staff be reorganized to come to grips with the issues now beyond its control? In all large organizations, the first cut at control problems created by size or technical expertise is to make a distinction between policy and procedure. The top level of the organization determines the direction the organization will go and why, and then authorizes the management to determine ways to get there.

If a medical staff were to make the same distinction and eliminate a mixing of the two, as well as recognize the differences between hospital administration and medical staff administration, it would be one giant step forward. It is not easy to accomplish.

The first step toward the separation of policy and procedural authorities in a medical staff is to recognize that the hospital charter and the board of trustees establish the outer limits of where the organization is going. Within these parameters, the medical staff has a role and mission. The focus of medical staff policy making should be the top organizational unit in its structure, typically, its medical executive committee. The membership must be accountable for carrying out adopted policies.

One caveat should be noted at this point. The bylaws of the hospital should be amended to remove the typical statement that "the medical staff is responsible for medical care in the institution." That statement is so broad that its significance is questionable. The statement should be changed to read either that the medical executive committee or the chief of staff is responsible, depending on the form of the organization.

Organization Chart, Committee Descriptions, Individual Job Descriptions

The second step is the use of a medical staff organization chart, committee descriptions, and individual job descriptions. A functional organization chart must define, in detail, reporting relationships and leadership positions in the medical staff, and how they are care coordinated.

To back up a functional organization chart, detailed committee and job descriptions are necessary to define the specific authority and responsibility of each position, to determine to whom that person reports for different activities, and what reports are to be issued and received.

In doing this, there should be a wide scope of procedural authority granted to subordinate leadership positions not tied to a committee structure. Once a policy has been promulgated, physicians should not be encumbered and restricted by continual review of their decisions, as long as they remain within the limits of approved authority.

In addition, the redistribution of authorities and responsibilities should recognize the constraints imposed by the absence of fulltime decision makers in the medical staff. Within defined limits, intermittent action should also be authorized by the hospital staff based on procedures clearly defined and easily understandable.

Data Accumulation

Another basic management tool for an effective medical staff is an adequate information system that accumulates needed data. The data collected should be the responsibility of each department and the function of the medical staff, even though the actual work may be done by members of the hospital staff. Comparable units of measurement should be used throughout the department or function to the maximum possible extent. The time periods used for summarizing data should be intervals of time that can be easily combined.

The fundamental criteria used for inclusion of data should be its usefulness for current and future medical administrative decisions of the medical staff and must be consistent with its organization structure. Control and assessment of operations and physician performance require a data collection system that identifies gaps in service, and good or poor performance.

As a corollary, hospital departments must also develop a complementary set of procedures. Many malpractice claims today arise out of the lack of articulation between medical and hospital staff activities. However, until the process just outlined has been accomplished, lack of coordination of the two major components of a hospital will contribute to confusion and evasion of responsibility. Poor management practices by either the hospital administration or the medical staff, or both, will eventually create patient care situations that result in medical malpractice claims.

Physician members of a medical staff have a right to expect clear lines of institutional authority and responsibility. If they do not exist, physicians cannot be faulted for making unilateral decisions. When the lines of authority are clearly stated, physicians at least know the risks they run by ignoring them.

Looking Ahead

Medical malpractice issues of today have highlighted past organizational failures. In the days ahead, management practices of medical staff, as well as those of hospital administrations, will need to improve. Careful attention will need to be focused on areas of discretionary behavior and more refined ways of control developed.

The usually used technique is to eliminate the individual physician member of a medical staff if there is a failure to conform to unstated but desirable behavior patterns. In geographical areas where there is an abundance of hospitals and medical staff appointments easily come by, this has been an acceptable practice in the past. However, it removes a problem in one hospital and transfers it to an unwitting second hospital. In essence, the hazards of malpractice claims have been shifted from one insurance policy to another.

CARING LEADERSHIP

To eliminate undesirable physician behavior in a hospital, the best solution is that followed in the past: use quiet, private, and firm leadership by the staff. Staff members must be their sibling's keeper if individual performance standards that have been cited as necessary to avoid malpractice claims are to be achieved. It is really the easiest way to go. If the senior physician approach is not tried, the alternatives that will be considered by trustees and administrators will be harsher and less equitable, but undertaken as a matter of survival.

In terms of physician personalities, physicians with more than usual pressures on them from their personal lives, such as marital or financial pressures, are most likely to be the staff members who abuse the permissive areas of discretionary behavior. An open attitude that projects a willingness to help staff members with any of their problems when asked is a good management practice. Deviant behavior that leads to sloppy medical practices is better handled by concerned interest through informal ways than by reliance on active professional standards committees. However, a caring leadership cannot be mandated; personalities with characteristics consistent with caring leadership as a standard for the office must be selected.

In outlining why a medical staff is responsible for the acts of individual members and what can be done to strengthen control mechanisms, there remains a nagging question. Do medical staffs that exercise effective controls over individual members in fact have lower medical malpractice claims? To the authors' knowledge, there have been no studies that might answer this question.

In fact, hospitals with the worst medical malpractice experience are often urban hospitals with more developed medical staff organization structures than suburban and rural hospitals with better experience. However, the issues previously discussed still exist, to a large extent, in urban hospitals. It may be that the factors that increase claim incidence are concentrated in city areas, and the claim picture would be even worse than it is without a strong medical staff organization.

As a last observation, it may be worthwhile to look at the present medical malpractice issue as a blessing in disguise. If it sufficiently disturbs administrators to face the long-ignored organizational matters of better coordination of hospital and medical staffs, and to improve necessary control mechanisms of the total organization, then increasing intrusions of government in the future may be forestalled through an improved hospital organization.

Chapter 23

Managing Physician-Directed Hospital Departments

In the past three decades, changing medical technology and patterns of practice of private physicians have created a steadily growing demand on hospitals for more and more physician positions in its organization structure.

Thirty years ago a typical community general hospital was adequately staffed if there were radiologists, pathologists, and anesthesiologists supplemented by nurse anesthetists on staff. Today, they are still in the hospital organization, and many other hospital-based physicians have been added. Emergency service, intensive care, coronary care, newborn nurseries, respiratory therapy, renal dialysis, medical education, nuclear medicine, psychiatry, physical medicine, and directors of medical affairs have significantly expanded the number of physicians directing hospital departments.

As each specialty developed, the chief executive officer faced a loss of his traditional organization control. Unless an administrator adjusted his management strategies and developed new ones consistent with the dual relationship of physician-directors, as a member of both the administrative and medical staffs, organization control was weakened.

ELEMENTS OF ORGANIZATIONAL CONTROL

Authority, responsibility, and accountability are the typical terms used to describe the elements of organizational control that were abridged. As the need arose to add physician-directors, the chief executive's role changed

---

Reprinted from "Managing Physician Directed Departments" by Everett A. Johnson from *Hospital & Health Services Administration* 1979 (formerly *Hospital Administration*), Journal of the American College of Hospital Administration.

because of the intrusion of medical staff prerogatives on these three concepts.

Authority

It was clear to chief executive officers that there was a difference in authority of the physician-director vis-a-vis the nonphysician director. The differences in authority of the physician-director were caused by the following four factors:

1. The appointment of a physician-director customarily included the approval of a contract that defines the scope of authority to be exercised in the direction of a department.
2. Professional autonomy was granted in clinical areas and assured through appointment by the board of trustees as a member of the medical staff. In addition, it is frequently reinforced by membership on the medical executive committee.
3. The certification of the physician-director by a specialty board in medicine typically added prestige to his opinions and judgments.
4. Within specified limits, physician-directors were consulted on the setting of professional fees for their service.

These four changes in traditional grants of authority and the physician's informal power through the medical staff created a new authority relationship for the chief executive officer. If the administrator did not recognize the significance of the changed authority of the physician department director, he was creating a situation of prolonged confrontation with the medical staff.

Responsibility

In addition to a difference in authority relationships, a physician-director has responsibilities that are more direct and less elusive than a nonphysician department director. There are four factors that operate to make his operating responsibilities different from the other hospital department directors. These four factors are:

1. State licensure and board certification create a personal responsibility for maintaining medical standards and the quality of patient care services provided.

2. Statutory and common law judicial decisions fix greater responsibility on a physician-director for administrative negligence than other directors.
3. The greater complexity of procedures and systems operated within a physician-directed department increases their responsibilities because of the unique technical knowledge required.
4. The knowledge and skill levels required by the technical staff of a professional department create a need for more direct control over technical staff decisions and consequently greater responsibility for actions and judgments of the departmental staff than for other hospital departments.

Where a physician-director does not carry out his responsibilities as completely as administratively necessary or desirable, the chief executive officer has great difficulty in both identifying the problem and finding a remedy because the different authority relationship often precludes a direct order. Frequently, a physician-director will attempt to shift his responsibility to that of a failure of the hospital administration by alleging that salaries are too low, instrumentation is inadequate, or that there is not a sufficient number of technical personnel. He garners support from the medical staff for this position.

Accountability

Such actions underscore the change that has occurred in organizational accountability and is sensed by the physician-director. He knows that accountability is shared between the medical staff—or physician-director—and the chief executive officer in these departments. Medical care is a continuum on which there are no totally separate and distinct parts.

A professional department must integrate its operations with the flow of patients and the operation of other hospital departments if efficiency and cost containment objectives are to be optimized. To establish totally independent departmental operations generates greater costs than when there is a mutual sharing of joint services. Since the physician-director is more likely to emphasize patient care concerns, then cost consciousness differences of opinion are commonplace between hospital-based physicians and administrators.

The physician-director has another reason for his lack of primary concern for cost. He knows that the medical staff expects accuracy, reliability, rapid reporting, and a wide array of services, and that attending physicians often attempt to hold the hospital-based physicians responsible for their failure in patient diagnosis and treatment. In addition, physician-directors are in more frequent contact with patients, families, and visitors than are administrators, and will strive to provide convenient services in a pleasant and attractive environment.

The differences in authority, responsibility, and accountability of physician-directors from other hospital department directors are confounding to chief executive officers because they know that these physicians frequently gain support from part of the medical staff by the use of emotional rather than rational statements. At times, these physicians attempt to cover their lack of management skills by projecting the cost control concerns of administrators as a desire to reduce the quality of medicine practiced. At other times, physician-directors attempt to compromise the chief executive officer's position through direct relationships with members of the board of trustees.

If a chief executive officer is to cope adequately with the uniqueness of the physician-director positions in a hospital organization, the skillful use of management techniques is necessary.

Since the authority relationship is the most difficult aspect to change, administrative efforts should be concentrated at a more detailed level.

ELEMENTS OF MANAGEMENT DIRECTION

Three management tools are basic to exercising reasonable administrative direction in a physician-director department.

Departmental Organization Charts and Job Descriptions

The first is the use of a departmental organization chart and job descriptions. A functional organization chart must define in detail reporting relationships and supervisory positions for each shift in the operation and how they are coordinated. Frequently, organization charts in professional departments simply identify each section with the department and do not clarify how evening and night shifts are controlled or the role of the chief technician, as well as many other functions that need coordination.

To back up a functional organization chart, detailed job descriptions are necessary to define the specific authority and responsibility of each position and to whom it reports for different activities, as well as what reports are to be issued and received.

Management Information System

The second basic management tool is an adequate management information system that accumulates both operating and financial data. Financial reports should report revenues by inpatient and outpatient sources, and by major clinical activities within the department. The expense statement should collect data for each area of major activity within the department based on a detailed chart of accounts.

Operating data should be consistently collected as a daily responsibility of each section and for the department. Comparable units of measurement should be used throughout the department to the maximum extent possible. The time period used for summarizing data should be intervals of time that can easily be combined for all parts of the system.

The fundamental criterion used for inclusion of data should be its usefulness for current and future management decisions, and it must be consistent with the organization structure of the department. Control and assessment of operations requires a data collection system that identifies gaps in service, or overloading and underloading of sections for the department.

The most important use of financial and operating data is its management use for developing performance and financial budgets. Financial budgets should include projections of revenue and expense and planned capital equipment purchases; details of estimated changes in revenue and expenses, such as new tests and their pricing rationale; as well as detailed expense estimates including such things as replacement personnel for vacation and holiday time.

Performance budgets should be prepared defining the productivity level expected during the next fiscal year. It should include such ratios as total procedures per technician man-hour, total procedures per clerical man-hour, actual man-hours versus authorized man-hours, and costs and revenues per admission or per diem.

Statement of Annual Objectives

The third element of management direction is the use of a statement of annual objectives. The physician-director should report in writing during the budget preparation period what improvements in instrumentation, new services, educational activities, and training are planned for the following year.

With the use of these three management tools, a chief executive officer will have sufficient routine data and operating commitments from the physician-director to control the management of a professional directed department.

To keep these departments current with medical advances, each physician-director should be asked to annually submit in writing to the chief executive officer an annual assessment of the professional competences of his physician associates in the department and how he plans to strengthen their capabilities. He should also be asked to do the same for the senior technical personnel in the department.

With these management tools, a chief executive officer has an adequate basis for administrative control of physician-directed hospital departments. However, he must still cope with the committee structure of the medical staff and their attempts to make decisions in administrative areas of the organization. Too often physician-directors, who are members of standing medical staff committees, use the committee structure to upend administrative decisions. If a chief executive officer is to counter such actions successfully, he must persistently defend his right to make administrative-type decisions. A failure to do so will open the door to end runs on his prerogatives by the medical staff.

Managing physician-directed hospital departments is a challenge for hospital administration. To integrate these positions into a hospital organization successfully requires skill and sophisticated management techniques. To fail to do so will place the chief executive officer in a position of endlessly justifying and rationalizing poor management practices.

Chapter 24

Medical Staff Responsibilities in Hospital Financial and Construction Issues

INTRODUCTION

In the "good old days," medical staffs and hospital administrations rarely had a partnership viewpoint on mutual responsibilities for hospital financing and construction matters. The effects of today's institutional environment of rising regulations will be moderated and costs better controlled only if there is a shared responsibility and accountability between medical staffs and hospital administration.

The key words here are "shared responsibility and accountability." Accountability is widely used in society and often inappropriately applied. The larger the organization the more likely its misuse. In multimillion dollar annual budgets in hospitals, it is obvious that accountability and responsibility are out of phase with each other.

Today the marginal value of continually increasing medical care expenditures is rapidly decreasing. Past medical successes have led to current medical failures. As life expectancy has increased and as formerly fatal and disabling diseases are overcome, an older population increasingly faces diseases difficult to treat. The rapid expansion of nursing homes, high energy radiation centers, and transplant programs is an example of a costly response with a low cost/benefit ratio.

In a simpler time responsibility in medical care was much clearer. Before the widespread use of third party reimbursement programs physicians did care about hospital rates.

Responsibility is now diffuse, and a much larger cast of people deliver care services. Regulations on PSROs, HSAs, HMOs, and medical care evaluation are efforts to reinstitute a larger sense of personal and institutional responsibility. Along the way to reinstituting responsibilities, incentives for accountability have been warped.

If the medical staff is to become a meaningful element in the fiscal processes of a hospital, individual physician members need to understand existing hospital reimbursement processes.

FINANCIAL ISSUES

Reimbursement Formulas

Without a doubt, the most pressing problem facing hospitals today is the use of federal reimbursement formulas by Medicare, Medicaid, and Blue Cross plans. The formulas do not fully cover a hospital's cost of providing care to a patient. Typically, these reimbursement formulas pay the lesser of costs or charges.

Many Blue Cross plans have negotiated contracts with hospitals that reimburse only for the exact cost of services rendered and do not allow any surplus for the development of new services. Medicare formulas include discounts so that they pay the hospital so many dollars for the care rendered, less "x" percent.

Two examples that have further strained a hospital's financing stability are the proposed elimination of the 8 ½ percent nursing differential without any utilization studies relating to patients 65 years of age and older, and the actual reduction in routine services payments from the ninetieth to the eightieth percentile without any studies to justify the shift.

Charges for hospital services that are not reimbursed must be madeup somewhere; most often, from commercial insurers and self-pay patients who pay full charges. Essentially this represents an outright subsidization of the federal government and Blue Cross by those patients paying charges. It is, in effect, cost shifting rather than cost savings.

Hospital-Physician Relationship

Another problem in reimbursement is the inability of the federal government to recognize the relationship that usually exists between hospitals and physicians. Physicians are not agents of the hospital. Yet, HHS persists in trying to control physicians' prescriptive practices by placing sanctions on hospitals.

One example is the utilization review regulation. Another the maximum allowable drug cost program; both of which place financial penalties on a hospital for physician decision making.

Rate Review Commissions

A third financial problem of major proportions is the movement toward the establishment of state review and control over hospital rate structures. At first glance, the idea seems attractive; once in place, it becomes a bureaucratic nightmare. Some states have established these commissions, while other states are contemplating their operation. Most administrators in rate-controlled states believe that the financial solvency of their institutions has decreased by actions of these commissions.

Basically, these schemes require a hospital to submit its operating budget for the coming year to a state-designated agency for approval. Rates of reimbursement are determined, and the hospital is notified of its authorized rates for the coming year.

The usual habit is to call such a system prospective reimbursement. It is, in fact, a long way from such a concept. The financial stability of a hospital is lessened because state rate commission programs have the following inequities:

- Interest expense on borrowed funds is not recognized at the rate the hospital must pay.

- Bad debt costs are not adequately recognized.

- Increased salary costs not budgeted in a hospital's original submission to the rate review board and that occur as the result of arbitration, areawide negotiations, and unanticipated results of bargaining cannot be passed through during that year.

- Arbitrary guidelines are applied to percentage increases in annual salary costs.

- Deadlines frequently are not met by the rate review board, so that a hospital may be several months into its fiscal year without knowing whether or not its budget has been accepted.

- Decreasing amounts of funds are approved each year for educational programs, such as intern and resident training or other training programs.

Another problem for hospitals is the widespread use and misunderstanding of the term "not-for-profit hospital."

Not-for-Profit Status of Hospitals

No hospital can afford to continue operating and literally be "non-profit." Each fiscal year, a hospital must show an excess of revenue over expense.

This margin is needed by the hospital to purchase the necessary capital equipment for new and/or expanded services. Also, with today's rate of inflation, historical depreciation does not set aside money fast enough to keep up with inflation or the rate of new technology.

Hospitals must have a margin of revenues over expenses in order to maintain dynamic growth. The common term for this operating margin is profit. Hospitals reinvest their margin or profit in new equipment, modern technology, and skilled personnel so that the margin or profit of the hospital is spread across the community.

INTERNAL FINANCIAL REPORTS

Financial Reporting System

From this quick overview of the major financial issues today in third party payments for hospital services, the question of the institutional role and responsibilities of the medical staff needs to be asked and answered.

Before defining a meaningful medical staff role, several comments about the internal financial reports of hospitals are needed. The basic reports of such a system include the 13 following elements:

1. budget preparation reports, initial and final
2. monthly revenue and expense statements
3. monthly balance sheet
4. daily cash balance
5. accounts receivable breakdowns by category and aging
6. cash flow statement
7. annual financial audit
8. monthly service statistics
9. position control and staffing pattern
10. wage and salary classification
11. monthly man-hours report
12. capital equipment budget
13. rate structure

If any of these elements are missing, the financial reporting system is deficient in essential control information that should be routinely reported. Larger hospitals will additionally have subsets of control data within each element to provide basic data for control purposes.

Hospital Budget

The basic report for establishing the anticipated financial direction of a hospital is its budget. Based on gross patient service statistics, such as average patient daily census, case mix, percentage of collection, number of surgical procedures, and number of deliveries, a historical trend of the past two to three years is used, with modification for inflation, alteration in reimbursement, regulations, and projected operational changes.

The key to accurate budgeting is accurate historical data and estimates of the average daily census of patients. Incidentally, the current emphasis on zero-based budgeting in the federal government is probably more fad than long-range fact. Once the budget is established and adjustments in rate structure are accomplished, a projected cash flow statement is developed that will include proposed capital equipment expenditures.

Because hospitals are typically controlled in their amount of net surplus or profit to about 3 or 4 percent annually, the margin for error in budgeting is small. For example, if a 200-bed hospital estimates an average daily patient census of 180 patients, or 90 percent occupancy, and at year-end winds up with an average census of 173 patients, the profit that was planned to purchase new types of equipment or pay down a mortgage will not be available, and the medical staff will believe the hospital administrator is once again poor-mouthing the hospital's financial position.

Hospitals are highly sensitive to patient census fluctuations. In today's environment there are no hidden corporate funds left to cover errors in financial judgment, or to fund unexpectedly the unplanned demands of a member of the medical staff in the middle of a budget year.

A hospital budget is basically a financial planning and forecasting technique. Standing alone it is simply a method for predicting where institutional dollars will be spent for the next year, not how wisely they are to be spent. An approved budget should be the culminating document of a series of interrelated reports involving the best judgments of a hospital organization. To tamper with budget projections during the year is to initiate a ripple effect that can easily upset the predicted results.

A major responsibility of institutional management is to forecast the financial future of an organization accurately. Therefore, it is reasonable to expect managers to have a sufficient grasp of the future to be able to predict events eighteen months ahead accurately. Consequently, budgeting is a serious organizational affair that can either promote or disrupt the hospital's future if poorly done.

This is particularly true in today's environment of unanticipated shifts in reimbursement regulations, retroactive post-audit adjustments, new regulations, slow-ups in government payments on accounts receivables, and hospital rate commission actions.

In a $20,000,000-a-year hospital operation, it is not unusual for a hospital chief executive to receive a year-end revenue and expense statement and believe the hospital has earned a profit of $600,000, only to have a government audit and find that the auditors adjustments have converted a profit into a $300,000 loss.

One major hospital in this country had a $95,000,000 budget and was faced with a $13,000,000 postaudit adjustment. Obviously that hospital is out of business unless some reimbursement rules are bent or invented to keep it in operation. Clearly, the rules will be modified, probably on a political basis in a way that is unpredictable to the hospital administration.

In past years a good budgeting procedure could come within a one percent error for projecting anticipated revenue and expense. In the current capricious regulatory environment, errors in budget estimates of five to ten percent are not unusual, even if difficult to explain to boards of trustees and medical staffs.

A particularly difficult budgeting problem for hospitals is the matter of case mix of patients. In all reimbursement formulas and in rate regulation programs, such as the unlamented Economic Stabilization Program of 1971 through 1974, no methods of measuring the financial impact of changing case mix of inpatients were developed. The best that was done was to provide for an exceptions appeal to existing regulations if the hospital could prove a substantial change that affected its financing.

Theoretically, the case mix impact on hospital finances is difficult to handle. However, if cost containment programs, or revenue caps, are ever going to be meaningful and equitable, a solution must be developed.

Typically, a hospital implicity assumes the same case mix next year as last year for budgeting purposes, except where an expansion or development of a new clinical service has been planned. In most instances, such an assumption is reasonable because the effort and medical staff upset required to obtain the necessary data ordinarily is not justified. But surprises do occur.

The usual budget planning assumption is that other cases requiring approximately the same dollar amount of hospital services will fill the emptied beds. This event may or may not occur; in the current situation of decreasing census in inner-city hospitals or an overexuberant expansion of beds in many hospital service areas, the anticipated replacement patients will certainly not cross a hospital's doorstep.

Because many physicians make independent decisions about their practices and do not stop to think about an impact on their hospital, the revenue side of a budget often takes an unexpected bounce that jangles administrative nerves.

Performance Budgeting

A good hospital budget is based on reliable input data and a judicious planning of expenditures. Few hospitals have, as yet, adopted performance budgeting techniques. This method of planning relates dollars to performance and productivity. For example, a hospital department such as the clinical laboratory projects the following data:

- *For revenue*: volume of tests by clinical sections, such as chemistries and hematology and average charge for each test

- *For expenses*: total worked and paid man-hours by clinical section and average rates of pay by employee category plus other major expense items, servicing, and reagent costs

- *For performance budget*: projected number of tests per man-hour by clinical section, revenues, and expenses per man-hour

Even when no variance between gross revenues and expenses occur, the targeted productivity norms by clinical section may vary and will quickly identify areas for administrative intervention. As a further refinement of performance budgeting techniques, quality control elements can be added, such as the number of repeat tests, quality control test variances occurring, and percentage of autopsies.

This kind of a system will come to be used sooner or later in hospitals. As it is developed and refined, medical staff participation will not only be desirable, but necessary.

Much effort is currently being spent on promoting cost containment by hospitals and physicians. From the viewpoint of hospital administration, the action to date in this arena, except in a state like New York, is mostly blowing smoke. No chief executive with a sense of the future and an understanding of the present state of affairs will seriously work at cost containment. If the present national administration manages to pass a cost containment bill, any cost savings previously achieved simply reduces an institution's chance for survival when cost caps are screwed down tightly.

Likewise, under cost-based reimbursement formulas where 85 percent of a hospital's revenues are controlled, a savings of $100,000 is, in fact, a net savings of only $15,000. It is a rare administrator who will take on the necessary struggles to achieve a $100,000 cut in expense—which is a major, bruising, accomplishment—only to see a final result of $15,000. The disparate between the two figures is so great it is not worth the fight.

Unfortunately, as long as savings from cost containment efforts do not stay in the hospital, there will be little real effort to accomplish much. In essence, there is no benefit; rather, there is a loss for a hospital that is serious about voluntary cost containment efforts. The incentives and pay-offs are misdirected.

ROLE OF THE MEDICAL STAFF

Hospital Financing

With the major elements of hospital reimbursement, the financial reporting system, performance budgeting, and cost containment reviewed, the unanswered question is still the role of the medical staff.

Historically medical staffs have not had an important role in hospital financial decisions, even though they were essential for institutional financial stability. They often recognized their collective financial impact, however, by organizing a hospital boycott to achieve a particular objective, and they generally succeeded.

The role of a medical staff in the days ahead will be different if a hospital is to maintain financial stability. The looseness in past financial planning must be replaced with a coordinated approach and a commitment by a medical staff to be responsible and accountable for helping to carry out a jointly planned budget.

A medical staff has several essential functions in a hospital's budgeting process: (a) assisting in a prediction of the projected number of inpatient days and the case mix of patients; (b) determining the needed medical equipment, order of priority, and levels of service to be provided; (c) developing new and expanded patient care services; and (d) reducing services when needed.

These budgeting inputs are irresponsible if they are shoot-from-the-hip personal opinions. To be valid and reliable budget inputs, they must be systematically developed, in a deliberate, objective manner. They must be balanced in terms of the total needs of a medical staff, and rational choices must be made when hospital revenues do not stretch to cover all improvements proposed.

Some of the major reasons that hospital chief executives previously avoided medical staff involvement was their past experiences that surgeons grind the surgical axes, obstetricians want their needs attended first, radiologists talk a technical equipment language understandable to only a few, and each physician believes his or her needs have a higher priority than all of the other members of the medical staff.

Budgeting is not a 90-minute, once-a-year chore. It is an involved, complex process with hard choices for those involved. Medical staff participation that does not recognize the total needs of the organization, such as new laundry equipment, salary increases for housekeeping maids, or new lobby furniture, is bound to put a medical staff's budget involvement back in the deep freeze. Discipline and balanced judgments are the keys to successful participation.

In addition to the role of the medical staff in the financial affairs of a hospital, they must be involved in construction and capital planning.

Construction and Capital Issues

With the development of certificates of need, 1122 reviews, and bulging construction costs, medical staffs have come to play a large part in any planning for hospital expansions, remodeling, and major capital expenditures. These issues come together when a hospital is working on a master long-range plan.

The unpredictability of future reimbursement levels is sufficient reason to forget about developing a master plan. The best hope for institutional survival in periods of great uncertainty are planning activities. They may need to be more sophisticated and require more complex methods, but not to plan for a variety of contingencies is to invite future trouble.

Historically, long-range planning involved the medical staff only to the extent of vaguely defining future hospital clinical programs and working with an architect on the functional design of a proposed department or service. Programmatic planning was handled on an *ad hoc* basis. With the enactment of PL 92–603 and Section 1122 reviews for both construction and substantial changes in service, program planning became a necessity. A new element was added.

Today a long-range plan must include changes in the scope and type of service a hospital offers. With the passage of PL 93–641 and the establishment of health systems agencies, long-range planning was mandated for each institution.

After the passage of PL 93–641, the typical viewpoint of a medical staff became outdated. In the past a medical staff wanted its hospital to be a full-service institution, with back up from a broad spectrum of physician specialists, modern equipment reflecting the latest technology, and an attractive workshop staffed by ever-smiling and highly skilled nurses and technicians.

The expectations of other groups must be considered. Trustees seek to maximize institutional resources, maintain a financially stable operation, deliver high quality service, and meet community needs. The community has different objectives; low cost care available day and night; convenience; pleasant surroundings; a wide spectrum of health and social services; and prompt, courteous treatment.

In the HSA arena now operating, the dissenters do not go away, they seek hearings provided by government regulation. What used to be a lackadaisical planning process is now much more internally complex and laced with a plethora of forms and reports to be filed.

Developing a master plan that promotes the delivery of quality medical care has become a real test of a medical staff's understanding and leadership skills. The first step is to develop an understanding of the approval process and its complexities.

An effective hospital planning process must rest on a well-defined statement of institutional goals. Statements about providing high quality care or treating the needy were fine in the days of low budgets, limited technology, inexpensive construction, and patients paying their own bills. Today such generalized statements are meaningless.

A hospital is no longer "all things to all people" for health care. As medical services in a community continue to integrate, hospitals and medical staffs must have a clear statement of what part of health care they are intending to service. A physician must be aware of how his hospital fits into the spectrum of health care and why.

Practicing modern institutional medicine necessitates a growing interdependency of physicians, nursing staff, engineers, lawyers, insurance experts, mortgage bankers, architects, and administrators.

For program development, the hospital administration must start with a collection and analysis of data. This information must then be organized and implications defined for consideration by the medical staff. Alternatives need to be spelled out, types of clinical programs defined, methodologies explained, costs delineated, and results anticipated. Physicians need to be involved in this process.

Once the initial program is defined, calculations must be made on financing, construction, remodeling, and operating costs, and must be evaluated in terms of reimbursement formulas.

At this point, the administrative staff frequently begins to wish they had never been involved in the project because financing capabilities usually fall short of providing sufficient funds. This is also the time when medical staff members begin to feel that the promises of the administration are ringing falsely. No matter how many times they have heard that the planning is only preliminary, they usually believe their task has been completed when the initial recommendations were prepared. Typically, an administrator is told that he never said the plan was only a preliminary program.

A choice must be made; either try to take a piece out of each program or adopt projects in order of importance. Typically, taking a portion out of each program fails because of construction or operating constraints. Usually, the decision is to ask the medical staff to recycle their work and put in order of priority their needs.

Once the medical staff has completed their review and are satisfied that it is the best possible solution within the financing restraints, they have a responsibility to help lobby the project through the board of trustees. Too often, the physicians who did not get a high priority for their project will make an independent approach to the trustees to salvage it. Such actions are disruptive and slow up final approvals by the board and the HSA.

For a good master plan to evolve, medical staff inputs are essential and must be organized. If adequate participation of medical staffs is to be useful and effective, they will need to understand the current complexities of institutional financing and planning, and to participate as a partner in the process. To be independent, uncompromising, and unbalanced is to assure themselves of ultimate institutional deterioration. To participate with wisdom, objectivity, and interest is to assure themselves of a future in an outstanding hospital.

Chapter 25

The Role of the Physician in Hospital Management

Both public expectations for hospital service and the regulatory climate have been expanding at a rate never before experienced in the hospital field. As a result, the governance and administrative requirements for hospitals have generated a new set of imperatives that are influencing traditional organizational structures of hospitals.

One of the most disturbing changes was the decision by the federal government to use the local hospital as the control mechanism for affecting the private practice of medicine at the community level. Over the past several years, physicians have increasingly resented their local hospital, its governance, and its administration, because they limit the past freedoms of medicine.

It is now foreseeable that hospitals that will best survive this existing national climate of excessive regulation and unreasonable expectation will be those institutions that have provided an administrative structure that appeals to both the hospital staff and physicians of the medical staff.

A QUIET REVOLUTION

A quiet revolution has taken place in the past decade in the composition and leadership of hospital boards of trustees. Today, a substantial majority of boards include physican members, and quite often, they are influential policy makers. At the administrative level, the situation remains mixed, with some hospitals increasing medical staff input on key operating decisions, while other administrations have continued the traditional complete separation of clinical and administrative affairs.

The typical organizational structure of today's hospital is generally the result of past accommodations to specific pressures of the moment, earlier

Reprinted with changes with permission from HOSPITAL PROGRESS, November 1977, © 1977 by The Catholic Health Association.

compromises agreed to for accommodating different points of view, and no concerned effort to create a well-defined, carefully organized medical-administrative structure.

A hospital will survive only if the major elements of its organization structure—governance, medical staff, and administration—can learn to work in partnership. The three issues of the day requiring cooperation are to assure solvency of the institution, to contain the costs of medical service, and to control the quality of medical care.

It is not sufficient to preach or plead for a partnership or cooperation. It is necessary to design lines of authority, responsibility, and accountability, so that, in fact, a partnership of cooperation and coordination occurs.

A large, complex hospital organization must operate in, and respond to, the realities of the day if it is to be successful in the future. The four facts of life today that a medical staff must, and too often do not, recognize are:

1. Regulation by the federal government and the JCAH is here to stay and must be followed.
2. Institutional solvency is more important than prestige, popularity, and amenities.
3. Labor unions will not go away.
4. Private practicing physicians in their spare time cannot run a large modern hospital by the traditional committee system.

DIFFERENCES BETWEEN HOSPITAL-BASED AND ATTENDING PHYSICIANS

When the role of physicians in hospital management is considered, the distinction between hospital-based and attending physicians must be considered. In terms of management relationships, each group requires separate consideration. Frequently, physicians espouse the position that in the hospital all physicians are due the same privileges and are equally free of organizational restraints. This is not so, yet there are current movements to debundle hospital-based physician fees and to promote the open staff concept, even in medical staff departments where it is sure to impair organizational efficiency.

Hospital-based physicians are an essential element of a large modern hospital and are, in fact, a part of the hospital administration; whereas, private practitioners are individual entrepreneurs for whom the hospital is a workplace. Private practitioners have privileges, and hospital-based physicians have contracts.

These differences mean that there are distinct medical-administrative authorities and responsibilities for each group of physicians.

Hospital-based physicians are placed throughout the hospital organization structure, from subdepartment director positions to second and third line executives at the top, with administrative authorities and responsibilities supposedly similar to nonmedical managers at the same hierarchical level. Typically, physician-managers have greater authority and responsibility than their counterparts, but their accountabilities are often not enforced to the same degree.

Private practitioners' organizational roles are usually quite loose, and they operate almost without any medical-administrative accountabilities.

For example, suppose three out of four urologists decide to attend a urological meeting in Miami, Florida, in late winter and also sign up for the ten-day Caribbean cruise offered to the attendees. For a two-week period, unknown to the hospital budgeters, the urological census will drop by three-fourths. Or assume three senior surgeons independently decide that next year they will begin to taper off their surgical procedures and will only do one-half the cases they performed this year.

The usual budget planning assumption is that other cases, requiring approximately the same dollar amount of hospital services, will fill the emptied beds. This event may, or may not, occur; in the current situation of decreasing census in many hospital service areas, the anticipated replacement patient will certainly not cross a hospital's doorstep.

AREAS FOR PHYSICIAN INVOLVEMENT

Institutional Financing and Planning

If participation of medical staffs is to be useful and effective, physicians need to understand the current complexities of institutional financing and planning. If they participate on the basis of independence or are uncompromising and unbalanced in judgments, they are assuring themselves of ultimate institutional deterioration. If they participate with wisdom, objectivity, and interest, they assure themselves of a future in a well-functioning hospital.

Too often today a few administrators and controllers are using the complexities of reimbursement to win an ego struggle with their medical staff. If physicians have traditionally practiced a snobbery of medical expertise, the institution's financial managers now practice a snobbery of financing issues.

Hospital financing applications are complex, but the concepts are reasonably clear. Rather than flaunt its complexities, the smart administrator promotes conceptual understanding of reimbursement matters.

Master Plan and Design of Facilities

The other major area of involvement of physicians is in the development of a long-range master plan and the subsequent design of facilities. Generally, physicians enjoy participation in planning and design activities, and the way this is done is straightforward. Only rarely, though, do hospitals spend time and effort reviewing and formally deciding an institutional role and mission; consequently, physicians usually do not have an opportunity to think carefully about what part their hospital plays in the local health scene.

Management Functions

While most hospitals have increased physician involvement in management functions, the approach has been piecemeal, on an issue-by-issue basis, rather than an analytical look at internal relationships.

Organizationally, a medical staff has a difficult time meeting its responsibilities because its decision making is handled through a committee structure, and its actions depend on the goodwill and unpaid time of individual physicians.

Organizational integration of a medical staff is not a will-of-the-wisp technique full of ambiguity. As the complexities of operating hospitals grow, and as medical and administrative functions become increasingly intertwined, inadequacies of the traditional medical staff control structures will become apparent gradually. Until that issue is recognized and faced, the participation of physicians in management decisions will not be optimized.

MEDICAL-ADMINISTRATIVE POSITIONS

When a hospital has reached the point in development where greater physician input is necessary, and it is beyond reason to expect unpaid service from individual members of the medical staff, the usual response is to establish one or more full time paid chiefs of service, a vice-president of medical affairs, or a medical director position. This is always an expensive decision because of the level of physician incomes, which also impedes the establishment of additional medical-administrative positions as other needs arise.

Decisions to create fulltime administrative positions for physicians, other than for the direction of professional departments and programs, may be the most expensive way possible to provide for a decision-making capacity. Rather than opt for additional positions, it makes more sense to reorganize the decision-making process of the medical staff between policy and procedural decisions.

What will gradually emerge is a medical staff organization that has a variety of functions related to quality of care: peer review, infection control, utilization review, and tissue review. Their administrative functions will be handled largely by hospital-based physicians operating programs, and the remainder of decisions will be folded into a variety of internal committees from departmental levels, to administrative activities and committees within the governance level.

The difference in outcomes in decision making will be significant. The present day medical staff committee structure dealing with administrative matters ties up the organization when they do not make timely decisions or refuse to reach a decision. In the future, when these administrative decision areas are assigned to mixed physician-administration committees, their absence or delaying tactics will be overridden by the total committee. The choice for the medical staff will be to participate on schedule or have decisions made in the open without their input.

As organizational changes unfold in the future for the medical staff, governance, and hospital administration, the day of the backroom decision-making hospital administrator or trustee will be limited. Physician involvement means honest participation; not structured inputs to committees not smart enough to know what is missing. It will be a time requiring greater competence in hospital administration. It will be a time when medical staffs have come of organizational age.

Part VI

Control and Appraisal

Chapter 26

Appraising Performance at the Top

Thanks to the shift from a limited form of government to a pervasive one that wishes to limit rigidly the health field, there is bound to be increasing interest in Washington in performance criteria, consequences, and controls. Like it or not, performance appraisal takes on new meanings in such an environment.

Performance appraisal has previously meant a system of formal or informal ways of judging managerial performance. Employees were judged by their supervisors, who in turn were judged by the department director, who was judged by the administrator, who was judged by the governing board, who was judged by no one. The board itself, however, is now being judged in this overgoverned society through a plethora of measuring mechanisms.

The JCAH has also developed an interest in the governing authority, its composition, and the kinds of information it regularly receives. The courts have increased their interest and are holding governing boards accountable for everything that goes on in the hospital. Meanwhile, HHS has its Medicare auditors, OSHA has its interests in physical safety standards, and the environmentalists have their share of clout. At the state level, there is a growing number of review boards and regional health systems agencies who are mandated to determine the future of hospitals. All are looking through their own set of interests at the hospital, invoking their own criteria, controls, and consequences if institutional performance fails to measure up.

Under such circumstances, traditional performance appraisal systems stop short of what is now needed. At the top, performance appraisal is needed as well as the traditional managerial review that has become part of a progressive organization. Measuring the performance of the chief executive and the governing board is a different process but should become

standard operating procedure for hospitals. Not to do so is to court unexpected public disclosure and possible embarrassment as a result of one
of the outside agencies' interests in the hospital. Governing board members
of hospitals who have experienced unexpected newspaper publicity over
conflict of interest are attuned to the need for careful board appraisal.

THE NATURE OF GOVERNANCE

Before focusing on trustee appraisal, a quick look at the nature of governance sets the stage. Governance is a collective process that is slow and
deliberative; the objective is to develop the best guidelines possible for the
operation of the institution. It requires the majority of the participants to
be in agreement before a policy can be adopted. Conceptually, the governing board role stresses:

- a grasp of the societal forces at work in the institution;

- the application of the highest obtainable levels of judgment in shaping
  the role of the institution in response to the societal forces;

- a preference for cool, deliberative approaches in shaping the role of
  the institution;

- the use of objectivity in the decision-making process, recognizing,
  however, that individual board members must be sensitive to the feelings and concerns of others and giving consideration to these nonquantifiable aspects;

- a willingness on the part of each participant to maintain an open mind
  on each issue until all of the data, opinions, and conversations have
  been heard.

THE ROLE OF THE BOARD

In addition to the nature of governance, the role of the board has also
changed. Clearly, the primary responsibility for the modern hospital's governing board is no longer fund raising. Of a scale of importance, the issues
of quality of patient care, third party reimbursement, decisions of health
planning agencies, interest rates, bank loans, and share of the market are
all of greater importance than fund raising.

HOW TO APPRAISE BOARD PERFORMANCE

Individual Performance

Inherently, performance appraisal at the board level must be treated differently than managerial appraisal. The purpose of an organizational structure is to pinpoint responsibility and accountability for performance so that the individual manager can be measured. At the board level, the purpose of the structure is to provide a mechanism for deliberative group action in a way that minimizes the impact of individual performance. Yet, to measure the board only in a collective manner and not to discriminate between individual board member performance denies that any real differences can exist between levels of individual board performance.

Any board watcher knows there is often a wide range of levels of performance and there are effective board members as well as ineffective ones. Yet, individual performance cannot be treated as separate and apart from the collective actions of the board. For example, it would be unrealistic to say that an individual has demonstrated outstanding performance as a board member, while at the same time the hospital files for bankruptcy. The two can neither be totally divorced, nor can they be totally integrated.

Outputs and Inputs

The measurement of board performance must, therefore, involve two elements that are *equally important*: (a) the quality and timeliness of board decisions (the output); and (b) the degree of participation (the input) by all of the members of the board. Both elements are required for a satisfactory rating of performance. For instance, suppose that a review of the last ten years of decisions made by a governing board leads to the conclusion that, on balance, the decisions were timely, imaginative, forward looking, and have led to a hospital regarded as outstanding. Also assume that the board has 28 members and is dominated by a brilliant, dedicated chairman who hasn't bothered to use the board structure, except to ratify his decisions.

Under such circumstances, what conclusion is reached about the performance of the board? Certainly the public and the institution haven't suffered, overall performance has been superlative and might well have been something less under other forms of leadership. Yet, as the organizational structure was designed, it failed to work as planned. On that score, under appraisal, a glaring weakness was revealed. The board was a deliberative body where 27 members failed to carry their share of the load. The fact that one person was outstanding in individual performance did not offset 27 failures.

There is a tendency in the health field not to be too critical of individual board performance on the basis that these are persons giving of themselves for community service, and it is unfair to measure them by the same rules that apply to corporate directors. Yet, as times change and boards come under increasing scrutiny by outside forces with prescribed, detailed standards, it is going to be difficult for trustees to get off the hook for poor performance on the grounds that this is a voluntary community activity that they are engaged in out of the goodness of their hearts. While true, it is unlikely to be sufficient grounds for defending a hospital caught in a substantial lawsuit or in justifying its course of action to the many government officials charged with securing compliance with their regulations.

Size of the Board

If there is acceptance of the concept that the governing board is a deliberative body whose members are expected to influence the shaping of the policy decisions reached, then the size of the board must be such that each trustee/director has the opportunity for making a contribution as an input during the discussion state of policy adoption. When finally acted upon, the individual trustee's vote should reflect personal conclusions. There must be an opportunity and sufficient time allowed for *all* of the board members to provide input. When governing boards grow in numbers to 15, 20, 30, or even 75, inputs are bound to be strictly limited, in the interest of concluding meetings. As simple and straightforward as this seems, many boards still carry on with the charade of using a small group for making decisions and talking as if all the board members of a large board are effectively making contributions to the development of policy.

Many an administrator or a board member defends a large-sized board on the grounds that the executive committee is really where the decisions are made. Large boards rarely exist without an executive committee that meets more frequently than the board and, in actual fact, operates as a *de facto* board. The truth of the matter isn't even honestly dealt with in hospital bylaws. Typically, the section dealing with the executive committee spells out its size and composition of membership and states that it shall meet between regularly scheduled meetings of the governing board to act on matters requiring immediate attention. Yet, members of the board who are not on the executive committee understand that at board meetings they are not to question seriously the decisions of the executive committee. These decisions are dutifully reported by a spokesman of the executive committee, who usually prefaces the remarks in a way that indicates these decisions were reached on behalf of the nonparticipating trustees in order to lessen their onorous burdens as board members. With institutional performance increasingly being scrutinized by big brother, there is going to come a time when nonparticipating trustees will recognize the perils of playing such roles.

Required Organizational Structure

Measurement of board performance includes answering the question, "Does the governing board carry out its functions in the way in which the organizational structure, as defined in the bylaws, requires?" Answered openly and honestly, large boards simply cannot stand up under such scrutiny. Inevitably, they are dominated either by a single trustee or a handful of trustees who call all the shots. This sham is usually aided and abetted by chief executives who go along because it reduces the amount of time they have to spend with individual trustees. As individuals charged with managing the hospital, administrators know the more time they spend on governance, the less time they will have available for operating matters. Because of this time factor, they tend to build personal relationships with this inner circle as a way of ensuring the adoption of their recommendations. In addition, they play up the importance of this small decision-making group in their own mind, which continually reinforces the gap between the inner group and the rest of the trustees. Instinctively, chief executives recognize that if others are to become deeply involved in the real decision-making process, the demands on their own time for governance activities (on an individual basis) would increase, thereby leading to a further reduction in time for operational activities. In doing so, chief executives become a part of the conspiracy that is dedicated to not operating in accordance with the responsibilities of trusteeship as defined in the bylaws.

Two Types of Inquiry

In evaluating the performance of the governance level of a hospital with a board, two types of inquiry have to be made; the questions deal with the inputs to policy making and the outputs in terms of appropriateness of the policies reached.

Input Questions

The input questions include the following:

- Does the board carry out its responsibilities in the organizational framework outlined in its own bylaws?

- Have position descriptions been written and followed by board members, chairman, and chief executive officer?

- To what extent do all trustees exercise their responsibility for providing inputs into the decision-making process?

- What periodic and formal review is made of individual trustee performance?

- What periodic and formal review is made of the performance of the chief executive?

Output Questions

Output questions that should be studied include:

- From a careful review of board minutes, to what extent do they indicate the adoption of timely courses of action?

- To what extent does the regular reporting system provide trustees with a clear picture of the quality of care being given in the hospital?

- Do trustees receive appropriate financial information?

- Can it be demonstrated that the board acts appropriately on the reports it receives?

- Does the board periodically review the objectives and goals of the hospital and determine to what extent performance has met them?

There are many advocates for large, consumer-oriented governing boards in hospitals, who believe that a broad representation of community viewpoints leads to increased responsiveness on the part of the operating organization. This may or may not be the case, but if it results in large boards with nonparticipating trustees, it leads away from organizational effectiveness, not toward it. Consumer dominated boards are usually not of a common mind but are made up of small enclaves of quite different viewpoints that offset each other and stalemate effectiveness.

WHO PERFORMS THE APPRAISAL?

If the questions just outlined are to be used, who applies them? If a committee of physicians on the medical staff answers them, the weighing of some questions will be greater than others in the physicians minds eye. Likewise, with administrators and trustees, each will see the questions through their own set of experiences and insights and weigh each question accordingly. How then to bring about measurement of trustee performance?

Basically, there are only two approaches to this kind of performance review, either externally by some outside organization or from within. An external review would not be too useful since the outside group would lack familiarity with the hospital and its problems, which can lead to a superficial analysis and conclusions. This leaves internal review as the only practical road to follow.

Since overall governing board performance is the collective result of individual trustee activities, evaluation of each one on an annual basis would seem to be in keeping with sound organizational practice. Medical staff members are expected to review individual physician performance annually, and hospital employees are reviewed on at least the same time frame as well. As the organizational landscape is surveyed, there is no reason to think that this shouldn't be an appropriate period for reviewing trustee performance. But who should do the measuring?

Since this review is missing in nearly all hospitals, finding a logical base for it does not infringe on past practice or tradition. Because the nominating committee is charged with recommending trustees, as well as the slate of officers at the annual meeting of a hospital corporation, it is the most suitable for undertaking this task as an extension of its existing responsibilities. As the definition of the functions of a nominating committee is reviewed in hospital bylaws, it becomes obvious that a careful and thorough formal review of each trustee's performance annually would be an invaluable asset in determining whether or not to reappoint for another term. Written reviews by such a committee would be a first step in bringing about a minimum standard of performance for all trustees.

VALUE OF GOVERNANCE APPRAISAL

The value of a properly structured performance appraisal of governance is that it balances the output factors with the input ones. All too often the fact that organizational structures are simply mechanisms for accomplishing the hospital's goals and objectives is forgotten. Structure is a means to an end and not an end unto itself. Also forgotten is that more than half of the hospitals in this country have small boards or no boards at all, and that the largest system of hospitals, the Veterans Administration, has no governing boards for its hospitals. It is only after the goals and objectives have been determined that the organizational structure that is appropriate can be realistically determined.

When hospitals had to rely on philanthropic funds for covering annual operating deficits and for the majority of capital funds, it was easy to justify large boards of potential donors. As accountability for hospital perform-ance is mandated, trustees will come to appreciate that large governing boards are as obsolete as large luxury automobiles. As nonfunctioning trustees find the heat in the kitchen uncomfortable, they will leave gov-erning boards. Those that remain will be fewer in numbers but will be tougher and more demanding of administrative performance. This will change the dimensions of the chief executive's role as it relates to both the governing board and the internal operations.

CHIEF EXECUTIVE APPRAISAL

Traditionally, chief executives of hospitals have been manipulators who carefully orchestrated their boards, never bringing up sensitive subjects before carefully laying a foundation for such a discussion. The strategies employed depended on having a keen ear for emotional traps and a nose for timing so that they could lead board members to their desired decision. So long as there were no serious constraints on the time element, board decisions could be delayed for months or years until board attitudes were successfully harmonized.

Today, this key to board strategy no longer can be freely used. The time that is available to respond to the pressures of outside forces cannot be stretched to meet the needs of board strategy. Because of the complexity of the problems now being dealt with at the governance level and the speed with which they have to be resolved, chief executives simply must bring up unpleasant situations and problems, and avoid straddling the fence on difficult issues. Circumstances are forcing them to tell it like it really is, whether or not board members are ready to hear bad news.

The focus of measuring chief executive performance has shifted away from skills of manipulation to those of administrative courage. Facing reality and standing tall in the saddle are basic requirements though the temptation remains strong to avoid this approach because it may lead to difficulties and jeopardize relationships. Many chief executives of hospitals tend to believe that formal performance appraisals apply to the rest of management but not to themselves, thinking that the test for chief exec-utives is overall institutional performance as presented in the monthly board statistics and their recommendations at such meetings. This is similar to college football coaches who, when asked why their salary is higher than members of the academic faculty, responded that they are the only person in the university having their performance reviewed at weekly intervals in the fall before 50,000 people. Certainly there is a continuing informal review that goes on through casual comments among individual board members before and after meetings. Occasionally, a board chairperson may drop a remark to the chief executive about his performance on a particular matter, but it is rare to find an organized feedback system to chief executives about their performance.

Persons who have been chief executives for only a few years often ask key board members, "How am I doing?" But those with more experience in the position usually come to believe they are sensitive enough to be able to read and interpret board thinking and modify their own behavior accordingly. While there are a small number that possess this ability, those that possess this skill are far fewer in number than those who believe it of themselves.

Chief executives are in a unique organizational position as the bridge between the deliberative and the operational sides of the hospital. They are managers and can be appraised as such, but they are also more than that; they are trustees, either in name or in a *de facto* way. Not only do they possess more information about the hospital and the health industry than anyone else at the board table, but they also are the only ones who have the authority to direct the activities of all those employed in the institution. This makes it particularly difficult for them to accept a formal performance review for themselves. The longer they hold a chief executive position, the less likely they are to listen carefully to others, some of whom they have maneuvered onto the board. Even top flight health care executives fall into the trap of believing they should be evaluating their management staff and trustee performance, but they will shun one for themselves.

Several years ago the author naively used to think that chief executives should sit down periodically with trustees and be willing to review trustees' individual performances as well as having their own performance reviewed at that time. This does not work. It is too much to expect chief executives to be candid and frank about individual trustee performance. They are likely to phrase their remarks so carefully that their impact is lost on the trustee. Telling it straight from the shoulder to a trustee is not reasonable, even though chief executives frequently rate trustee performance in an informal way in conversations with key subordinates. Hospital executives dissect trustee performance far more often than trustees concern themselves with administrative performance.

Purpose of Chief Executive Appraisal

The purpose of a formal appraisal system for the chief executive is the same as for other subordinate managers, to bring about modifications in behavior. Performance appraisal and a review of salary should not be treated separately. Together they act to reinforce each other with respect to modifying behavior. It is the application of a penalty or a reward system that should financially recognize good performance more than poor performance.

Measuring the performance of the chief executive is more complex in a hospital than in other kinds of industry because of the medical staff. In a very real sense, they lie outside the control of the chief executive. As the unabashed critics of hospital activities, they are often vocal in their feelings about administration to individual trustees, who in turn have no real basis of judging the validity of their criticisms. Not being part of the medical staff and spending only a few hours per month in the hospital boardroom, trustees lack any basis for judging for themselves the extent to which the chief executive has failed to deal appropriately with matters of patient care.

How to Measure CEOs' Performance

From a financial reporting standpoint, there is also an unusual degree of complexity in determining the chief executive's capability. Most trustees do not conceptually understand how cost reimbursement differs from a pricing system—such as they may use in their own businesses—though they accept the fact that there are real differences. Because they do not feel comfortable about it, they are often unsure of how to measure the competence of the chief executive on financial matters.

The net result of these differences is to make it difficult to apply definitive yardsticks of performance. This does not mean that formal evaluations of performance cannot be made. Rather than the typical performance appraisal, a different format for reviewing chief executive performance is indicated. Basically it should be a peer review, taking place at stated intervals in a manner that can best be described as a loosely structured meeting with as much room as possible for candid, honest, and open discussions among key governing board members and their chief executive. Such a conversation assumes a confidence in this person; therefore, it should be conducted in a positive direction toward improvement. Obviously, if confidence is lacking, the conversation will, and should, take on an entirely different tone. Sugarcoating of major deficiencies of performance leads only to more problems. Straightforward discussion is a necessity under such circumstances. It may not be pleasant, but it can prevent reaching the point of no return where the only solution is for the chief executive to move on to another hospital.

The difficulty with performance appraisal is that it often gets in the way of social relationships. Much of the action between a chief executive and board members is carried on in a semisocial situation. Board meetings may be preceded by a dinner with the chief executive acting as host. Or the chief executive may meet several trustees for lunch on varying dates throughout the month to discuss individual matters with them. Chief executives usually see themselves in the same peer group as trustees, with the result that this pattern of social interaction acts as a deterrent to the kind of objectivity needed in the annual or semiannual performance appraisal.

Because performance appraisal at its heart is criticism, thoughtful people, be they trustees or administrative personnel, do not take easily to the use of this organizational tool. Improperly applied, it can be destructive even though it was meant to be helpful.

Chapter 27

Hospital Productivity

There are many ways of looking at the concept of productivity. Quite often it is thought of as input divided by output, which yields the efficiency of the activity. It may also be expressed as the physical output per unit of effort or as the degree of effectiveness of industrial management in utilizing facilities for production, particularly labor and equipment use. Whatever definition is used, it is assumed that the output of the system can be measured so that productivity can be gauged. This is, of course, a debatable point.

To illustrate the problem, assume a person is asked to make a decision as to whether IBM or Remington Rand is the more efficient and effective corporation. However, in reaching a conclusion, the following data could not be used:

- earnings per share
- units produced
- share of the market
- net profit

Without this data, the problem is similar to making a determination about a hospital. This is why there is a lot of heat being generated about hospital costs and little light being shed. Each group is defining the end product as they see it, and there is no agreement.

THE DELIVERY SYSTEM OF HEALTH CARE

Rapidly Rising Expenditures

In general, hospital productivity is of interest because the public, the carriers, and the government are all concerned about rapidly mounting

279

hospital costs and, to a degree, they believe that hospitals are inefficiently managed. They feel that, if modern American management methods were applied, hospital costs could be contained, and the public could go to hospitals without worrying about facing bankruptcy. This feeling about hospital costs has been repeatedly expressed at all levels of society. The public also believes that hospital performance has been so poor that some actions should be taken.

The problem of rapidly rising expenditures for hospital care is not unique to the United States. As long ago as February 1969, an article in *Hospitals,* pointed out that other countries are experiencing the same difficulties. "These rising expenditures are taking place regardless of the ownership of the hospitals, the sources and control of funds, the degree of centralized control over the total operation, and the hospital staffing patterns."[1] As they also point out, the total expenditures for hospitals have risen 131 percent in an 11-year period in the United States, while in England they rose 128 percent and in Sweden 223 percent.[2] Data from the other developed countries of the world reveals the same conditions.[3] This is not to say that in the United States there should be no concern about hospital costs. Rather it is to say that the difficulties in achieving the desired results may be much greater than most people appreciate and in the final analysis may defy reaching a solution satisfactory to the public and its representatives.

Certainly the public is concerned about hospital costs and wants steps taken to prevent cost increases. If this means keeping people out of hospitals, then this should occur. Again in 1969 in *Today's Health,* the secretary of HEW, when asked about some of his long-range goals, responded by saying:

> There are many, but I'll mention just one that comes to mind. That is, the delivery system I've talked about has to be able to cope with the urban explosion. This means that if we're going to try and get better coverage for more Americans, health facilities will have to be in the inner cities, not just in the outer white suburban belts.[4]

At that same time, Tom Tierney of the Social Security Administration made the additional point that the federal government was interested in the fact that the Kaiser system of delivering health care has resulted in lowered admissions per 1,000 population and a shortened average length of stay.[5] Every year since then representatives of the federal government have favored changing the delivery system of care.

It is difficult to believe that the insiders in the health field will make such changes voluntarily. This must come about through the efforts of outsiders, that is, government and third party carriers. To open deliberately the question of the delivery system is to examine the problem of (1) who receives the care; (2) how much care each person is to receive; (3) who is to provide the services. In attempting to build a rational health care system, many deficiencies will be found as answers are sought to these questions. As these are recognized and programs are developed to correct them, the overall costs of the health care system will continue to rise. In this process the average length of stay continues to shorten in the acute hospital part of the system. To state it in a slightly different frame of reference, the per unit cost of some of the services may be reduced, but the total cost (units produced times unit cost) will be much higher, because the number of units of all services produced will have greatly increased and will more than offset any decrease in the unit cost of a hospital service. The moving of various parts of the health system from one pocket to another is going to lead to discovering all of the holes in the pockets. As these holes are mended, the costs will rise and lead to speculation about the ability to afford the repair job that is being proposed.

Personnel

Before leaving the subject of the delivery system of health care, a moment should be spent on manpower aspects. In spite of the current criticisms about hospital costs and inequities in service to lower income groups, no public voice is being raised claiming that physicians are dogging it or that nurses are loafing on the job.

To the contrary, many staff members will be expected to cope with the sudden increase in demand. Labor costs will spiral upward as personnel recognize the economic advantages that have been created for them. Because of the scarcity of personnel, in contrast to the demand for health services, concern for productivity will not be much of a factor in the scramble to attract sufficient personnel. In a labor intensive industry producing only units of service, such a situation should prove to be extremely interesting to economists.

IMPROVING PRODUCTIVITY

Turning away from the overall problem, the question might be asked, "What improvements can be made in the existing hospital system to improve productivity?"

Incentive

Far and away the most important consideration is putting some incentive in hospitals to become more efficient. The cost reimbursement formula works against improving efficiency. In hospitals, approximately 36 percent of the patient days is paid for by Medicare, a cost reimbursement program. Another major group ranging from 10 percent to 50 percent is paid for by Blue Cross, another cost reimbursement program. Together they provide from 40 percent to 80 percent of all hospital revenue from operations. In most hospitals this will fall between 60 percent and 70 percent. Under such a system, there is little or no incentive to improve labor efficiency since the result is a lower reimbursement from the prepayment agency. Also there is no advantage to substituting a capital investment for a labor cost. Hospitals are limited under reimbursement formulas to recapturing capital costs from depreciation payments tied to historical costs. In an industry where obsolescence is more of a factor than worn-out equipment and buildings, the rational decision for a hospital administrator is to incur costs that can be recaptured through the reimbursement formula. Given a choice of using automatic equipment or a manual system, the forces at work give preference to increasing the labor cost. In spite of this bias, which is built into the reimbursement system, the extent to which administrators substitute equipment for people whenever possible is surprising.

Technological Advances

Because of technological advances that have been made in the last decade, the public has come to place a great deal of faith in the systems approach. The Apollo 11 space shot will stand for all time as a monument to American ingenuity in engineering. Logically, the public is curious about what adaptations can be useful in hospitals and the extent to which automation can be useful and can be applied in hospitals. A number of such approaches have been brought forth by manufacturers. Among these are automatic transportation systems. When a cost benefit analysis is made, it usually turns out that the payoff takes 40 years or more. This often comes as a shock to those who advocate hospitals automating their activities as rapidly as possible. The payoff periods simply did not justify the expenditures involved. Such a result is understandable. The systems approach has its greatest usefulness in those functions that are high volume, uniform activities, and the least payoff in low volume, wide variety activities. The characteristics of the hospital industry are of the latter type.

Unit Costs

Unlike industry, the larger the hospital, the higher are its unit costs. In a typical manufacturing process the more units produced, the lower the unit cost. This is the hallmark of American ability. Not so with hospitals.

Table 27–1 indicates that the costs of operating the 400- to 499-bed hospital is 32.1 percent higher than the cost of operating the 25- to 49-bed hospital. The 500 + -bed hospital uses 8 percent more personnel per patient than the 25- to 49-bed hospital. Looking at the raw numbers, the conclusion might be drawn that the larger the hospital, the more inefficient it is. Such a judgment would not be valid. In reality, comparing a 25-bed hospital to a 500-bed hospital would be like comparing apples to oranges. As hospitals become larger, they add to the range and comprehensiveness of services they provide to patients. It is this increased scope of services that is reflected in Table 27–1.

Not only do the larger hospitals offer a broader range of services than the smaller ones, but the typical hospital of today, even if it has the same number of beds it had 20 years ago, offers a broader scope of services. Table 27–2 reveals some trend data for the last three decades.

Average Length of Stay

Over the last 14 years, the average occupancy of hospitals has decreased 3.2 percent. When it reaches 80 percent it is close to being as high as it can go. There is little slack in the system, at the most 7.5 percent.

Table 27-1 Average Cost per Patient Day by Size of Community Hospital—1979

Size	Per admission	Adjusted average cost per patient day	Fulltime personnel per patient
6 - 24 beds	760.13	151.22	3.23
25 - 49	888.87	151.90	3.31
50 - 99	995.86	148.77	3.03
100 - 199	1,209.76	171.54	2.84
200 - 299	1,381.24	186.94	2.98
300 - 399	1,548.83	200.70	3.10
400 - 499	1,633.55	207.89	3.38
500 or more	2,036.45	228.53	3.57

Source: AHA Guide to the Health Care Field, published by the American Hospital Association, copyright 1979.

Table 27-2 Selected Factors—1946-1978—Voluntary Nonprofit
Hospitals

Year	Fulltime personnel per patient	Average occupancy-percent	Average length of stay-days
1946	1.56	76.7	8.8
1950	1.91	74.4	7.7
1958	2.24	75.7	7.4
1966	2.64	78.5	7.9
1968	2.76	80.0	8.3
1978	3.36	73.5	7.5

Source: AHA Guide to the Health Care Field, published by the American Hospital Association, copyright 1979.

The average length of stay is interesting in that it bottomed in 1958 at 7.4 and has not decreased much since that time. When Medicare came into operation in 1966, a large influx of older patients began coming to hospitals. These patients usually stayed 12 or 13 days, so that the average length of stay moved back over the 8-day level. The combination of an increasing average length of stay and a rising cost per patient day had a double-barrelled effect on the average case cost for several years.

At the national level, patient statistics on the average length of stay have not been kept by clinical services, but just for the overall. The drop in the average length of stay that has been going on for many years may, in large measure, be attributable to changes in the length of stay of obstetrical and pediatric cases. Prior to World War II, obstetrical cases typically stayed ten days. Today the stay is between three and four days, which is also the pattern of pediatric cases.

In spite of all the comments about the impact on hospital costs of reducing the average stay, this average stay is far superior to what can be found in other countries and in federal hospitals in the United States. In these other hospital systems the average length of stay is three to five times greater. In the rest of the world, it is rare when the average length of stay drops below 20 days. The control of hospital costs does not lie in the direction of limiting length of stay, utilization committees not withstanding.

Effect of Minimum Wage

Hospitals are a labor intensive industry where salaries represent two-thirds of the operating costs, unlike manufacturing where they are one-third. Since hospitals employ many personnel at the minimum wage level, the changing of that level by congressional action has a pronounced effect on the hospitals. This can be seen from 1966 on, when hospitals came under the federal minimum wage and hour act. In the succeeding years hospitals' costs annually increased by 15 percent to 16 percent rather than the 6 percent to 7 percent that had been typical for the prior two decades.

KEEPING PERSONS OUT OF HOSPITALS

Like all other American industries, hospitals can be more efficient. The use of industrial engineers is now recognized and growing. However, the opportunities for cost reductions are not nearly as great as a person might believe when listening to the stories about hospital inefficiencies. It is rare to find a hospital where reductions in excess of 15 percent can be made in operating costs.

To pin hopes for containing hospital costs on increased productivity is not in the cards. The problem is to keep persons out of hospitals. This is where the real gains will be made.

NOTES

1. Odin Anderson and Duncan Neuhauser, "Rising Costs Are Inherent in Modern Health Care Systems," *Hospitals*, 43 (Feb. 16, 1969):50-52.
2. Ibid.
3. Ibid.
4. Robert H. Finch, "Inside Look at Health, Education and Welfare: What Are the Health Goals?" *Today's Health*, 47 (August 1969):16.
5. Ibid.

Chapter 28

Staffing—The Importance of Control

End-product measurements have only limited usefulness in determining year-end results. In citing earnings per share, net profit, or total patient days (units produced), hospital people are acutely aware that these kinds of numbers say nothing about the quality or comprehensiveness of the service provided. A concern about any given profit center usually finds the defense rallying around the quality and comprehensiveness factors. Where end-product measurements do not reflect the whole picture, attention must be devoted to measuring and monitoring the way in which the organization goes about its work. This requires far more detailed information on a routine basis. Because hospitals are labor intensive, control of the staff-hours worked and the productivity achieved is of utmost concern.

EXERCISING CONTROLS

Controls can be exercised on a highly informal basis where managers make all of the decisions with regard to staff-hours and by direct observation on a daily basis, monitoring both quality and productivity of the services rendered. Proponents of MacGregor's theory X and theory Y wince at the thought of organizations being managed in this fashion. Yet, most small firms or operating units perform well with this philosophy. However, as the size of the organization increases, such an approach becomes weaker and weaker as the need for decision making outpaces the manager's time. By the time a firm has several departments, more than 100 employees, and the complexity of the modern hospital, this approach must be restricted, and other forms of control must be introduced that are more formal in nature.

Using Statistics, Management Tools, and Reports

While every hospital, regardless of size, should collect and utilize statistics for all departments, all hospitals do not require the same number of statistics. Statistics should be related to the complexity of the organization and to size. (See Figure 28–1.) The ability of a hospital to maintain efficiency will be determined by the statistics it keeps. Statistics, properly developed and utilized, based on up-to-date, complete information make possible sound decisions that ensure the judicious use of men, money, and materials.

In a 50-bed hospital, there are fewer departments and subdepartments than in a 400-bed hospital. There are also more layers of supervision in the larger hospital. As size and complexity of the organization increases, management is forced to resort to an increasing reliance on the formal tools and techniques of management, and less and less on direct personal supervision of activities. Consequently, more detailed reports must be used in order to achieve coordination. For example, in the 50-bed hospital, one figure of total amount of laundry processed may be adequate, but in the 400-bed hospital, this may be subdivided into obstetrics, surgery, nursing divisions, or other appropriate groupings. In many hospitals, the controlling and coordinating functions of management, based on the kinds of statistics and reports used, have not kept pace with the growth in the complexity of the organizational structure.

Historically, hospitals have faced a chronic problem of underfinancing. Dollars spent on activities for other than direct patient care have been grudgingly provided. As a result, the reporting system in many hospitals is inadequate, not solely with regard to service departments. As hospital costs continue to rise and the organization becomes more complex, greater attention and allocation of dollars will, of necessity, have to be provided for reporting purposes.

Figure 28–1 Statistics and the Complexity of Organization

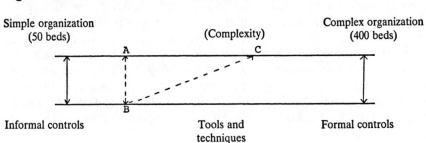

The challenge is the development of objective standards of work performance for personnel, of reports that accurately reflect the volume of departmental activity, and measurements of efficiency that fairly evaluate the department and thereby the managerial skills.

Personnel Cost Containment

Cost containment has to be a major consideration for hospitals in the years to come. The escalating costs of hospital services emphasize the need for health care administrators to initiate controls on the rapid inflation of costs. Certainly, many of the variables affecting higher costs are necessary and beneficial to the health of the population. New technology, equipment, and medical innovations are all costly but necessary in the evolving health care environment.

Some costs are unnecessary. They represent sacrifices to efficiency in order to generate effectiveness, with the incorrect assumption that efficiency and effectiveness are counterbalancing concepts (when one is increased, or decreased, there is a directly opposite reaction by the other).

All too often arguments that oppose measures instituted to create efficiencies center around the sacrificial nature of cost reduction programs as in the following: (1) "Reductions in staffing automatically decrease operational effectiveness"; or (2)"The quality of patient care will decrease if staffing is reduced."

At one time or another, most administrators have heard these arguments and found themselves unable to refute their validity completely. Usually the defense consists of "let's give it a try and see what happens." This does not persuade department directors who are convinced of the negative effects of personnel reductions. Ideally, the decision to institute personnel controls should be based on sound criteria and with a relatively clear view of the expected results. Better yet, a system should be adopted that requires the attention and participation of department directors so they can become better managers by participating directly in the operational review of the department.

Manpower cost containment in hospitals is often cited for the growing use of management engineering techniques in hospitals. The initial consideration for the implementation of personnel control activities certainly should be one of cost control with costs related to staffing being a primary candidate for review and analysis.

THE BUDGET AS A TOOL FOR CONTROL

Once a budget has been adopted, it can ensure a systematic and orderly manner of effecting change. The effectiveness of the budget, however, depends to a great extent on the respect with which it is held by management. If the chief executive officer and key executives ignore the budget during the fiscal year, the inevitable results. The budget will be ignored by the rest of the organization as well.

Measures Performance

For example, if a new position is created and the funds required for staffing it are not shown on the budget, the impression is created that the budget is not being regarded as a measurement device of performance. Discussions concerning changes in line items in the budget should always be confirmed by memo so that a formal record is available for reference at a future date. A budget, once approved, is a contract between the departments and administration that says in effect: "Department director, you have x dollars to spend for the coming year. With these dollars you are expected to provide Y units of service or of production, and to maintain, as a minimum, the quality of the units produced in the present fiscal period. Further, as the head of this department, your performance as an individual will be gauged by how well you live with this contractual relationship. In the event some unanticipated activity arises during the course of the budget year, the management reserves the right to renegotiate this contract." With this implied understanding, a base line is established that permits a realistic, objective evaluation of performance.

Prevents Organizational Inefficiency

The approach just outlined rests on the assumption that both parties to the contract—administration and the departments—will act in a logical, objective manner when dealing with problems of the organization. Unfortunately, this may not be the case. Top management may quickly approve a new activity or an expansion of present activities but may be unwilling to discuss providing additional resources with which to meet the new objectives. The initiator of the proposal may then be in a quandary; the project is agreed to, but the wherewithal is lacking. To go back to management may result in a reversal of the hard-won decision.

Other equally distasteful results may occur. Management may infer that subordinates are not trusted, which, although it may be true, is not a position that is usually a suitable stand for a subordinate, or the initiator of the change may discover that this new project has been added to the program for which he is held accountable and that he is expected to accomplish it with present resources. To do so may be an admission to management that he has been operating in an inefficient manner. Frequently, the result of this kind of decision-no-decision process is that subordinates become wary of management and tend to shy away from suggesting any change that requires the allocation of additional resources. When followed by management, this technique eventually results in a loss of organizational effectiveness. A formal budget, realistically developed and employed, is useful in preventing this form of organizational buncombe.

Fosters Objectivity

The countering of nonlogical viewpoints is a skill that can be acquired. Subjectivity is a luxury that must be avoided by management in favor of utilizing as objective an approach to the organization as can be made possible. The budget is one such method that contributes to this end.

Ensures Organizational Thrust

When persons in an organization become adept at using a budget, which may require three to five years for those with no previous experience, it becomes possible to achieve a greater follow through on the implementation of new projects and programs. Departmental personnel will recognize that when additional funds are provided, they will be called upon to answer for any deficiencies that may occur between budgeted goals and actual achievements. The threat of this accounting provides a continuing spur to keep an eye on the progress of the new program. This, in itself, is one way of ensuring organizational thrust.

Measures Achievement

The achievement of budgeted goals of performance within allocated funds is a basis for providing recognition if taken advantage of by management. The administration should be willing to reward more amply those persons who meet goals than those persons who do not meet them. This requires managerial courage to reward and penalize performance in accordance with the degree to which each responsible person has contributed to meeting the objectives of the institution. Weak administrators will back away from making such judgments. The extent to which they engage in this backsliding is the degree to which the organization will fail to meet its potential. The budget provides a tool for making such measurements possible. The courage to use it in this manner will vary in direct proportion to the firmness of mind of administration.

Program Planning

The heart of budgeting is program planning. Dollars are attached as the last step in this process. When a new activity is contemplated, serious attention should be focused on attempting to determine realistically the amount of units of service or production that are anticipated. The time span should be projected on both a short-range and a long-range basis. This long-range estimate should be made in order to determine the ultimate effect on the total program and space allocations of the institution. The short-range estimate should be subdivided into steps, and estimates should be made for each step. Personnel required, space needed, and the translation of these into dollar amounts of expense and income provide guideposts to the development of the program. Such a breakdown into short periods of time permits corrective action to be taken rapidly when there is failure to achieve the estimates that have been projected.

Before any new activity is undertaken, consideration should be given to the formal reports that will be made to management at periodic intervals. Frequently, no thought is given to this need at the time a project is initiated. In order for management to exercise control, it must have reports that clearly reflect both the quality and quantity of usage. By neglecting this phase of planning, management openly invites a lack of attention to the project. By insisting on a report, the feeling is imparted to the responsible department that management is going to watch closely for results.

Strengthens Emotional Maturity

The budget is an excellent device for management to use in strengthening the emotional maturity of departmental directors. It provides a framework for critical analysis of problems by subordinates and, in so doing, permits associates to stand up to managers with differing opinions. This will force managers to examine their decisions to see if they were made because of bias or if enough facts were present to support the decision. The budget assists in developing the ability to think logically and objectively, placing all factors in proper perspective. Without it, executives and department directors are not inhibited from wearing their emotions on their coat sleeves.

A Tool to Create Interest

The use of a budget is an art. In the hands of a skillful administrator it can be used to create interest and a willingness to accept challenge by subordinates. The stimulations and satisfactions of work come from meeting new problems, conquering them, and, in the process, acquiring new skills and understandings. This willingness to accept challenge is a characteristic of a vigorous, dynamic organization. When personnel are imbued with this spirit, organizational change presents no difficulty.

Vehicle to Measure Error

The budget permits managers to maintain a clinical interest in organizational problems. Thus, in any discussion between managers and subordinates, by citing the budget, managers can show that they are concerned with reaching organizational goals, not in affixing blame. Both parties can concentrate on examining the prior estimates made in compiling the budget in order to determine where honest errors of judgment were made, rather than upon defending present positions.

BUDGET MISUSE

While the budgeting process can provide an orderly and systematic way of effecting change and assist in maintaining organizational thrust, it can also be misused. Because it provides a frame of reference for decision making, it offers a tempting avenue for those persons in the organization who are responsible for compiling financial information to insert themselves into the line organization. Since many changes that are proposed require additional funds, comptrollers may review the merits of the proposal rather than restricting themselves to recommendations concerning financing. When top management fails to prevent this, there may be a "drying-up" of worthwhile ideas coming from the various departments to management. No one will deny the necessity for carefully scrutinizing the financing of any project, but this alone is not a satisfactory appraisal. Other factors must also be taken into account, and these lie beyond the organizational competence of the financial personnel. These must remain between the department involved and the administration; they are line decisions.

"No Funds Available"

The financial arm of an organization may, upon occasion, be unfairly criticized by others in the organization because of a tactic that is frequently used by management to forestall accepting or rejecting a proposal or a new activity. To delay making a decision, the administration may inform the initiator of the project that it is a good idea, but that there are no funds available in the immediate future for this purpose. Since there are, in nearly all situations, at least some elements of truth in this statement, the administration unduly emphasizes it in order to avoid saying no. Thus, without knowing it, comptrollers find themselves taking the blame in the organization and regarded by others as being a proponent of the status quo.

"The Budget Has Already Been Approved"

Another tactic sometimes used to "stall" a decision is for management to take the position that nothing can be done for the current fiscal period since the budget has been approved and is in operation. Such a statement implies that administration is a slave to a tool of management. In fact, the budget is no longer a tool; it has become the major objective of the enterprise. Under such circumstances, the message to departments comes through clearly: changes in the ongoing pattern of activities are not looked upon with favor.

Other Abuses

There are other abuses of the budget that could be cited. To do so is unnecessary since the purpose of listing a few of the hazards is to highlight the fact that it is a tool that must be used with discretion. The budget is only one of a number of managerial tools and techniques used by skilled executives. Effectiveness can be enhanced and goals more readily achieved in those organizations that attack their problems in a systematic manner.

The lack of a formal budget in an institution does not mean that the enterprise will fail. It does mean that personnel will be required to solve problems primarily from an expediency base, and may, because of this, make more errors in judgment than are made in comparable organizations that have a well-developed, orderly manner of planning the utilization of resources.

Organizational change goes on continuously in any form of enterprise. Management cannot prevent its occurrence. It can speed up change or impede it. It can give direction to change or permit it to transpire without guidance. Good judgment dictates that management should rely on those mechanisms that assure the enterprise of the greatest chances of realizing its objectives. The use of a formal budget is a major factor in effecting organizational change that contributes toward this end.

A GOAL WORTH ACHIEVING

Like all other American industries, hospitals can be more efficient. The use of industrial engineers in them is now recognized and growing. However, the opportunities for cost reductions are not nearly as great as one might believe when listening to the stories about hospital inefficiencies. It is rare to find a hospital where reductions in excess of 15 percent can be made in operating costs.

When management engineering approaches are applied to a hospital to improve its efficiency and it is possible to come away with 10 percent savings on operating costs, and if these savings are applied to construction projects, 15 percent savings can be realized. Usually much of these savings will be reinvested in the interest of improving patient care, so that the 10 percent may become two percent or even zero, and the 15 percent becomes something less. This represents the world of reality, not the myths currently surrounding the hospital system. The obligation to improve patient care dominates, but maximizing productivity is also a goal worth achieving.

Chapter 29

Elements of an Internal Management Audit

An internal management audit is a sound way either to locate the loose ends in the organization or to find out that it is afloat without a helmsman. Typically, the loose ends in the operation of a group are of greater concern to its individual members than major issues.

Little problems are daily annoyances, such as charts not being available on time, instruments that don't work, unbalanced workloads, and the hundred odd issues that can make the workday a nightmare. The big problems are not as imperative to individuals since they have to get through the day first, and then they may be too frustrated or tired to want to think about the major issues ahead. Further than that, the solution to big problems may tear apart physician relationships or let the powers that be know that everything is not as they think it is.

An internal management audit at its heart is criticism. Thoughtful people do not take easily to the use of this kind of organizational tool. Improperly applied, it can be destructive, even though it was meant to be helpful.

The real thrust for an internal management audit is seriously seeking to evaluate performance from top to bottom. It means that a hard look must be taken at the chiefs as well as the indians. It is not an exercise to find convenient scapegoats; to improve efficiency only among nursing, clerical workers, and junior physicians; and to allow the top dogs to go along as they choose. If an audit is to be useful optionally, without a backfire, top to bottom in the organization must be included.

Reprinted with changes from "What are the Elements of a Good Internal Management Audit?" by Everett A. Johnson in *Medical Group Management* with permission of Medical Group Management Association, © 1978.

There are basically two ways to do an internal management audit: (a) instruct an internal organizational member to do the audit, or (b) spend some money and bring in an outsider. There are no comparisons in results between the two ways.

The internally staffed audit knows the existing relationships in the group and the limits of their willingness to accept either indirect or direct criticism. There is the further problem that they know the trees, but may have difficulty in seeing the forest. Beyond these problems there is the issue that the report may be biased because of personal opinion and less than forthright because reprisal can be directly applied. All of these reasons argue that only an externally performed audit will accomplish the purposes for which an internal management audit is undertaken.

HOW DOES AN INTERNAL MANAGEMENT AUDIT WORK?

Given these caveats about an audit, how does an internal management audit work? There is a generally accepted way of doing an audit in any organization, whether it is commercial, industrial, or medical.

Establish the Purpose of the Organization

The starting point of all internal audits is to ask a direct, but often overlooked question: What is the purpose for operating the organization? In other words, what are its goals and objectives?

Frequently, when this question is raised with presidents, they simply reach for the corporate bylaws and read its purpose clause. This leaves the auditor no place, since the clause was generally written by a lawyer, perhaps a dozen or more years ago, to fulfill a legal requirement of the state for incorporation.

The question implies a much deeper issue, the major purpose.

- Is it to provide primary care medical services to a specific population or geographic area?

- Is it to provide primary and secondary medical services to a defined population or areas? What percentage of effort goes into each activity?

- Is it to be a single specialty group for a certain area?

- Is it to be a group of compatible physicians who really have not defined a specific objective?

These questions raise issues that are often ducked by the board of directors. By not facing them, life can continue as it is, and no planning or evaluation of present performance is necessary. In effect, the hard decisions about what is being done and where it is going are postponed. Unfortunately, that is no way to run a railroad, and that is why the railroads are in their present strait; no one wants to understand or face the effects of jet planes, trucks, and automobiles.

Likewise, with medical care, board members must be sensitive to changing patterns, forms of organization, technology, and public expectations.

Goals and Objectives

A statement of goals should be meaningful. It should state what part of a community is to be served and in what medical ways. How often has a wave of enthusiasm swept through a group of professionals who wish to offer new services that will cost a substantial sum of money to set up the instrumentation and train the necessary personnel, without even a sideward glance at the risks and demands on the existing organization? Too often the new service is bought on the basis of it being better medical practice or because a new intellectual challenge is needed around the shop.

A careful examination of goals and objectives not only establishes a standard by which current performance can be measured, but it can be used as a stimulus to open up new programs of service in different organizational forms that would not have otherwise been considered. But the point really is, by doing an audit there is an organized way for risks and benefits to be assessed objectively and the *raison d'être* has been established before a costly mistake has been made.

When the goals of an organization are reviewed, the topics of concern are organizational goals, not individual goals. Both must be compatible for success; nevertheless, individual goals do not override group goals. Individual goals must be considered in the establishment of corporate goals, but accommodation can only go so far. If individual goals predominate, then it might as well be acknowledged that the purpose of the group is to serve one or more individual's goals and that the effectiveness and efficiency of the group is secondary to this objective.

Objectives are a suborder of decisions that relate to group goals. In effect, objectives establish targets and dates to take specific steps that lead to fulfilling the goals. In essence, they are tactical steps to implement strategic decisions.

For example, if a medical group has a goal of providing comprehensive primary medical care to a defined geographic area and has only one obstetrician, while national norms indicate that the population of the area being served requires a total of three obstetricians, then an objective of the group would be to add two obstetricians to the group within the next year.

Examine Planning Activities

Once the goals and objectives have been clearly defined, the next step is an examination of its planning activities. The questions in an outsider's mind are:

- How systematic is planning work being done?
- What documents support its planning function?
- Does the group systematically pursue its plan?
- Are all elements covered in their plan?
- How well does their planning program mesh with their established goals and objectives?

The issue today is no longer whether to plan or not to plan. With the current rate of change, not to plan is to court ultimate disaster. The real issue is only that of "how to plan."

The Master Plan

A reasonable master plan should include a definition of the service area that the group has decided to serve. The demographics of the population, such as ages, sexes, levels of education, incomes, and future population projections for a reasonable period, should be in the plan.

With basic past, present, and future population data available, there should also be an inventory of available manpower within the service area. How many physicians by age and specialization are there, and what are the physician to population ratios for each grouping? This data should then be projected to determine the number of physicians needed for medical care by specialty and the surplus or deficit in physician personnel.

Beyond this data, there is another set of issues that needs to be spelled out to relate facilities, personnel, relationships to other medical practices, and financing. The following issues raise questions about the marketing strategies.

- What share of the total medical market does the health care facility serve, and why?

- In terms of objectives, will its share of the market increase or decrease in the next five- and ten-year periods?

- Are satellite facilities a future program?

- How will national health insurance and other foreseeable insurance and social welfare programs affect the share of the market?

- What type of public image is desirable?

- What will be the financial results of its marketing strategy for the next three years?

Community Attitudes

Frequently ignored are external issues that may have serious effects on internal operations. That is, the effect of the relationship of the facility to the community is ignored. A group of physicians, even when few in number, has a disproportionally high visibility in its community. What people think has indirect, but real impact on the facility's operation. Public attitudes are reflected by the ease or difficulty in hiring unskilled employees, the amount of vandalism in its facilities, the attraction of new patients, the degree of difficulty in recruiting new physicians, assistance from government agencies when needed, the number and amount of malpractice claims, and a host of other incidental events.

These community attitudes come out in two ways during a management audit. The obvious way is, of course, by conducting interviews in the community, with its leadership, the press, and patients. Internally, it is easily picked up through private interviews with employees and staff members.

The meaningful interrelationship between the outside world and the facility is at the governing authority level. It is their responsibility to lead the organization within the constraints and opportunities of the larger world around them.

Examining Corporate Records

A management audit undertakes this next phase of the job by initially looking at the records of the corporation. What meetings are held, how often, who attends, what decisions are reached in what amount of time, and what is the quality of these decisions? Other questions in the mind of the auditor are: (a) what committees are in use; (b) do they stay within their area of responsibility; (c) how are committee chairmen selected; (d) what is the tenure of membership on the committee; and (e) do committee members deal with substantive matters in their area of committee responsibility?

Later on, as the audit progresses, the committee and board of directors' decisions are traced out in the organization at the department level to determine to what degree and how well these policy decisions were executed. An eye is also kept on the committee activities audited to determine the quality of work going into reports that are prepared for a committee discussion.

Properly organized facilities, like other complex forms of corporations, require chief executives who are responsible for operations and accountable to their governing authority. At this level, coordination of major functions is a prime responsibility. As such, chief executives' scope of authority should extend over all functions, including those necessary to assure the quality of medical care. Unfortunately, it is not often seen that way in a large organization by the physicians.

Physician Appraisal

Too often, medical responsibility is interpreted to mean that the entire physician staff is accountable for the quality of medical care. While it is clear that physicians have a direct responsibility for the care of their patients and must have the authority necessary to direct the diagnosis and treatment, the way in which accountability is maintained is through the organization structure of the facility.

One of the audit elements for the governing authority is a check on quality control measures in use for medical practice. In the present climate of watching the medical halo becoming burnished, any reasonable-sized institution already has, or soon will have, a need to demonstrate to outside agencies that they carefully and periodically evaluate the competence with which an individual physician exercises clinical judgment. The key words are "to demonstrate," and this means written review of records.

There are three elements involved in the performance appraisal of physicians:

1. an evaluation of their clinical capabilities for rendering medical care;
2. a review of their improvement in professional knowledge and skill within a defined period of time;
3. an evaluation by their department heads of their administrative performance as a part of the group.

Administrative Principles

Once these steps are reviewed by the management audit, a more typical path lies ahead. These steps arise out of a series of administrative principles that must be followed if the organization is to be both effective and efficient. These principles are as follows:

- The governing authority should carry out its corporate responsibility for all activities related to the achievement of its corporate goals and objectives, which include all elements of medical care rendered under its auspices.

- To discharge its corporate responsibilities, the governing authority should organize all elements of the organization in such a way that accountability is maintained throughout the structure. This means that (a) specific functions are assigned to each organizational component and that appropriate delegations of authority are commensurate with the responsibilities assigned; (b) all delegations of responsibility and authority are clear-cut, without overlaps, gaps, or duplication; and (c) the assignment of functions and the delegation of authorities is contingent upon evaluation of performance and modes of accountability and may, as a result, be changed or even revoked.

- Final approval and adoption of all policies, including those of medical care are the responsibility of the governing authority.

- The function of the governing authority is deliberate in nature; therefore, the governing authority should appoint a chief executive who is responsible for the operations and accountable to the governing authority. This means that (a) the chief executive, as the operating head of the organization, is responsible for all functions, including those necessary to assure the quality of medical care; and (b) the governing authority, in consultation with the chief executive and medical chairperson, should appoint the clinical chairperson.

Examine Organization Functions

The management audit within this framework then examines the functions of planning, organizing, supervision, control systems, information flow, cost controls, and productivity.

One of the easiest ways to carry out these tasks is to examine the internal information records. What kinds of clinical, financial, and administrative records are kept on a regular basis? By sitting down with each clinical chairperson and each department director, and reviewing each reporting form used in its functioning, a reasonable approximation of the other elements of the organization can be made. There are almost an endless variety of issues that might be examined. However, it is more useful to look at major activities, either by dollars involved or clinical importance.

The Weakest Link

At this level in the organization, it would be pleasant to find a coherent, articulated management system in effect. This is seldom the case. A common experience is to find bits and pieces developed within subdepartmental systems, but rarely coordinated into a total system.

An example of this is a detailed, well-thought-out patient appointment system, but a medical records system that is continually failing to have a patient's medical record at the right point at the right time. Another example is a laboratory or x-ray requisitioning system that promptly delivers the requisition, but the final report wanders around the organization for prolonged periods of time before reaching the attending physician.

The auditor will more frequently identify problems developing in functions that overlap two or more departments than in activities that take place totally within one department. Coordination of interdepartmental work is typically the weakest link in any organization. The more cavalier the approach, the greater the lack of effective coordination throughout the organization.

Parts of the organization may be tightly controlled because of the manager's tastes and drives, while other parts may look like a Chinese puzzle.

Reporting Systems

An organization or corporation exists to direct its resources toward the accomplishment of specific objectives, whether they are written or implied. Consequently, the reporting systems of the organization are similar to the nervous system of the body. They are a tool for notifying the top about what is going on throughout the organization, when, and where. If the system is not tracking the major activities in an organized fashion, programs will gradually get out of balance.

A usual experience of this type of problem is the "that's my turf syndrome." Translated, it means that managers and physicians practice eminent domain over a definable square foot area within the facility. If they aren't there to use the space profitably, it will sit there unused until they desire to put it to use. If some type of productivity statistics and standards were routinely collected and evaluated, the expense of this attitude and how much it takes out of the total hides of all would soon become a major issue, that is, if the organization could stand the shock wave that this type of data collection produces.

A well-thought-out management audit often points up the 'fact that a well-developed management information system would bring together on a regular basis meaningful measurements about how well the institution is using its resources of manpower, money, equipment, and buildings. By generating output statistics, reporting both volumes and quality of services being produced, it can be related to the input required. By the use of simple comparative ratios of inputs to outputs, measures of effectiveness and efficiency are easily come by.

Patient, Physician, and Staff Satisfaction

Since a health care enterprise is a service operation, three groups of people must be satisfied if success is to be achieved. Obviously, patients are a major concern. If their dissatisfaction is rising for a prolonged period of time, it will eventually affect the monthly revenue statement. If physicians or staff members have increasing levels of dissatisfaction, the expense statement will sooner or later reflect this attitude, as expenses increase without a satisfactory explanatory reason. Too often the rise in clerical costs may be explained away on the basis of increased employee turnover or a necessity to raise salaries higher than expected to attract new personnel. These explanations are, in fact, symptoms of more fundamental dissatisfactions that are showing up in these particular ways. A well-worked-out management system would identify such problems long before they hit the revenue and expense statement, and corrective action would be started before monthly net profits drop into the bargain basement.

THE ULTIMATE GOAL OF AN AUDIT

Obviously, every operational problem faced on a day-to-day basis is a potential for inclusion in an internal management audit. However, that is not the ultimate goal of an audit. The audit is aimed at sorting out and identifying the good from the not-so-good, in order to achieve the goal of delivering quality medical care in a reasonably efficient and effective manner. How the job gets done is less important than getting the job done. Every organization in existence has a style of its own, but the fundamental issue is: "What is the organization accomplishing?"

It is one thing to see the number of laboratory procedures per patient visit increasing, and quite another to decide to what extent the increase is medically justifiable. Quality and quantity issues are inevitably intertwined in the operation of an institution. What is desirable on the one hand may be an anathema on the other hand. Fortunately, they sometimes go hand-in-hand, and those are the days when management looks like it might be worth a try for another day.

In reviewing the elements of an audit, the focus has been on certain activities that may be beyond the scope of the usual thinking about audits. Deliberately omitted is the spelling out in any detail of the nuts and bolts of exactly what should be reviewed, what specific data might be useful, and what kinds of audit reports should be prepared. Productivity could have been discussed, the effects of financial incentives, distribution of workloads, unit supply costs, personnel practices, overhead costs, and the other numerous ways of measuring an operation. These questions are part and parcel of an internal management audit.

Their fundamental importance, however, is within the framework of responsibility and accountability that has been defined. All parts of an organization find their real importance only in juxtaposition to the other parts of the organization. Good auditing procedures, therefore, establish a method for reviewing the activities of an organization within a logical framework that traces out the systems of accountability and responsibility. Each question that is raised in the audit is there because it ties one more piece of the operation into the overall control mechanism.

Perhaps there is a feeling that each health care institution is uniquely different than other organizations because of the administrative difficulties created by the individualism of physicians. Before finally arriving at that conclusion, let's look at the real world.

The primary mission of an institution is to provide medical services to people. When physicians join a staff they implicitly and explicitly agree to accept the goals of the organization and the governing authority's right to direct the organization in its accomplishments. This means that a physician member must deliver medical services within the organizational limits of the structure. If this were not the case, there would be no need for an organization. The setting of priorities by a governing authority means that individuals do not have the prerogative to claim unilaterally a separate set of priorities in goals. Each person is committed to the priorities and agreements that have been negotiated at a higher level.

Of course, the real world issue in daily life is not who has a right to establish goals and priorities, but whether those in the authority positions will act when organizational limits are exceeded. Both activities take nerve. An internal audit will help to identify the consequences of not blowing the whistle when it should have been blown. An audit will summarize the scope and depth of damage done over a period of time when there has been a failure to act appropriately within the organizaton.

THE IMPACT OF AN AUDIT

Too often, the day-to-day ignoring of organizational limits is forgiven on a rationalized basis that looks at each issue separately and never stops to add up its cumulative effects. This is one of the hazards of a management audit. The final audit report will bring to a head the problems that are continually swept under the rug by *ad hoc* management and will present a strong rationale for taking corrective action.

This is one way of saying that an internal management audit is at best a useless procedure and at worst a dangerous tool to use in an organization if administrators are not committed to following through and implementing its recommendations.

An audit by itself can be dangerous to an organization because the mere act of interviewing key people and asking meaningful questions can detonate hidden feelings of insecurity and animosity. The result may not appear on the surface to have been caused by the audit, since skilled incompetents, who are good infighters in organizations, are smart enough to mask their real concerns by raising a whole series of peripheral issues. In other words, if enough sand is heaved into the machinery, it can grind to a halt.

At best, an audit report that rests on the chief's desk for weeks on end will create a sense of insecurity in the organization. The whole outfit knows that something out of the ordinary has taken place, and they are waiting for the other shoe to drop. There is no point in needlessly generating feelings of insecurity. Better to leave well enough alone and continue to go about business than stir-up the organization with fears that lead nowhere.

A management audit will not solve problems because it is an organizational tool that identifies less than optimal performance. The final report may suggest that, for the well-being of the institution, certain problems be worked on, but the audit will not tell administration how to get the job done. A good audit and a well-intentioned drive to achieve improvement in performance are not sufficient to optimize organizational effectiveness if the leadership is inept. If leadership cannot cope with the findings of the audit, it is better to forego an audit than to invite the chaos and difficulties that follow an audit when there is a left-footed general.

These observations add up to the fact that for an audit to be successful, the organization must be prepared ahead of time for it, and there must be competent leadership to undertake the changes that will ensue. To spring an audit unannounced is to invite total failure. People need to know the purposes and procedures involved in an audit and why it is necessary at this time. They need to have time to prepare for the audit.

One of the values of a proposed audit is the fact that it provides an incentive to deal with problems that have been hanging around the organization for a long time because there was no initiative to work on them. It is naive to undertake an unannounced audit to find out what really is going on in the organization. If administrators do not already know, then their existing information system is inadequate, and they have missed an opportunity to motivate their organization to better performance.

The purpose of an audit is not to trap people in their inadequacies, but to provide a stimulus to try to do better and to extend a helping hand in doing so. It is not a device to get rid of the incompetent; that is a regular, ongoing responsibility of any healthy organization.

Competent outsiders doing an internal management audit will walk away from the study if they believe that its major objective is to get rid of "old Joe." It is a total organizational tool for improving performance through appraisal. To that end, it is a useful technique, if appropriately applied.

If administrators want to evaluate the effectiveness and efficiency of their operations and have the motivation and security to help make changes, then they should consider the use of an internal management audit. They should be prepared to find out, as the great pitcher Sachel Paige used to say, "that it will jiggle your mental juices."

Chapter 30

Effect of the Labor Movement on the Hospital Pharmacist

Hospital pharmacists are strange animals. They are a minority among their peers in pharmacy, where they are vastly outnumbered by their colleagues in retail pharmacy. In the hospital they are also in the minority, being only a handful amidst a host of other professions and technical personnel. If numbers are important, their clout does not count. Yet in spite of their numerical disadvantage, they have two attributes in their favor: they deal regularly and routinely with the full range of the medical staff, and their department is a profit center that makes substantial contributions to the financial well-being of the institution, a significant factor in the game of "let's squeeze the hospital" that is now being played by the third party payors.

Given this set of circumstances, is the hospital pharmacist better off participating in the labor movement or remaining outside of it? Are there any other groups that can be examined that will benefit pharmacists in determining the answer to this question?

LABOR MOVEMENTS IN HOSPITALS

The labor movement, which was in the doldrums for a decade or more, has come to life with the passage of federal legislation removing the exemption of hospitals. In effect, Congress has said that hospitals are no longer different from other forms of enterprise, be they profit or nonprofit. In *Fisher B. Sibley Memorial Hospital*,[1] handed down by Judge Gerhart Gesell in a federal court in the District of Columbia, this same thread of thought was followed holding that trustees are bound by the rules of conduct of corporate board members, not of true trustees. The public's attitude is clear; hospitals are going to have to accept the fact that they are going to be held legally to the same standards as other corporations, including those that relate to collective bargaining. Even if the legal hurdles no longer exist, social attitudes may still be negative.

The occasional strikes of interns and residents that have taken place indicate that young physicians see advantages to collective bargaining through unions. Among physicians they no longer stand alone, many older physicians are examining joining a union as a means of protecting themselves from the encroachment of third party payors and the federal government.

For a number of years, the American Nurses Association (ANA) has favored collective bargaining for its membership. In the San Francisco Bay area and in the twin cities of Minnesota, there is a long history of negotiations between hospital management and nursing staffs.

Within the pharmacy profession itself, there is a track record of negotiations between retail drug chains and their professional employees. Social attitudes as well as legal positions have shifted. Stated from a slightly different perspective, the environment now favors an aggressive union program to enroll professional and technical personnel in hospitals.

THE FUTURE FOR HOSPITAL UNIONS

Strength in Numbers

The future, however, will be different from the past in some respects. The ground rules that have been pragmatically worked out through the turbulent labor-management negotiations and arbitration history will be found to be lacking when applied to a professional group. A new dimension will be added when the classic model is varied. This professional movement is not the classic work clothes versus vest and suit, the less well educated versus the college graduate, the hourly paid versus the salaried executive, the monotonous job routine versus the variety of work experiences, or the loud racket of machinery at work versus the quiet serenity of a well-furnished office.

In spite of these differences that result in an imperfect fit in labor history, there are subtle similarities that will lead hospital pharmacists to joining unions. Pharmacists, like their predecessors in the labor movement, recognize there is strength through numbers. They believe that formal negotiations over salaries and fringe benefits lead to better results than individual salary increases. They are aware that a staff pharmacist is an identical position in most hospitals.

Professions

Despite the similarities and the differences, there is a third dimension for professionals, their profession. This will cause difficulty in the years ahead and is going to become a headache for the National Labor Relations Board (NLRB). The NLRB has defined broad bargaining units for hospitals with the intent of avoiding proliferation of bargaining units in institutions, which is in keeping with the intent of Congress. The NLRB has found that a bargaining unit composed entirely of registered nurses (RNs) is appropriate. Likewise, service and maintenance employees constitute an appropriate bargaining unit, which also includes ward clerks and other clerical personnel not part of the business office. On technical employees, the board held it appropriate to have all technical employees except licensed practical nurses (LPNs) in the same unit. At the state level, the New York labor board found five units appropriate, RNs, LPNs, clerical, technical, and service and maintenance employees. The residual group, all other professionals, were excluded in New York, though the NLRB uses this catch-all category. However, it is not clear where interns and residents belong.

As the lexicon of labor jargon is applied to hospitals, problems arise. Where pharmacists have received a special type of education at the collegiate level and have passed state examinations to qualify to practice their profession, it is difficult to believe that a substantial case cannot be made for their being treated separately, as are the RNs. The only difference seems to be that there are many more nurses than pharmacists in a hospital.

As the NLRB gets it feet wet in the health field, it is going to have to come to grips with the fact that pharmacists are different from physical therapists, who are different from clinical laboratory technicians, who are different from inhalation therapists. Even within nursing the NLRB will eventually have to recognize the differences between emergency room nurses, special care unit nurses, operating room nurses, psychiatric nurses, and floor duty nurses. All in all the advent of the professional in the ranks of labor is going to force much rethinking about the collective bargaining process.

Direct Bearing on Patients

In the face of this complexity, still another aspect will need to be dealt with that traditionally has not been a factor in labor-management relationships. Hospital professionals, for example, pharmacists, have a direct bearing on a patient. They can, in an unthinking moment, create a major liability for a hospital. As the experts on drugs, it is part of pharmacists' professional responsibilities not only to see that all prescriptions are accurately filled, but that inappropriate dosages are not permitted to be given to patients. Where this kind of responsibility fits into the labor-management scheme of things is probably not yet settled, but there will come a time when it will become a major point of discussion in NLRB considerations. Not only does case law define a hospital's responsibility for patient care, but it may include inappropriate acts by professional employees. How is this kind of responsibility going to be taken into account in the collective bargaining setting? Does this type of consideration put the pharmacist on the side of management, on the side of labor, or in some other frame of reference?

Salaries

In those states where hospital rate review commissions have been established or where prospective rates are in force, there is an added incentive for all personnel to participate in a union. In attempting to control hospital costs, these agencies are prone to determine what is "reasonable" cost. As part of having to deal with an inflationary economy, they are aware that next year's salaries will be higher than the current year's. Since their objective is keep the lid on hospital costs, they may be tempted to fudge on the amount of inflation that can be included in salary increases. Since hospitals receive the majority of their revenues from cost reimbursement formulas, any increases in cost automatically become reimbursable. Given a guideline to go by, a hospital is likely to do all it can to stay within it, even though the hospital management may recognize that the guideline is less than the rate of inflation. In this kind of situation, unorganized employees will be less well treated than those represented by unions. In all likelihood a salary settlement as a result of collective bargaining that exceeds agency guidelines will have to be recognized as part of "reasonable cost." The fact that hospitals cannot be told to take any settlements over guidelines out of profits, since there are none under cost reimbursement, puts the agency in a tenuous position. By sticking to their guidelines, agencies would, in effect, be telling hospitals they cannot bargain in good faith with a union representing an employee group.

MAJOR AVENUES FOR PHARMACISTS

"All Other Professionals"

Assuming that hospital pharmacists decide to unionize, there appear to be two major avenues open to them at the moment, to become part of

"All Other Professionals" in the hospital or to affiliate with a local of retail pharmacists. In either case they are at a disadvantage.

As part of a mixed group of professionals, they are apt to discover that their matters of importance for negotiation are not those of the others in the group and that in effect two levels of negotiation take place. The first level will take place among the various professions represented in the group, where compromises have to be reached in order to determine the priorities for bargaining with management. The second stage will be that of the formal negotiations itself. In the course of working through the first stage, pharmacists are going to be asking themselves if they have more leverage or less leverage than others in the group. If they conclude their leverage is greater, they will be more insistent on their priorities being brought to the bargaining table. If they don't succeed in arranging the list to their satisfaction, they will be caught in the dilemma of staying in and going along, of backing out and going it alone, or of joining up with the retail pharmacists.

The Retail Group

By becoming part of the retail group, the problem of the hospital pharmacist remains: they are still only a small percentage of the total. In addition, what may be of prime concern to the retail group may only be of secondary interest or no interest at all to the hospital members. For instance, in a chain drugstore operation a matter for negotiation might be the moving of pharmacists from one store to another, hardly a matter of import to the hospital pharmacist.

The major flaw in joining such a group is that the hospital probably would not recognize the union for collective bargaining purposes. The negotiations that would occur between the retail management and pharmacists would not be binding on the hospital. The best that could be accomplished would be to take the accords reached on salaries and fringe benefits to hospital management and plead the case from the standpoint that these should be adopted by the hospital for its pharmacists if the hospital wants to remain competitive for the services of pharmacists.

The ANA Model

Some may believe the model of the American Nurses Association is a good one to follow. It is a professional group that encourages and supports collective bargaining for its members. However, it is different in one significant respect: most of its members work in hospitals. Therefore it is able to become a recognized bargaining unit. Here again the "All Other Professionals" grouping puts hospital pharmacists in a setting that precludes the ANA as a model to be emulated.

Hospital pharmacists who want a collective bargaining mechanism face a difficult situation. They are so small in numbers in any one hospital that they cannot reasonably expect to receive recognition as a bargaining unit on their own. They cannot expect recognition by the hospital as a part of a larger pharmacists group either. As part of a category of "All Other Professionals," they are in a grouping that is a mixed bag of interests, expectations, and attitudes. What then can they do?

ALTERNATIVES FOR PHARMACISTS

Professional Corporation

Several alternatives can be suggested for consideration. Taking a cue from single specialty physician groups, a professional corporation might· be formed, such as often occurs among pathologists and anesthesiologists. A contract is drawn between the two parties, the hospital and the professional corporation. From the standpoint of hospital pharmacists, this probably would have considerable appeal. The drawback to such a course is that the hospital is under no compulsion to enter into such a contract. Given the manpower supply of pharmacists, the probability is that a hospital would seek to employ other pharmacists, most likely employed in retail drugstores, rather than enter into such an agreement. Hospital pharmacists do not have the leverage enjoyed by hospital-based physicians.

Employee Association

Within the hospital organizational structure, the pharmacists might spearhead the formation of an employee association whose function is to provide a communication channel with the hospital management that goes around the hierarchical departmental structure. Such a forum could be utilized to bring up grievance matters, wages, and fringe benefits. However, an alert management is unlikely to let this kind of organization develop or be used for such purposes.

Pharmacy and Therapeutic Committee

Another avenue might be to gain the support and enroll the assistance of the pharmacy and therapeutic committee in going to bat for the hospital pharmacists. Rather than restricting this medical staff committee to drug recommendations, its purpose would have to be broadened. This approach is not too promising since it would be regarded by the hospital administrator as being one step away from blackmail.

The Management Reporting System

The remaining method is for hospital pharmacists to be sure that the management reporting system accurately, and in a timely manner, reflects the contribution of their department to the financial health of the institution. With that in place and properly functioning, an informal occasional chat can be had with administrators where they are reminded of the pertinent facts. The extent to which this approach is viable can be readily determined at budget time when salary increases are discussed.

Become an Entrepreneur

There is, of course, one other alternative: become an entrepreneur and open up a retail drugstore.

A RIGHT THAT CANNOT BE DENIED

Recognizing that none of these pathways rate an Oscar, one is left with a feeling that Don Quixote must have had when he was tilting with windmills. The opportunity to join and participate in a labor union will probably be exercised by a growing number of hospital pharmacists in the years ahead. This is a right that cannot and will not be denied.

NOTE

1. Fisher B. Sibley Memorial Hospital, 403 A.2d 1130 (D.C. App. 1969).

Chapter 31

Thinking Conceptually about Hospital Efficiency

What do critics mean by hospital inefficiency? By what criteria are they deciding what is efficient or inefficient? The chaos caused by the indiscriminate use of the concept of efficiency has made today's national hospital scene appear more like a person trying to net elusive butterflies than an organized, thoughtful concern of an industry's acceptance of responsibility, even though a voluntary cost containment program is in place.

If the hospital field-at-large is to thwart the stigma of inefficiency successfully, it will be necessary to promote a common concept of efficiency and its general acceptance.

WHAT IS HOSPITAL EFFICIENCY?

To find a working definition of hospital efficiency is difficult. More than that, it is a greater struggle to understand that such a concept applies only to the hospital as a whole and not to separate programs and departments.

The unique purpose of a hospital is to provide clinical services to patients as directed by physicians. Efficiency of the whole hospital, therefore, means developing a measure that reasonably reflects the totality of clinical services provided by a hospital to all of its patients, both inpatients and outpatients. Effectiveness is frequently interchanged carelessly with the word efficiency. Their meanings, however, are quite distinct.

Effectiveness is concerned with the degree of medical benefits patients receive from the rendering of clinical services. How the services controlled by the physician benefit the physical and mental conditions of patients is a medical judgment and does not relate to the efficiency with which a hospital delivers these services. Appropriate measures of effectiveness for a hospital as a whole would be the number of patients admitted or the amount of clinical services ordered by physicians.

317

This is an uncommon viewpoint because concepts of efficiency and effectiveness between hospitals and physicians are not commonly separated; yet each has a unique, but articulated role in medical care. Often overlooked by critics is the fact that patients contract with attending physicians and pay a fee for these services, and the physician acts as the patient's agent in ordering a hospital's clinical services. This relationship is similar to the one that exists between attorneys and clients in the courtroom.

Literature in the field of management is typically generalized and fuzzy about the meaning of efficiency. In management books several different ideas are often used to define efficiency. Some of these are:

- progress toward organizational objectives at the least possible cost
- personal efficiency in individual performance
- work output above normal expectations
- doing work right
- satisfaction of individual motives when operating jointly toward a common goal
- productivity
- reduction in unit cost of output

Cost Reduction

In the hospital field at the present time, the idea of a reduction in cost is often used two ways: (1) to mean a slowing in the rate of increase in hospital charges, such as a decrease in the annual rate of increase from 14 percent to 12 percent from one year to the next; or (2) to mean an absolute lowering of hospital charges, such as decreasing patient day charges from $300 to $275 per day.

Each of these ideas has a ring of rightness in expressing the meaning of efficiency, but they are, likewise, less than a total meaning.

The Concept of Productivity

The use of the concept of productivity as a measure of efficiency is more sophisticated than merely cost reduction. Productivity is generally used as a ratio measurement to compare inputs to outputs or as a measurement between input costs and the required productivity for a given level of output. Expenditure can be measured over time by the summing of inputs and outputs.

Productivity is, however, less than a whole concept of efficiency, except for one firm producing one product. In this situation, productivity and efficiency are identical. However, in one firm with many different outputs, productivity is meaningful for one product, while efficiency is related to the total outputs of the firm.

Two difficulties are encountered when productivity and efficiency are used as synonymous terms. One difficulty is that the input elements of capital, labor, and plant are diverse and must be reduced to a common measurement to be additive. The unit commonly used to make these elements additive is to measure each in terms of their cost or in dollars. Multiproduct or service firms, however, require a distribution of overhead dollar costs to each output to determine the total cost of one specific product or service. To accomplish this kind of distribution requires the use of reasonable but artificial rules for indirect and overhead cost distributions. Thus, there often is less or more than an equitable distribution of input costs to each item of output. In addition, the time period used can unevenly affect the distribution of these costs. Parsimonious decisions of the day often increase productivity in the short-range of a firm and sacrifice long-range productivity increases.

The other difficulty with using productivity and efficiency terms interchangeably is the difficult problem of output definition for hospitals. A diagnostic patient is a different output than a gall bladder patient, while an appendectomy in a six-year-old is different than one in a sixty-eight-year-old. The work on diagnostic related groups now being started is only a first step in developing the kind of knowledge needed to group hospital outputs into standardized units of output.

If the concept of efficiency is more than cost reduction, productivity, satisfaction of individual motives, personal efficiency, or doing work right, then what is hospital efficiency?

Definition by Example

The inherent difficulties of finding a commonly accepted definition of hospital efficiency can be visualized by contrasting two different hospitals operating in circumstances at opposite extremes in their institutional characteristics and local environment.

For example, one hospital might be a 400-bed, suburban hospital with comprehensive medical services, a physical plant that is five years old, high occupancy levels throughout the year, and no indigent patients. Professional personnel are in adequate supply, and there is an abundance of specialized physicians. Patient day charges are $300 per day, and patient day costs are $280 per day. Its annual surplus is $2 million.

The other hospital might be a 400-bed, inner-city hospital with comprehensive medical services, a 35-year-old physical plant, and an average occupancy of 60 percent. The professional staff is chronically in short supply, and the medical staff membership is steadily decreasing in numbers and increasing in age. There is a ten percent contractual allowance and bad debt write-off rate. Patient day charges are $300 per day, and patient day costs are $315 per day. The hospital is losing approximately $2 million annually because of below cost Medicaid reimbursement and caps on revenue increases.

Which hospital is more efficient or more inefficient?

Management activities in these two hospitals are quite different. The suburban hospital administration is busy planning additional programs of care, introducing new technologies into the operations, and has an expansionist frame of mind. The inner-city administration is actively retrenching programs, increasing security, jerry-rigging major repairs, juggling accounts payable, and is reductionist in thinking.

The board of trustees in the suburban hospital is busily reviewing ways to finance the next building program, buying all major capital equipment recommended by the medical staff, and increasing executive salaries to assure a stable management. The inner-city board of trustees is continually hearing complaints from the public and medical staff members, who wonder what is wrong with their chief executive officer, and resisting every effort to raise any salary, even with a high level of inflation in the economy.

The medical staff of the suburban hospital is regularly developing new recommendations for expansion of services and equipment, complaining about HSA restraints, and pleasing the PSRO with a low average length of stay. At the inner-city hospital, members of the medical staff are always threatening to transfer their appointment to other hospitals because of old equipment, outmoded facilities, inadequate nursing staff, reductions in programs of care, and are unaware of the HSA and fighting with the PSRO because of the above average length of stay.

Which hospital is more efficient in the short run and in the long run?

The way things are today, there is no way to identify quantitatively either hospital as efficient or inefficient. To compare these two hospitals a common criteria must be used to make judgments about their efficiency.

LIMITATIONS IN THE DEFINITION OF HOSPITAL EFFICIENCY

A workable application of the concept of efficiency requires a person to focus only on the organizational resources under the control of the hospital.

To achieve such a focus, three limitations must be recognized and accommodated in the definition of hospital efficiency.

A Firm with Multiple Outputs

The first limitation is a recognition that a hospital is a firm with multiple outputs and not a simple organizational entity producing one standardized product or service. A hospital provides nursing services to surgical, medical, and obstetrical patients, plus laboratory tests, operating rooms, and many other functions over a wide range of services. Each completed test and clinical procedure is an output of hospital services. Conversely, dietary services, medical records, the business office, administration, and other activities support clinical services, but not the essence of medical services to patients. The only hospital services that really count are the clinical services. Therefore, all clinical tests and procedures are part of a hospital's output.

Lack of Control of Proscriptive Medical Practice

A second limitation is the fact that hospitals do not control proscriptive medical practice, except at the outer edges, of a range of tests and procedures. The control of the number and scope of diagnostic and therapeutic measures, and their mix, is controlled by the physician and not the hospital. Therefore, the efficiency of a hospital does not encompass attending physician decisions. This means that the concept of hospital efficiency is limited to whatever type of patient is admitted and to all specific tests and clinical procedures under the control and direction of the medical staff and its members. For example, if the appropriateness of admission or length of stay is to be evaluated, it is a question of the effectiveness and efficiency of physicians, and not of hospital operation. In essence a physician is the customer, and the patient is the consumer of hospital services. It must be assumed that the customer, the physician, is always right, and if he or she is not, then the organized processes of the medical profession must deal with the problem since it is not a matter of hospital efficiency.

The Variety of Pricing Mechanisms

A third limitation arises out of the necessity to measure hospital inputs or dollar costs in different ways because a hospital uses a variety of pricing mechanisms. Hospitals set rates for services on both a specific test and clinical procedure basis, such as $17 for an anterior/posterior and lateral chest film, and also on a collective basis, such as a daily services charge of $210 for a two-bed accommodation.

As all hospital administrators know, rates charged for any particular service are adjusted annually with two criteria in mind: (1) how departmental costs have shifted since the last budget period; and (2) an estimate of the difficulty to be faced in collecting the adjusted departmental rates in the next budget period. In essence, hospitals try to maximize reimbursement and minimize difficulties in the collection of revenues.

An ultimate restraint on hospital operations is the total dollars of revenue anticipated for services provided to patients. This means that forces external to a hospital control the dollars needed for hospital operations and affect any given level and scope of service. This may appear to be an overestimate of the actual situation, but, in fact, if hospitals did not perceive any ultimate income restraint, both formal and internal hospital prices might be several times their present levels.

However, a dilemma exists. In a free market economy, a firm may be highly efficient, but if the market does not buy its output, the firm will fail. Hospital services do not face this restraint. The market need for medical services has, historically, exceeded an ability to produce and finance these services. Because of the existence of third party cost reimbursement, critics of the hospital field argue that issues of efficiency do not motivate hospital administrators.

EFFICIENCY CANNOT BE MEASURED

Lost in the debate of "yes, it does" and "no, it doesn't matter" is the understanding that hospital productivity is only measurable at the department level and that statements about its efficiency are value judgments or personal opinions, not sustainable by a rational, organized set of data.

No Methodology for Measurement

Today, efficiency is only personal opinion because the many different clinical service outputs of a hospital are not additive. The present state of knowledge provides no methodology for measuring the efficiency of a single hospital. Output measures for a physical therapy department, such as modalities per man-hour, cannot be added to nursing man-hours per patient day, plus laboratory tests per man-hour, and on and on to reach any sensible conclusion. Technologies and processes of each clinical department in a hospital are unique and nonadditive.

Levels of Quality of Service

Also ignored are issues about the levels of quality of service. Over the last 30 years, measures of quality of care in hospitals have been steadily developed by the JCAH, state boards of health, Commission on Professional and Hospital Activities, various specialty boards in medicine, and individual hospitals. Because quality of care is a most fundamental matter in hospitals and medical care is generally understood by diagnosis and treatment as well as aseptic concepts, separate and minimum acceptable standards are established by each procedure. Because quality of care is the heart of the matter, there are many vigilant enforcers in each hospital. This persistent quality of care concern is further reinforced by medical malpractice concerns, so a pursuit of efficiency, which forces quality of care below levels acceptable to either the medical or nursing staffs, will not long be tolerated. This means that every hospital is restrained in its administrative ability to lower quality standards to a much larger extent than in other industries.

On every nursing station in a hospital, be it medicine, surgery, obstetrics, pediatrics, or any other specialty service, the internists, surgeons, obstetricians, and pediatricians establish a hospital's quality level, not the administrative staff. The quality of care in all hospitals varies by the quality of its medical staff, and not by the impact of its administrative staff.

Range of Services

Concerns about the quality of hospital care are reflected not only by adherence to a variety of medically developed criteria, but also by the scope of services available in a hospital. This fact is demonstrated by an awareness among health professionals that two hospitals of the same bed size may have significantly different clinical services. One hospital may treat patients mostly at a secondary care level and have few clinical services beyond nursing services, laboratory, radiology, operating rooms, and an emergency service. Another hospital may have dialysis, several specialty intensive care units, stress and gastrointestinal laboratories, and a whole host of other special services aimed at patients needing tertiary levels of care.

These differences are frequently accommodated by reimbursement plans through categorization of hospitals by the number of clinical services operated, with each service equally counted. Such a practice is a crude method for identifying differences in hospitals, but is a step in the right direction.

No generally accepted reimbursement program has, as yet, recognized the differences inherent in specific clinical services. For example, a clinical laboratory in one hospital may routinely offer 200 different kinds of tests, while a second hospital's laboratory may offer 400 separate tests. This same situation applies to every clinical department and service operated by a hospital. To compare hospitals without identifying the total range of services routinely available in each clinical department is to count a Piper Cub and a Boeing 747 as equivalent because each one is an airplane and can fly.

Physician Freedoms

Often overlooked by critics of hospitals is the fact that attending physicians must have sufficient freedom in diagnosis and treatment decisions to use their professional judgment in the care of patients. Such legitimate freedoms mean that hospitals can control the number of tests and clinical procedures ordered by attending physicians only at the outer margins of medical care. Consequently, whatever is ordered by a medical staff should be included as an output measure for hospital efficiency purposes, which will also reflect the differences in the range of tests and procedures for every clinical department in a hospital.

Different Organizational Arrangements and Processes

Hospitals have organizational arrangements and processes that are significantly different from organizations typically used to demonstrate an accepted economic concept of efficiency, where long-run equilibrium of price through pure and perfect competition is assumed. The past practice of economists has usually been to ignore any differences and proceed with a traditional economic analysis. The hospital field has typically ignored economic analysis and concentrated on productivity analysis at the department level, on the theory that all savings are worthwhile. In both instances, efficiency opinions remain only as value judgments of the individual expressing a view.

WORKABLE CRITERIA FOR HOSPITAL EFFICIENCY

However, despite current day practice it is desirable to try to find a way of gradually moving toward a more workable criteria for hospital efficiency. At the present time, productivity measures of hospital performance cannot be added together to reach a meaningful conclusion because the units of measurement are different and therefore not additive. To the degree that different departmental units of measurement can be made additive, there will be a more accurate approximation of a measurement of hospital efficiency. If all clinical departmental unit output could be calculated in standard terms and added together, the result would be a reasonable estimate of the efficiency of a hospital.

A Common Unit of Measurement

By thinking about finding a common unit of measurement for all clinical tests and procedures through an examination of departmental productivities, it should be possible to find one. The basic ratio used to express clinical departmental productivity is outputs divided by inputs. For the total hospital, where there is a common unit of output measure for every clinical department, an approximate measure of efficiency would be:

$$\text{Hospital Efficiency} = \frac{\text{Nursing output}}{\text{Nursing input}} + \frac{\text{Lab output}}{\text{Lab input}} + \frac{\text{X-ray output}}{\text{X-ray input}} + \text{etc.}$$

By separately thinking about the various elements in each departmental numerator and denominator, it may be possible to find ways to improve present day practices.

By developing a numerator for the total hospital and a measure of departmental outputs in a standardized way, a count of the total number of physician orders for each patient can be used as an estimate of total hospital services to a given patient. This is a step in the direction of developing a total hospital measure, but it is limited by the fact that a laboratory white count has the same weight in the count as a radiological gastrointestinal series, and these are two entirely different procedures in terms of hospital resources. Furthermore, this type of measurement does not include standing orders and routine procedures in a hospital that trigger many patient services without any physician entry on the order sheet.

Because the meaningful workload of a hospital is its total output of clinical services to patients, a useful efficiency measure should include as many clinical services as possible and on a basis that reflects as many differences in resource use as are in reality consumed.

Clinical Service Units

A way to develop a unit of measurement for hospital operations, which would allow different clinical services to be additive and also measure total usage, would be to calculate an average for the number of manpower minutes needed to perform each specific clinical procedure. For example, pathologists directing hospital clinical laboratories have separated all laboratory functions into detailed, discrete items, such as specimen collecting or performing a white count, and assigned relative values to each activity. By knowing the total number of functions performed, a total output measure for laboratory services can be accurately estimated. Whether it is done automatically or by hand, the workload unit value remains the same.

The kind of approach used to estimate clinical laboratory output can also be used as a model for other professional groups to develop similar workload units. By using the lowest possible whole number—one, or multiple of one—for procedures that take longer than one minute, a series of values can be developed for each test and clinical procedure in every clinical department.

To calculate clinical service units (CSUs) for a hospital, the total CSU units of every clinical department can be obtained by multiplying the annual volume of output for each test and procedure by their estimated values and adding them together to give total CSUs for the department. For example, a laboratory white count might have a CSU value of 4, and a radiological gastrointestinal series a CSU value of 50. If there were 10,000 white counts done in a year, the CSU value would be 40,000, and for the G.I. series, where 500 procedures were completed, its CSU value would be 25,000.

The total CSUs for all hospital clinical departments could then be added together because there is a common unit of measurement, minutes of time. The total CSUs for a hospital would then be a reasonable estimate of its total clinical effort for a given period of time. Further than that, a standard unit of measure common to all hospitals would be established, and thereby would provide a basis for comparison of institutional clinical outputs between all sizes and types of hospitals.

Accumulation of this kind of data can easily be accomplished since all clinical departments routinely maintain these kinds of service statistics. By multiplying each service statistic by its CSU value, the total clinical effort could be rather closely approximated.

The one clinical service in a hospital that would require a new service statistics system would be the nursing department. However, a few hospitals are using service statistics similar to the categories of analysis used in nursing audits.

A CSU system of this kind should be focused on departments because the goal is to arrive at an estimate of total hospital clinical output. For research purposes, a CSU system could be used on a patient-by-patient basis to obtain a measure of individual service requirements or on a diagnosis-by-diagnosis basis similar to a diagnostic related grouping.

A CSU system could also help resolve the age-old problem of combining inpatient and outpatient volumes for the same test or procedure. For example, the workload value for a white count would be the same for the actual performance of the test, such as a value of four; however, the additional value of three would be added for inpatient white counts because of the need for a phlebotomist to travel from the laboratory to the patient and return. Therefore, the CSU value for an inpatient white count would be seven and for an outpatient, four.

The use of CSU values would also provide a way to account for the differences between hospitals in departmental range of services, since the hospital with a more elaborate service would generate a higher total CSU value. A hospital with a clinical laboratory offering 200 different tests might have an inpatient annual CSU volume of 4 million CSUs, while another hospital with 400 different tests, including some exotic types, might have an annual CSU volume of 9 million.

Another way to demonstrate the difference between these two different types of laboratories would be to calculate an intensity ratio for laboratory services. If each hospital annually had 10,000 inpatient admissions, the CSU values of 9 million and 4 million could be divided by 10,000, and the intensity index would be 900 for one hospital and 400 for the other hospital.

By repeating this logic for each department and then adding the CSU outputs together of all clinical departments, a total CSU for a hospital could be found. Even though the CSU value for any specific test or procedure was not quite accurate, it would still provide a general index of the clinical outputs of a hospital, because all hospitals would be applying the same CSU value to each clinical output.

The total CSUs for a hospital would be in the range of a million or multiples of a million. A 400-bed hospital would probably be 60 million to 150 million. This number could be reduced in different ways to make it easier to understand. One simple way would be to divide the total CSUs by 1,440 for minutes per 24 hours, so that the result would be average CSU units per patient day.

Efficiency Ratios

The elements used in the denominator of an efficiency ratio are the input measures for the use of capital, labor, and plant expressed as dollars for a specified period of time identical to the numerator.

The elements of inputs to be used in the denominator should be determined by the kind of efficiency index desired. Depending on the particular purpose, three different input measures might be selected: total revenue, net operating revenue, or total operating expenses.

From a third party reimbursement point of view, total revenue would be the choice for a denominator. Hospital rates charged for clinical services to patients when billed to third party carriers become a cost to the carrier and are of primary concern to them. However, hospital rates are a function of the total monies received from all third party carriers. Whenever a third party carrier, such as Medicare and Medicaid, has a reimbursement formula that covers less than total cost, plus a reasonable surplus, a hospital increases rates to other carriers to offset this below cost reimbursement and total revenue is overstated.

From a hospital perspective, net operating revenue as a denominator is a more reasonable choice. Contractual allowances and bad debts, which are deductions from total revenue, are not within the control of the hospital and are properly excluded if a concept of efficiency is to be a measure of management's judgment and skill in the use of its resources.

Another way to look at hospital efficiency would be to use total operating expenses as a denominator, which would most accurately reflect the operating judgments of management. This would be a more direct comparison of resource use to output measures. Capital expenses would be included to the extent of depreciation charges. Since the basic goal of management is to create the lowest possible cost mix between capital and labor, depreciation is properly included.

The argument would, of course, be raised that a new hospital would have much higher depreciation charges than an old hospital and would therefore have a lower efficiency. This is what would happen, but the rational economic argument would be that the departmental productivity of a new hospital would be higher and should offset the increased depreciation costs. If this does not occur, then to the extent of the difference, the new hospital is inefficient.

Total operating expenses would include all of the service and administrative functions of a hospital, because institutional efficiency is achieved by the way management rations total dollars to specific departments through the budgeting process.

Table 31–1 illustrates the application of CSUs in the measurement of hospital efficiency between the old and new 400-bed hospitals previously described.

In Table 31–1, the number 2.92 is an index of the efficiency of the old hospital and 2.64 of the new hospital. On a relative basis, the old hospital is 10.6 percent more efficient than the new hospital in the way it uses its input resources (dollars) to deliver clinical services to patients.

EFFICIENCY IS RELATIVE

No absolute scale of efficiency for hospitals can be achieved, because maximum hospital efficiency is unknown. Efficiency is therefore relative

Table 31-1 CSUs as a Measure of Hospital Efficiency

	Old hospital	New hospital
Total beds	400	400
Annual patient days	87,000 (60%)	130,000 (90%)
Annual operating expenses	$27,400,000	$36,400,000
Average CSUs per patient day	920	740
Annual hospital CSUs	80,040,000	96,200,000
	(920 × 87,000)	(740 × 130,000)
Hospital efficiency	$\dfrac{80,040,000 \text{ CSUs}}{\$27,400,000}$	$\dfrac{96,200,000 \text{ CSUs}}{\$36,400,000}$
	2.92	2.64

between hospitals. However, the efficiency number of many hospitals could be arranged in rank order, and their range and efficiencies could be related to operating conditions for new insights into management decisions and hospital characteristics that improve efficiency.

One adjustment would be required for use of any of the three suggested denominators. The economic concept of efficiency is based on an equilibrium model that assumes that the price of inputs is the same for all firms in an industry. Since this is not a real world fact, a price adjustment would be required for different regions of the country, through the use of the consumer price index, the wholesale price index, or some other appropriate index. Within the same city, in most instances, no price adjustment would be needed.

Another major use of total CSUs would be the opportunity to compute an intensity of service index for hospitals. This could be done by, as in the example, computing the average patient day CSUs by dividing either total patient days or number of admissions into total inpatient CSUs.

BENEFITS FROM AN EFFICIENCY INDEX

If the development of an overall efficiency index were to be explored and developed by the hospital field, there would be a new way to respond more clearly to persistent criticism. Hospitals would benefit in three ways from the development of an efficiency index. The first would be the separation of hospital efficiency from that of the efficiency of physician responsibilities in hospitals. Second, by focusing on the use of either net operating revenues or total operating expenses to measure inputs, the impact of below full-cost reimbursement from third party reimbursers could be highlighted and used to respond intelligently to criticism. Third, it would provide a better way to make more reasonable comparisons of efficiency between hospitals because a uniform criteria for efficiency would be used in the same way by hospitals.

Part VII

Financing Services

Chapter 32

The Specter of Bankruptcy

The regulations promulgated in wholesale lots for the past decade have reached the point where the Chairman of the Board of a large voluntary hospital in the midwest commented that, in his judgment, hospitals are now a more highly regulated industry than his own. He is President of a railroad. The providers of health care are increasingly challenging the laws and their interpretations in court. Many of the suits being filed deal with one of two primary factors; attempts either to curtail the outflow of government dollars to health care providers through the introduction of new regulations, or to block individual hospital decisions on proposed capital expenditures. Behind these two factors is the basic issue: a government that has legislated into being programs of health care benefits to citizens that it now finds it can no longer fund at the enacted programmatic level.

While it will not change the course of events, hospitals need to understand (a) why they will remain one of the favorite targets of Congress and various federal agencies and (b) that no matter how hard the hospital field strives to be responsive it is confronted with an impossible task. The culprit in the hospital-government game is the Congress, not the agencies or Department of HHS. They are the agents of the decision makers and as such are forced to live within the boundaries specified by Congressional appropriations.

The Congress, by authorizing appropriations well in excess of revenues over a sustained number of years has fueled the engine of inflation. Though hospital costs have risen drastically in the last few years, it is not due to a devil-may-care attitude among hospital people.

Reprinted with permission from *Hospitals*, published by the American Hospital Association,© March 16, 1974, Vol. 48, No. 6.

Table 32–1 reflects what has happened overall to the cost per patient day. All of this increase is not due only to inflation, but neither is it due solely to hospital mismanagement.

It should be noted that federal hospitals are exempt from the controls placed on all other hospitals. Table 32–1 suggests that federal hospitals are substantially more in need of controls than any other category. Congress approves appropriation requests for all federal hospitals and is the responsible party for permitting this to occur.

Since hospitals are a labor intensive industry, the impact of inflation has a more profound effect on them than on many other industries. Yet the public hue and cry is aimed at hospital costs that keep going higher and higher. The hospital field is opting to do battle in the wrong corner, taking on the agencies and bureaus whose basic purpose is to protect the interests of Congress.

The sustained and chronic nature of federal expenses outstripping revenues can be seen in Table 32–2.

The Congress has been reluctant to trim benefits in programs when costs rise at an unanticipated rate. It appears they regard the imposition of limits on the initial benefits of a program as a way of committing political suicide and, therefore, something to be avoided at all cost. From the standpoint of the hospital industry the result is a no-win situation. Congress has passed health legislation guaranteeing citizens certain benefits to be provided by hospitals and physicians. Yet, it later backs away from total funding of these benefits. All too often this line of reasoning is obfuscated by charging hospitals with mismanagement and needlessly broadening their comprehensiveness of service in response to physician pressure for new and im-

Table 32-1 Comparison Of Hospital Expenses Per Patient Day, 1970-1978

Year	All U.S. hospitals	Federal hospitals only	Nongovernment not-for-profit hospitals
1970	$53.95	$53.10	$74.94
1975	$118.69	$116.74	$133.31
1978	$186.49	$192.12	$195.07
Increase in $	$132.54	$139.02	$120.13
Percent increase 1970-78	246%	262%	160%

Source: American Hospital Association, Guide to the Health Care Field, 1979 (Chicago: American Hospital Association, 1979).

Table 32-2 Selected Indicators Of Inflation 1960-1979

Year	Consumer price index all items	Consumer value of the dollar	Wholesale price index all commodities	Gross federal debt
1960	88.7	$1.13	94.9	290.9
1965	94.5	1.06	96.6	323.2
1967	100.0	1.00	100.0	341.3
1970	116.3	0.86	110.4	382.6
1973	133.1	0.75	134.7	468.4
1974	147.7	0.68	160.1	486.2
1975	161.2	0.62	174.9	544.1
1976	170.5	0.59	183.0	631.9
1977	181.5	0.55	194.2	709.1
1978	195.4	0.51	209.3	780.4
1979 (May)	214.1	0.47	231.6	839.2 (est.)

Source: U.S. Bureau of the Census, *Statistical Abstract of the United States, 1979* (Washington, D.C.: U.S. Government Printing Office, 1980).

proved diagnostic equipment and procedures. It should be obvious that there is much public support for this line of reasoning, but when the economic history of the recent past is examined with respect to hospitals, it turns out that inflation is the primary reason, not mismanagement or clinical fadism.

Since 1966 when the Medicare program became operational, it has been fashionable for government leaders to deplore the costs of the program, giving the impression they are pouring money into a bottomless pit. As a matter of fact, the costs of the Medicare program have been relatively stable as measured by the health care costs per social security recipient which reflects the impact of inflation rather than a higher and higher true cost. This is seen in Table 32–3.

The availability of the dollars per enrollee for health care has not kept pace if inflation is backed out. Even though the dollars expended per recipient remained stable, the total cost of the program has risen sharply, due to the number of additional persons becoming eligible each year. This has been accomplished through coinsurance and deductible changes as well as by further limitations on allowable costs paid to hospitals. The thrust of the governmental interest is to blunt the rise in spending though the number of eligible recipients is growing.

Before peering into the years ahead and seeing what is going to happen to the hospital industry as a result of these forces at work, a look at the

Table 32-3 Comparison of Enrollees in Hospital and Supplementary Insurance Programs

| | Hospital insurance | | | | | Supplementary medical insurance | | | | | |
	Persons 65 and over	Disabled under 65	Total enrollees	Amount reimbursed	Per enrollee	Persons 65 and over	Disabled under 65	Total enrollees	Amount reimbursed	Per enrollee	Total per enrollee
1966	19,082	—	19,082	824	43	17,736	—	17,736	63	4	47
1967	19,494	—	19,494	3,135	161	17,893	—	17,893	1,080	60	221
1968	19,770	—	19,770	3,947	200	18,805	—	18,805	1,342	71	271
1969	20,014	—	20,014	4,485	224	19,105	—	19,105	1,783	93	317
1970	20,361	—	20,361	4,845	238	19,584	—	19,584	1,751	89	327
1971	20,742	—	20,742	5,373	259	19,975	—	19,975	1,956	98	357
1972	21,115	—	21,115	5,915	280	20,351	—	20,351	2,227	109	389
1973	21,571	6,376	27,947	6,677	239	20,921	6,265	27,186	1,909	70	309
1974	21,996	10,081	32,077	8,341	260	21,422	9,579	31,001	2,933	95	355
1975	22,472	12,702	35,174	10,333	294	21,945	12,080	34,025	3,605	106	400
1976	22,920	14,721	37,641	12,647	336	22,446	13,977	36,423	3,915	107	443

Note: Enrollees in thousands, dollar amounts in millions (except where per enrollee).

Source: Social Security Administration, *Social Security Bulletin, Annual Statistical Supplement, 1976* (Washington, D.C.: U.S. Government Printing Office, 1976), pp. 175-176, 178, 180.

history of cost reimbursement in payment for hospital services is helpful. Cost reimbursement took hold in the mid 1930s with the introduction of the Blue Cross concept. This paid for the actual cost of patient services rendered, rather than on rates and fee schedules developed by the hospital. The advantages were twofold:

1. Blue Cross was able to market a policy with great public appeal since they would pay for the services used by a subscriber and not just to a dollar amount on an inadequate indemnity basis. At that time, existing indemnity levels were usually well below the actual costs incurred by a patient. This broadening of coverage was welcomed by the public.
2. Hospitals were delighted because Blue Cross plans negotiated cost reimbursement contracts that agreed to pay hospitals all of the costs they incurred in treating Blue Cross patients.

This promise to pay full costs was a breath of fresh air since they were typically being paid well below full costs by the third party payors of that day and age, primarily county welfare departments and various state agencies. Hospitals accepted contracts below full cost because the country was in the midst of an economic depression and hospitals felt that any payment, no matter how small, was better than none at all.

As the depression ended hospitals began to clamor for full cost reimbursement from public agencies since they were receiving this from a rapidly growing number of Blue Cross plans across the country. At first, the argument for full cost concerned itself with salaries and supplies, but later was expanded to include depreciation on buildings and equipment, which was a logical extension of accounting theories about costs and expenses.

By the time World War II approached, Blue Cross was making impressive strides. To hospitals this meant they were enjoying increasing support for full cost reimbursement. The first major federal government involvement in reimbursement resulted from the drafting of civilians into the army. Many of the draftees were married and responsible for their families. This led to the Emergency Maternal and Infant Care (EMIC) program to pay for their hospital care. The decision on the method of payment was made by representatives of the government who met with hospital representatives who had enjoyed the benefits of cost reimbursement. Having been impressed with it they argued successfully for its adoption by the EMIC program. In turn, this became the basis for payment for hospital services for Medicare and Medicaid when this legislation was adopted by Congress in 1965.

Today on the East Coast, it is typical to find cost reimbursement sources, Medicare, Medicaid and Blue Cross, accounting for 80 to 90 percent of all hospital operating revenues. Moving westward, cost reimbursement sources gradually decline to the 50 to 60 percent range in the midwest and 30 to 40 percent on the West Coast. Taking all hospitals together in the United States, it is probably fair to observe that the primary source of their revenues is now derived from cost reimbursement.

What was once regarded by hospitals as a Godsend has, in the course of forty years, turned around and become the central point of contention between government and hospitals. As the dollar has been eroded in terms of purchasing power, hospitals respond by raising salaries of their employees to keep pace with what is happening in the economy as a whole, which in turn forces the cost reimbursers to increase their spending in hospitals. This puts the administering officials of Medicare and Medicaid in a most difficult position when they appear before the appropriate Congressional Committees. Blue Cross executives have the same kind of difficulty where they have to secure approval of premium increases from State Commissioners of Insurance.

As implementers of Congressional decisions, the responsible agency personnel are reluctant to return to appropriation hearings year after year requesting sizable increases without being able to demonstrate they have pursued a vigorous program of limiting the outflow of monies to hospitals. From their point of view it would be folly to go to such a hearing and tell the members of a Congressional Committee that benefits cannot be maintained as long as hospitals are paid on the same cost formula. Rather than tilting with such windmills, and to avoid what could lead to some derogatory comments from committee members about an agency's lack of efforts to protect the public's tax dollars they substantiate their request by pointing their finger at hospitals as the problem. This is accomplished by detailing the steps they have taken to control hospital costs. They can point out that under cost reimbursement, hospitals are going to be paid the costs of their operations and that no incentives exist for hospitals to run a taut ship, playing on the publicly held attitude that hospitals are mismanaged and inefficient. This is music to the ears of a committee member who doesn't wish to cut back on benefits already enacted, knowing he has to go back to the voters the next time his seat is up for election. It is, and always will be, more palatable to an elected official to side with the vested interests of his constituency in continued government benefits than with legitimate needs of an industry, even though industry needs may also be in the public interest.

Those who serve in Congress or in the executive branch of government do not see where this leads. As yet, they do not recognize that a continuing of a tightening of the financial noose will ultimately endanger the quality of patient care and impair the ability of hospitals to respond to the needs of the public. Hospitals are on a one-way street named "Going For Broke."

Decisions reached by Congress with regard to hospitals are most likely to be based on the Medicare program since it involves a considerable chunk of money directly under Congressional scrutiny. Expenditures for Medicare are going to continue to rise rapidly in the years ahead because of three factors having nothing to do with hospitals: (a) a growing population which was approximately 216 million people in 1979; (b) a growing percentage of persons 65 years of age or older which had moved from 9.2 percent to 10.5 percent by 1979; (c) a continuation of inflation.

Should the Congress vote in a national health insurance plan the problem will be compounded. In a study conducted by the Rand Corporation and Tufts Medical School* the cost was estimated at $50 billion annually, excluding $10 billion paid directly by patients. If financed like Social Security a tax rate of 6.9 percent would be needed using an income ceiling of $15,300. Those earning $13,000 would pay nearly $900 per year. If general revenues were used, a 28 percent increase in personal and corporate income taxes would be needed, or $560 more taxes from a person in the $15,000 bracket. If premiums like private health insurance were utilized the family rate would be $850 per year.

As these numbers and approaches are pondered, it appears that such a step would only accentuate the present difficulties leading to higher rates of inflation, greater deficits in the federal budget, greater hospital and health care expenditures and ultimately the imposition of more and more stringent fiscal controls. The passage of a catastrophic insurance bill would have far less serious implications to the financial operations of hospitals.

The concern over the rapid and continuing rise in hospital operating costs has tended to focus on the item of wages and salaries since it is the largest single component of hospital budgets. As hospitals moved away from religious and charitable concepts towards an increasingly technological base, there was a growing recognition that salary levels would have to be competitive if skilled personnel are to be employed. Hospitals have been striving toward this end for the last quarter of a century. Playing catch-up with industry has lasted a long time and has led to the feeling that hospitals may be soft touches for securing large salary increases. When the average earnings are compared for a number of industries it seems that hospitals may have been running in place rather than leading the pack. This is seen in Table 32–4. In spite of this record of moderation, hospitals

---

Source: Chicago Tribune Editorial, October 18, 1976.

are still regarded suspiciously by public representatives even though government employees average $2,735 (37.5 percent) higher than that paid by health care institutions.

All of the tables in the world are not going to alter the direction of the present trends. The funding mechanisms, state agencies, or Blue Cross plans, are still going to be faced with securing appropriations from state or federal legislatures determined to keep the lid as tightly shut as possible on further inroads on tax dollars for health care provider services.

The pattern is unlikely to change in the foreseeable future. This suggests that the uneasy relationship of mutual distrust and suspicion is apt to continue. John C. Calhoun understood this tug-of-war between the public and the private sector. In 1850 in "A Disquisition on Government," he wrote; "The interval between the decay of the old and the formation and

Table 32-4 Wage Data by Industry Groups

Rank	Industry	Total payroll $
	Total, all non-manufacturing	$14,080
	Total, all industries	13,924
	Total, all manufacturing	13,808
1	Petroleum	18,239
2	Public utilities	16,619
3	Transportation equipment	15,607
4	Miscellaneous non-manufacturing industry	15,332
5	Chemicals and allied products	14,883
6	Machinery	14,501
7	Primary metal industry	14,123
8	Printing & publishing	13,802
9	Electrical machinery, equipment, supply	13,755
10	Food, beverages and tobacco	13,466
11	Pulp paper, lumber and furniture	13,404
12	Instrumental and miscellaneous manufacturing industry	13,294
13	Fabricated metal products	13,126
14	Stone, clay & glass products	13,005
15	Trade	12,869
16	Insurance companies	12,539
17	Banks, finance co., trust co.	12,464
18	Rubber, leather, plastic products	12,399
19	Hospitals	11,262
20	Textile products and apparel	9,674
21	Department stores	9,098

Source: Employee Benefits, 1978 Chamber of Commerce of the United States, 1979, Table 18, page 25; TriBrook Group, Inc.

the establishment of the new, constitutes a period of transition which must always necessarily be one of uncertainty, confusion, error, and wild and fierce fanaticism."[1] Whether or not the health field becomes fiercely fanatical is questionable. But certainly his concept of the effort required to meet the changing scene cannot be denied.

Preferable to this approach is the one suggested by Brooks Atkinson in his "Once Around The Sun," who wrote in 1951; "Bureaucracies are designed to perform public business. But as soon as a bureaucracy is established, it develops an autonomous spiritual life and comes to regard the public as its enemy."[2] Here he deftly puts his finger on the difficulties faced by hospitals. We are too busy dealing with the bureaucracy and have too long neglected the force behind them, the legislative bodies who write the laws and determine the appropriations.

Hospitals must now move to the more difficult task of bringing their thinking to bear on the legislative process, as a matter of top priority. To continue to passively watch inflation march onward and not put forth a sustained and continuous effort to guide legislative thinking on health care policies is simply going to lead to a bankrupt system. It will be unable to provide the quality and quantity of care the public has come to expect from its health care system. It is up to hospitals themselves to take the leadership required. Justice Robert Jackson understood this responsibility as he clearly stated in his opinion in the 1943 West Virginia State Board vs. Barnette when he wrote, "Freedom to differ is not limited to things that do not matter much. That would be a mere shadow of freedom. The test of its substance is the right to differ as to things that touch the heart of the existing order."[3] Many health professionals, particularly those in New York, Massachusetts and Maryland know where the existing order leads. Others in California, Arizona, and New Mexico have not as yet felt the heat, but the road ahead is clearly marked. The time for a national consensus on health policy is not when the end of the road has been reached, but when one can see the end of the road ahead.

Some of the steps that need to be taken are probably well beyond the reach of the health field acting alone. Yet a beginning is needed. The problems of inflation, of Congressional unwillingness to cut back on benefits of adopted programs, of representatives having to run for a seat every two years all work to the disadvantage of the public interest. These basic difficulties in the American way should be brought to the forefront and kept in mind. They are the backdrop against which policies and appropriations are, of necessity, being determined. Other industries must become concerned if these issues are to be seriously explored. Matters of defense spending, of taxation, of unemployment, of carrying the cost of the national debt, are relevant considerations to health policy determinations because tax dollars must be used for all.

Labor learned these lessons many years ago. The AFL-CIO built their national headquarters one block from the White House in order to exercise their prerogatives of free speech in our society. They often speak out publicly as well as testify on a wide range of matters coming before the publics' representatives. They recognize the way to be heard is to be present, to have their viewpoint taken in account at the time public policy is being formulated, and to have those making such decisions concerned and caring about the position of labor on any given issue. In contrast to labor, the American Medical Association, the American Dental Association, and the American Hospital Association maintain their bases of operation in Chicago with outposts in the nation's capital. This is in spite of the fact that the federal government is now the single most important influence on health care in this country. This influence is going to grow and expand in the decades ahead. A worthwhile step would seem to be to follow the example of labor and establish the base of operations at the place where the basic decisions are now made.

Whether or not this can be accomplished, the advice of Paul Ward, the President of the California Hospital Association, should be adopted. He points out that the health field is unique in that the regulator on the industry is also the major purchaser of the services unlike the relationship between the Federal Reserve Board and the banking industry. Today, the Department of HHS is not only deciding on the services it will buy from hospitals but is also making the determination as to what it will pay for these purchases. Hospitals should move vigorously with the Congress to uncouple these dual responsibilities. The agency that determines the rates to be paid should be free to make independent judgments about them without being directly concerned with the dollars to pay for the provider services. As it is now, decisions reached are not objective, but rather are intimately tied to the decision-making process of appropriations. This needs to be rectified.

Because of the multiple financing mechanisms now in use to pay for hospital care, each source feels at liberty to make those decisions regarding allowable costs that best answer its own needs. For example, Medicare does not permit the inclusion of the costs of operating an obstetrical service while Blue Cross plans often do not permit the inclusion of bad debts as a reimbursable cost. Many other examples exist and are increasing in number and variety as those who write the reimbursement procedures come up with new and different twists on their formulas.

As a result of each reimbursement program deciding for itself what is or what is not allowable as cost, the hospital finds itself with a widening gap between gross revenues and net revenues. As contractual adjustments become larger and larger the gap has become 18 to 20 percent in many eastern seaboard hospitals. For every dollar being spent on cost reimbursed patients, hospitals are receiving something less than a dollar in revenue. Even when depreciation dollars are used for operations hospitals often are losing money. Many are forced to use up not only interest but principal that has been accumulated through endowments and trust funds. Inevitably, when a dollar is spent and not fully replaced in some way or another, the hospital is on its way to bankruptcy.

To prevent each reimburser from determining for itself a definition of allowable cost an industry-wide standard definition of full cost is a necessity so that hospitals receive equal payment from all purchasers of service. To continue as at present can only lead to a demise of the voluntary hospital system.

If these legislative steps can be accomplished, hospitals stand a chance of surviving. They will still have major financial difficulties because of Congressional unwillingness to deal effectively with inflation and making modifications in program benefits to the public when costs far exceed appropriations. Facing reality by looking after doing those things that need doing has to become the criteria of measuring individual Congressional performance by the hospital field. And after making such measurements there must be a willingness to publicly state the suitability of incumbents in Congress for reelection. To date, the health field has shied from this degree of involvement. This must change if the public's interest in health care is to be protected.

Such an approach goes considerably beyond the activities now engaged in by hospitals. Having hospital leadership present prepared testimony at Committee hearings on matters of concern needs to be continued but it is not enough as judged by the events of the last few years. Hospitals should now go to the point of using political muscle, muscle that must be exercised fairly, honestly, and openly on behalf of the constituents of hospitals, the American public. To do this requires leadership of a high order, courage to work towards bringing about changes in our legislative process.

NOTES

1. John C. Calhoun, *The International Dictionary of Thought* (Chicago: J. G. Ferguson Publishing Co., 1975).
2. Brooks Atkinson, "Once Around the Sun," 1951.
3. West Virginia Board of Education vs. Barnette, 319 U.S. 624(1943), 87 L. Ed. 1628, 63 S.Ct. 1178(1943).

Chapter 33

The Impact of Prospective Rate Review on Hospitals— Setting the Stage

In 1969, the American Hospital Association (AHA) adopted a statement on the financial requirements of health care institutions and services. This was recognition that the health field had to pay heed to the financial viability of institutions. In 1971, the Economic Stabilization Program was undertaken by the federal government. By the time the controls were lifted three years later, the worst fears of administrators had been realized. They came to appreciate that rigid and inflexible rules were likely to be the wave of the future if the federal level was to be the prime mover.

STATE CONTROLLED RATE REVIEW

Prior to that time there appeared to be a choice between voluntary controls or no controls. This notion died with the expiration of the stabilization program and was replaced with looking at the question of mandatory government controls or voluntary controls. This has led to a steadily increasing interest in the concept of each state having a rate review mechanism, similar to the kind of controls applied to utilities. Further emphasis to this approach occurred at the AHA meeting in Washington on January 23–24, 1978, when the AHA adopted the following statement. "The Board supports federally mandated state-sanctioned budget review under federal guidelines, is dedicated to it as the best possible control structure, intends to push it philosophically in every way, and will introduce it at the earliest

---

Reprinted with changes from "The Financial Future of Hospitals," by Richard L. Johnson in *Hospital Financial Management,* with permission of the Hospital Financial Manager Assoc., July 1976.

possible moment when it is determined that the bill will be assured a fair hearing and broad support from the membership."[1]

On the surface, the AHA policy seems to be reasonable since it assumes rational people can arrive at mutually satisfactory decisions on a timely basis, given adequate data, and that the beneficiary of such a process is the American public. Testing the assumption by reviewing the experiences of selected states who have been operating under rate review for several years, as well as by hearing from some states that are just in the process of establishing a commission is being questioned. Finally, the experience of a state, Indiana, should be reviewed in an attempt to look at the possibility of a viable alternative, viable politically from the public's interest and economically from that of the individual hospital.

PROSPECTIVE RATE REVIEW

The Intent

The intent of prospective rate review is to preset rates of payments to hospitals based on their operating costs and financial requirements so that those paying for services can anticipate their expenditures in the coming year. The desire to do this stems from two factors: (a) an annual increase in costs for the same level of operations from the previous year; and (b) an increase in the amount of usage of hospital services.

To those who pay bills, the widespread use of cost reimbursement (Blue Cross, Medicare, and Medicaid) has led to a belief that paying allowable costs on a retrospective basis is a disincentive to hospital management. Out of this concern has developed the notion that requiring hospitals to submit budgets for approval prior to the coming year of operations will permit both the providers and the payers with a common understanding of the magnitude of dollars that are needed.

The Problem

Herein lies the problem. The hospital sees the program as having to agree to funding levels that provide the level of quality of care intrinsic to the institution, while the reviewing body sees it as a commitment to dollar levels of expenditures first and quality of care as something that can be accomplished by the institution once these dollar levels have been established. In essence, one talks patient care, the other dollars. Both are right, but neither is meeting the needs of the other party. Reviewing agencies want to know and approve the total costs of the hospital, and various methodologies have been employed to accomplish this. In all states with such a program there has been a recognition of the need for standard definitions and accounting methods so that reviewers know that they are comparing apples to apples, and not oranges to apples. One of the serious questions is the extent to which the adoption of such definitions and methods has been workable to both hospitals and the agencies involved.

Methodologies

A related question deals with the various methodologies that have been used. Is it to be line item approval? Is it to be the establishment of categories by bed size? Is each hospital to be judged by its total budgeted dollars and anticipated volume of activity? Finally, is there any experience that dictates one method over another?

The Use of Facilities and Services

A separate consideration that needs to be explored deals with the use of facilities and services of a hospital and how they can be controlled. When the budget of a hospital is approved by an agency, it implicitly, if not explicitly, is tied to the projection of patient days of care by clinical service and the projected use of all patient ancillary services. This, of course, is based on previous years' performances and a projection of the trend lines. This may be modified, upwards or downwards, by projecting a change in the market share or by estimating the potential effect in the coming year of some externally applied rules and regulations such as the application of PSRO. Or it may be significantly changed if new funding mechanisms are created, as pointed out in the *Special Report #1* of the Robert Wood Johnson Foundation.[2] In a sponsored study, "National Survey of Access to Medical Care," the principal investigator, Ronald Anderson, comments on the results: "The removal of financial barriers appears to have major impact on whether or not various groups have access to medical care."[3]

In the Institute of Medicine report that was used by HHS as the basis of its proposed standards for the number of beds per 1,000 population, it is interesting to read the dissents of two of the committee members, Shropshire and Cross. They point out that the use of hospital facilities is not under the control of the hospital corporation, but rests with the clinical decisions of the physicians who are members of its medical staff.[4] These comments were ignored, yet they are at the heart of the problem of attempting to control the costs of hospital operations.

Items Beyond Hospital Control

Those in Congress struggling with cost containment have come to recognize that there are items in a hospital budget beyond the control of the institution, such as utility bills, insurance charges, and the purchases of drugs, goods, and supplies. Believing there is a need to be fair and just in the application of ceilings, they found themselves in a dilemma, in favor of some kind of a cap, but thinking that all would be lost if legitimate pass-throughs were permitted.

Compounding the difficulty is the problem of a rising intensity of care. This has been ignored in congressional bills and is also being sidestepped by rate review commissions. From the regulator's shoes no one wants to tackle the physician-patient relationship, preferring to hide behind the PSRO as answering this need. Yet, the major concern is an ever-increasing demand for a growing variety of patient care services in the hospital. PSROs are directly concerned with the appropriateness of the length of stay and the diagnostic and treatment modalities after a patient has become accustomed to the horizontal position. From the standpoint of hospital economics, this is like locking the stable door after the horse has already vacated the premises.

The intensity of demand for service is the core of the issue of controlling hospital costs. If it turns out that this is really the case in those states that have had several years of experience with rate review, the methods for braking demand need to be described and an assessment made of their effectiveness.

The hospital field is moving into an arena where an attempt will be made to answer the question, "How much health care is enough?" Others may see the question somewhat differently. They may think the question of hospital resources answers itself, that the real issue is a fair and equitable distribution of care, since the resources are adequate to cope with any demands that may be placed on the system.

If, in fact, it turns out that the physician-patient relationship is the real issue, then the mechanisms for controlling this aspect need to be carefully considered. What has worked, and what has failed? Will physicians play a game where the ground rules are dictated by a central government, be it in the state capital or in Washington? What is apt to happen if a program is commenced and the doctors fail to play the game as defined in the regulations? Is it possible to go back to "go" under such circumstances?

THE PATH AHEAD FOR RATE REVIEW

One of the criticisms of the health field that is frequently heard in the corridors of Congress and the halls of HHS is that the hospital field is always against any proposal that is put forward. Also, hospital representatives never suggest any worthwhile alternative for consideration, and they always find reasons why any legislative program will not work, without suggesting ways for developing a program that will work. Frustrations, anger, and resentment on the one side are met by hostility, disbelief, and mistrust on the other. Clearly, any thoughtful observer would have to conclude that the present state of affairs cannot continue indefinitely.

The difficulty lies not with thinking things have to change; it rests in determining the pathway to be followed. Looked at from the standpoint of the next ten years, the proposed mechanism of rate review needs to be examined. Where will it take the hospitals of this country? Will the American public be as well served a decade from now as it is at present? Or is this question irrelevant when examining the issue of cost of health care? Will administrators find themselves in a Catch-22 situation where what they are doing cannot be afforded, but what can be afforded leads to doing things that are not in harmony with acceptable levels of quality of care?

Looked at from another perspective, there is a viewpoint that expresses alarm that the percentage of the GNP going for health services has steadily risen to where these services account for more than nine percent of the GNP. The argument runs that this country is spending a disproportionate share of resources on health and that it must not be permitted to become a higher percentage. On the other hand, there are those who take the position that who is to say what is the correct percentage? This argument goes further and says that the determination of the "right" percentage is a decision that should be made in a free marketplace where individual consumers should be permitted to decide how much they wish to spend for such services, and if these conditions are permitted to function, the answer will be obtained without government intervention. This approach is countered by others who maintain that to do this is to deprive lower income segments of society from having access to their rights for health care.

This country is not alone in its public debate over how much of the GNP is enough for health care services. It goes on in most developed nations even though the percentage varies widely, for example, 12 percent in the Soviet Union; 5 percent in the United Kingdom; 8 to 9 percent in Canada; 8 to 9 percent in Sweden; and 8.5 to 9 percent in the U.S.A.[5] The extremes are noteworthy because both the United Kingdom and the Soviet Union have strong central control of their health delivery systems, yet the Soviets spend 1.4 times more than Britain of their share of GNP. This would seem to indicate there is unlikely to be any one correct answer for the United States.

In a study published by the Government Research Corporation, the conclusion is reached that commissions on rates and budgets should be established. In an explanatory note, it is pointed out that "Total revenues per institution, rather than unit price is the object of regulation."[6] It goes on, "The focus on total revenues is designed to avoid the situation in which increased utilization offsets rate controls."[7] The next paragraph explains further:

> Including the rates charged to all payers is a second fundamental feature of the Proposal. To the extent that existing state rate review programs do not apply to all payers, costs may be shifted from those who pay regulated rates to those who pay unregulated rates. Not only is this inequitable, but more importantly, it subverts the objective of moderating increases in the total cost of institutional health care services.[8]

This seminar of the Government Research Corporation was cosponsored by Senators Edward Kennedy and Jacob Javits. It is interesting to note that the list of 27 participants included only 1 hospital administrator, but 10 persons from government, 2 from the AHA, 1 insurance consultant, and 13 from insurance or managers of employee funds.

As pointed out by Arnold Silver in the January 1978 issue of *Rate Controls*: "There was no correlation between the increase in hospital expenditures and the increase in the gross national product."[9]

When all aspects of underwriting the costs of the health delivery system are considered, it appears that there are two major elements: the demands for the services and the costs of meeting those demands. Both are integral parts of the same equation, but each has its own set of requirements. Demand is intimately intertwined with the physician-patient relationship and the established pattern of coverage paying first dollar costs of an episode of illness in the hospital. Hospital costs are woven into the fabric of the economy, reflecting the impact of inflation, the purchase of goods and supplies not under the control of the institution, and the continuing thrust of technology. Whether or not the restraining influence of rate review honing in only on the cost side of the equation can be effective for the long haul is what needs to be carefully examined before verbally agreeing to such an approach before the evidence is clear and compelling.

NOTES

1. American Hospital Association, Minutes of the Board of Trustees Meeting, January 23-24, 1978 (Chicago: American Hospital Association, 1978).
2. Robert Wood Johnson Foundation, *Special Report #1* (Princeton, N.J.: Robert Wood Johnson Foundation, 1978), p. 6.
3. Ibid.
4. Institute of Medicine, *Controlling the Supply of Hospital Beds, A Policy Statement* (Washington, D.C.: National Academy of Sciences, 1976).
5. Odin Anderson, "Comparative Health Delivery Systems" (Lecture delivered to Tri Brook Group, Inc., February 24, 1978).
6. Government Research Corporation, *A Proposal for State Rate Setting: Long Range Controls on the Cost of Institutional Health Services* (Washington, D.C.: Government Research Corporation, 1977).
7. Ibid.
8. Institute of Medicine, *Controlling the Supply of Hospital Beds.*
9. Arnold Silver, *Rate Controls*, 1, no. 1 (January 1978).

Chapter 34

Old and New Thinking about Hospital Payments

The present day extensive regulation of hospitals through the Medicare program is based on an assertion that federal dollars not be wasted and that accountability for government dollar expenditures is of first concern. However, the unstated objective in manipulating hospital payments appears to be to limit federal spending to Social Security Administration funds and congressional appropriations. Consequently, HHS continually defines and redefines allowable costs for hospitals.

After years of being directed and controlled through Medicare regulations, private hospital corporations are now almost as tightly controlled as military, veteran, and public health hospitals. The only significant difference is that HHS actions have not saved money, but have shifted unallowable costs to the total responsibility of non-Medicare patients. HHS has been practicing cost shifting, rather than cost saving.

If the federal proportion of patients is further expanded beyond Medicare and Medicaid and encompasses a national health insurance program, control will then be as strong as in government-owned hospitals. Currently, having an average of 35 percent of total revenues coming from federal sources allows the federal government to escape responsibility for deficits in operations as well as the freedom to carp about the high cost of hospital care.

To continue a federal program of cost-based payments to hospitals is to keep the cart before the horse. The principle is the same as the local supermarket permitting the federal government to control its accounting systems, pricing policies, profit centers, depreciation, expansion, and inventories, simply because it accepts federal food stamps from its customers.

The basis of the present dilemma arose in the original Medicare legislation. The American Hospital Association (AHA) encouraged the use of "reasonable cost" as the criteria for determining hospital payment. The

353

AHA should have used the concept of "cost plus." Any large contractor of the Department of Defense in the preceding 20 years could have quickly explained the differences and the necessity for such language in the legislation.

Experience with "reasonable costs" has taught hospitals that they are still receiving less than total cost for caring for the beneficiaries of government programs. There is growing belief by bureaucrats and Blue Cross executives that cost-based payment formulas for hospitals must be abandoned. Medicare and Medicaid bureaucrats, as well as an increasing number of Blue Cross executives, are now espousing prospective payment methods.

LOOKING FOR A NEW WAY

For the past several years, the federal government has encouraged experimentation with a variety of new payment approaches. The government hopes to find an effective way to slow the continual rise in hospital costs and payments. How realistic is this hope? Is it a good theory that works in the real world? What effect will recent federal planning legislation have on hospital costs and charges? Are there economic forces in hospital care that are beyond the scope of hospital control? Underlying the government efforts is a hope that hospital rates are controllable by hospital administration, rather than by external economic forces.

In the late 1940s, when Blue Cross had an explosive growth, rate setting was almost completely a private affair. A rate structure was established according to a hospital's own needs and goals. When hospital costs began to rise significantly in the early 1950s, cost-based methods increased in popularity. Even today a significant number of hospitals do not receive most of their reimbursement through cost-based formulas, despite Medicare and Medicaid programs cost formulas. Such systems require an audit and postaudit settlement when hospital revenues exceed a specific definition of cost.

Yet hospital costs have continued to increase rapidly in those parts of the country where there is heaviest reliance on cost-based systems. Obviously, cost systems have gradually become ineffective, or at least do not now make a significant difference for cost containment purposes.

With national health insurance being considered, it is worthwhile to review the rationale for prospective payment, since this will probably continue to be the most seriously considered method of paying for hospital services.

PHYSICIANS AND COMMUNITY REINFORCE MONOPOLY

In the hospital industry, market forces are not elastic because hospitals are a series of mini-monopolies. Why is this so?

In a community two major forces tend to reinforce monopoly conditions. The first is the physician. Today a majority of patients in hospitals are attended by specialists, since 82 percent of all physicians restrict their practice to a specialty. When a patient has more than one disability, is older, or is admitted for trauma, several physicians may be involved in the care rendered. Hospital care is now practiced by a series of related specialists who supplement the work of the attending physician. They are selected by the attending physician who uses personal knowledge of their abilities, judgments, and skills.

This kind of knowledge about a colleague's abilities is acquired over time and is limited by the range of earlier experiences. Until a patient's problem is recognized as clearly beyond the capability of locally available physicians, the patient will not be transferred elsewhere. Patients obtain their medical care locally, except for that small proportion of patients who self-refer to a "superclinic." In many communities less than two percent go elsewhere for care.

This is a reality of medical practice. It is reinforced by a public that selects and prefers to remain with one source of primary care. Economically, this practice tends toward a monopolistic hospital market condition, since a physician's knowledge of colleagues' competence is limited to those with whom he or she has frequent contact, typically to the hospital medical staff. Even if all physicians could attend their patients in all hospitals, this limitation would remain. The informal human restraint leads to referrals to local colleagues rather than distant medical centers.

THE COMMUNITY

Community attitudes are a second reinforcing element toward monopoly. Demographic studies on patient choice repeatedly report a preference for hospitalization near the patient's place of residence. This should surprise no one, even though some patients occasionally bypass the nearest hospitals.

Most patients are part of a family and want their relatives nearby in time of severe stress. The greater the distance to a hospital, the more difficult it becomes for a family to visit the hospital. Patients are also aware that in the local hospital their friends are on the hospital staff. This provides additional reassurance to them. Except for serious medical problems, patients do not readily accept distant hospitalization.

These two factors are sufficiently important to overcome any differences in hospital charges. Price variation does not effectively operate under these local monopoly conditions. In addition, third party payments, government programs, insurance carriers, Blue Cross, and Blue Shield provide coverage for more than 80 percent of hospitalizations. Consequently, price differentials are inconsequential for a substantial number of patients. The public is far more concerned with monthly insurance premiums than with the cost of a hospitalization.

In effect, hospital market behavior is what it is because physicians and patients make uneconomic decisions. Most people who have thought about these issues have therefore concluded that some type of price review and control is necessary for a hospital rate structure.

Most hospital administrators would not argue this conclusion. They would argue, however, for reasonableness in the use of any review mechanism and for a need to allow surplus retention, or profit, for well-managed institutions.

Within this setting, the implications of a prospective payment system need to be defined in terms of capital costs and operating costs of hospitals, as well as the effect of patient volume on hospital services.

The issues of capital cost have been faced by federal planning legislation. Because of local monopoly conditions in hospital markets, new services can be initiated or existing ones expanded that are unneeded or uneconomic, such as the current excess of open heart units. Planning agency approval must now be obtained for capital programs in excess of $150,000 if depreciation and interest costs are to be included in reimbursement from a federal program.

SOLVING THE PROBLEM OF EXCESSIVE DEVELOPMENT

The present thrust of mandated planning is to deter "excessive" hospital development. The implicit expectation is that somehow a process of attrition will gradually size hospitals to population needs. Unfortunately, mandated planning mechanisms still have to prove that this objective is achievable.

The real cure-all for overexpanded hospital facilities is a program that can use market forces to phase out institutions that have excessive charges for inferior services. As it is now, if planning agencies are responsible for this goal, they must face extremely sensitive issues because hospitals arouse local feelings of pride. In addition, planners are placed in the difficult position of making judgments on the competence of boards of trustees and hospital administrations, as well as on levels of medical care for which no generally accepted criteria exist.

Market forces that operate in a competitive industry are ineffective in the hospital field, and excess capacity remains available at higher than needed market prices.

There are at least two ways to solve this problem. One is to limit the annual amount of payment-on-debt service that can be included in a hospital rate structure. The other is to use rate ceilings to eliminate inefficient operations, that is, hospitals that make poor capital investment decisions, in terms of financing instruments or estimating market demands.

At this time, planning agencies seldom consider the interrelationship between capital and operating costs. High construction cost may mean lower than average operating cost, while lower initial capital cost may create higher operating cost. Life-cycle costing is the only logical basis for determining the financial cost of a new project, and it is rarely used.

The expanded, mandated planning process will substantially reduce future program flexibility and also delay the general use of new medical knowledge. The current situation of planning agencies is the fact that their planning has precedence over institutional planning.

In practice, the $150,000 exemption on hospital projects means a detailed control of hospital capital costs since most significant improvements in medical instrumentation or programming exceed this amount. It is an example of unequal control because, in a hospital with $1 million a year in revenues, there is a ten percent ceiling while in a $20 million hospital, the ceiling is 0.5 percent.

A planning agency, which is one step removed from the operating experience of hospitals, is more likely to attempt to plan future medical care schemes on the basis of "what ought to be," rather than "what the public will support," as outlined in PL 93–641 and PL 92–603. The efforts of the federal government to promote HMOs is an example of encouraging a particular model of ambulatory medical care that has as yet to gain much public or medical support and is now caught in many bureaucratic entanglements.

While authority from planning agencies may be a necessity, comprehensive, detailed control is a poor substitute for policy direction. The goal sought is a combination of concern for desired medical care programming and reasonable capital expenditures.

A major interest in medical programming is the administrator's concern about human behavior, particularly that of the physician. When a hospital does not go ahead and develop a new program, it may mean that some of the more competent and concerned physicians will shift their interests to another hospital where additional medical capability is available, depreciating the quality of care in their present hospital.

Rather than a nitty-gritty approach, it would be more sensible to set a sliding ceiling on capital costs to accommodate different volumes by size of hospital and inflation, and yet allow hospitals to proceed with plant expansion and new programs that are justifiable by market experience as reflected in hospital revenues.

LIMITING EXPENDITURES

There are two concepts that meet this criteria. The first is a limit on total annual capital costs, including leasing agreements, to between seven to eight percent of total operating revenues. For example, an eight percent ceiling for a $1 million annual revenue hospital could have a total annual capital expenditure of $80,000, while a $20 million annual revenue hospital would be authorized $1.6 million. Another is to set an indebtedness ceiling at 1½, or 1 times annual revenue. The total allowable long-term debt for a $1 million hospital at 1½ times annual gross revenue would be $1.5 million, and a $20 million hospital would be $30 million. Specific studies are needed to establish a reasonable range.

Reasonable ceilings for expenditures for annual capital equipment purchases and long-term needs are needed. Debt ceilings of those types would prevent gross overexpansion and would eliminate capital cost mismanagement without undue and unnecessary interference with hospital operational autonomy. Under special conditions, an appeals process should be developed for unique situations.

These concepts do not imply an elimination of approving expansion plans of hospitals. However, rather than use a fixed amount of $150,000, no matter what the size of an institution's budget, a more reasonable approach would be to require planning agency approval for all building capital expenditures that exceed ten percent of annual depreciation costs, or about one percent of revenue. This rule should apply no matter what the source of capital funds, operating surplus, mortgages, leasing, or gifts. In addition, the required approach for "any substantial change in service," as included in PL 92–603, should be redefined to remove subjective interpretation.

Such changes in present planning legislation would eliminate a substantial amount of planning agency detail, allow an increase in hospital initiative, and permit time to be given to the serious, more meaningful areas for planning future developments of the health care system.

If a hospital program is demanded or required by a community and cannot be supported by patient revenues, special Hill-Burton type government grants might be considered. Alcohol and drug addiction treatment programs are examples. These grants should pay both capital and operating costs over a long period of time. In the past and present, government programs have provided only a partial subsidy of capital costs and a gradually decreasing support for operating expenses. It is time for government to consider once again the desirability for block grant funding, even though the present federal fiscal climate will not favor this mechanism.

To facilitate competitive forces, well-managed profitable hospitals should be allowed to retain and spend their surpluses to increase working capital or one-time purchases of capital plant and equipment. This would encourage the well-managed institutions to improve their local market position gradually by acquiring new, more sophisticated instrumentation or to develop a stronger financial position. It would encourage rational hospital administrations to develop new programs of service that their markets would support, that is, where new revenues exceed new costs. Unmet need would quickly become apparent to planners, who would have a well-defined mandate to lobby the development and funding of new programs to fill existing gaps in service. To perform at this level of sophistication will require more improved quality and expertise than current planning agencies demonstrate.

Operating costs are another area of major concern in prospective payment. They are inevitably intertwined with the size and service volumes of a hospital, as well as its case mix of patients.

Within rather broad limits, a relationship exists between volume of service and cost per unit of service. This fact is often obscured by the use of gross measures of cost, such as patient day expense or case cost. At a department level, where individual cost data are maintained by test or procedure, a relationship to costs is much clearer. Gross statistics mask this relationship since it is generally true that the larger a hospital, the more comprehensive its medical care services and the greater its efforts to ensure quality control.

For example, the larger the hospital, the greater the likelihood that there will be programs such as a social service department, a rehabilitation service, health education programs, and medical education. Each program adds to the total cost of hospitalizing a patient, but expands a physician's ability to cope with medical problems. Quality redundancy is increased by an organized infection control program; safety, fire, and disaster program; security efforts; and a multitude of management and operational procedures that ensure hospital and medical staff performance.

KNOWING THE CASE MIX OF PATIENTS

The case mix of patients affects a hospital's operating expenses. If there are many seriously ill patients with shortened lengths of stay who must use a high level of diagnostic and therapeutic services, costs are higher on a case-cost basis. A cancer patient treated by surgery, rehabilitative services, and radiation is a much more expensive case than a patient treated for an uncomplicated gall bladder removal, length of stay being equal. The proportions of each type of patient in a hospital population substantially change operating costs. A hospital's case mix of patients will affect total costs, revenues, case costs, and per-patient day costs in a variety of ways.

Existing gross measures of overall measures of hospital costs and revenues are inadequate without a detailed knowledge of the case mix of patients.

At best, a community general hospital can control case mix only in a crude fashion. Three major ways are used by hospitals to exert a limited control, and none are in a patient's best interest. The first is to block admission of patients who will probably have an expensive hospital stay; the second is to prevent the appointment of physicians to the medical staff who have a preponderance of expensive cases in their type of practice; and the third is to limit the types of equipment and trained personnel available, or as a variation, to restrict the number of beds in that clinical service. A hospital's control over case mix is therefore more fantasy than fact.

In the past, the costing of hospital care by disease entity has frequently been tried. Since indirect costs are generally between 30 and 40 percent of total expense, the results of disease costing have been ambiguous.

PSRO PROGRAMS

As a result of federal legislation, PSROs are responsible for admission, concurrent, and discharge reviews for each patient, for the patient's length of stay, and for appropriateness of care. Useful disease-costing data can be accumulated through this program. Over time it is likely that the data will come to be used by PSRO programs to encourage the standardizations of diagnostic procedures and treatment modalities. Its ultimate effect will tend to promote a lock-step method of treating patients. When physicians ultimately perceive this effect, their resistance to this program will and should substantially escalate. It is also likely that the federal government will attempt to apply disease costing to hospitals through the use of case cost ceilings. An embryonic effort in this direction was made under Phase IV of the Economic Stabilization Program in 1974.

If a market price is not achievable because of local monopoly positions of hospitals, and since cost-based payment provides no incentives for cost containment, what will? No matter what the choice, *the desired goal is the maintenance of fiscally healthy hospitals needed to provide readily accessible services of a quality nature at a desired level of medical care, in a reasonably efficient manner.* At this time no federally-controlled payment program achieves this objective or recognizes that a majority of hospitals will never achieve maximum dollar efficiency, just as in the case of all other industries.

If a prospective payment system is considered, a hospital's rate structure would be established prior to rendering patient care. This implies that no postaudit settlements are a part of the program, only that operating experience is considered when a new set of rate adjustments is requested. If a postaudit adjustment is involved, the system would again be back to a form of a cost-based system because cost caps are used. Further, prospective payment means that an external, more powerful agency reviews and approves or adjusts a proposed rate structure. In essence, a hospital proposes, and a more powerful agency takes action on, a rate structure.

Several schemes have been proposed that fly under the banner of prospective payment, but are, in fact, a camouflaged variation of cost-based payments. Line item budget review systems are an example. Here rates are established based on an analysis of the costs involved in each department. The Medicare method of apportioning departmental costs, based on the proportion of revenue from Medicare to total department revenue, is another. Target rates are also cost based rather than prospective, because it is a system that uses group averages to arrive at approved rates. The systems are simply a bureaucratic rationale to justify cost-based payment systems.

Incentive rate systems that establish rates and then have the hospitals participate proportionately in profits or losses are also fundamentally cost systems. If the hospital kept all of the earned profits, this would not be true. At the present time, hospital financial reserves have been so seriously eroded that the existing prospective rate systems have in effect become cost based because there is no absorption capability left.

To date, no system is in use that requires performance budgeting. This type of system requires that departmental statistics, as a ratio of inputs to outputs, be measured and paid. Many such ratios, using man-hours per unit of output, are in regular internal use in hospitals. Unfortunately, certain areas of hospital operation can be calculated only in a gross fashion because they are variable as to meaning when quality control factors are considered.

Any external system is based either on a hospital's cost of operation or some form of averaging a group of hospital changes. Such devices imply that all hospitals within a category can achieve the same level of efficiency.

The ultimate goal should be to separate the efficient from the inefficient hospital and to reward efficient ones for superior performance or penalize the others for poor performance. The difficulty with this concept is that external forces determine a large part of the cost of operating a hospital. If a hospital is in a labor market where the minimum wage is $3 per hour and another is in a $2 market, it does not necessarily mean that the higher cost hospital is more or less efficient. The higher labor market rates would raise the overall costs of operations approximately 19 percent. With between 58 percent to 63 percent of hospital costs wrapped up in wage and fringe benefit costs, such differences have substantial impact.

DETERMINING EFFICIENCY

The size of a hospital usually correlates with the scope of medical services available. The larger the hospital, the greater the number of patient care services. It is therefore not logical to compare a 200-bed hospital to a 500-bed one. The smaller hospital is not necessarily more efficient because its average costs are lower. Marginal costs by service is a more meaningful way to analyze this issue.

Older hospital plants typically have higher operating expenses than newer ones. Generally an inner-city hospital is older and more expensive to operate, as well as to remodel, but has lower depreciation costs.

What is an efficient hospital? Even if performance budgeting were the basis of payment, older physical plants and out-of-date design will affect efficiency levels, as well as having clientele determining the breadth of service demanded. Furthermore, the volume of service rendered by a particular hospital department is not within the control of the hospital administration. A small intensive care or coronary care unit may be essential, but if the need for it is sufficiently small so that a reasonable productivity level is unattainable, what then?

The total complexity and interweaving of these variables are incompletely understood. Any system that attempts to categorize hospitals by these variables will produce inequities because the magnitude of the cumulative effects are unknown. As yet it is impossible to separate the efficient from the inefficient hospitals easily.

Furthermore, at any pont when a new payment system is introduced, hospitals will not all be equally situated. Any standardized approach will therefore fail to keep all needed hospitals fiscally sound, since efficiency in adversity will go unrecognized. Also, some inefficient hospitals will need to be maintained because there are no reasonable alternatives for the populations they serve. Whatever the system, its goal should be to improve performance even in the needed, but inefficient hospital.

The problem of the efficient but unneeded hospital is a political dilemma. Realistically, the only acceptable decision is to allow it to continue to operate but to prevent its expansion. Over a long period of time, the establishment of more modern services in other hospitals will gradually increase their attractiveness to physicians and patients and decrease that of the unneeded hospital. Eventually, the population base may increase sufficiently to justify expansion, or it will collapse because of a decreasing or static population base.

In the past, the main focus has been to erect a logic based on consideration of a hospital's operating costs or a limit of profits. Limitation on profits is an unwise policy when coupled with a rate reviewing process because it increases the penalty for increasing efficiency.

The public, however, needs protection from a hospital that sets its charges too high. Just because there may be a sufficient number of patients who will pay twice a reasonable charge for a service is no reason to ask them to do so when the hospital is operating at 50 percent efficiency.

Buried in the problem of equitable hospital rates is the issue of payment to hospital-based physicians for their services. The majority of these physicians are on contracts that are a percentage of the gross or net revenue of a hospital department, so that an individual charge for service, such as $10 for an x-ray flat plate of the chest, includes a radiologist's fee for interpretation of the film. In other instances, such as laboratory tests, there is no direct involvement of the pathologist. When a hospital increases rates, additional income is added to the hospital-based specialist because of the percentage arrangement.

In federal medical programs, private practice physician fees are "usual and customary." This is to reduce the effect of hospital-based physicians so that they are treated like other physicians on a fee-for-service basis where standardized fees have been established. As it is now, if one radiologist receives 25 percent of the gross revenue for a $10 x-ray, he or she will receive $2.50, where another one at 33⅓ percent would be paid 3.33.

National, regional, and local standardized hospital charges are an impossible dream because cost factors of production are significantly different between hospitals. Rates charged for services must reflect the uniqueness of a particular set of problems with which an individual hospital copes. To pay the same rates to two hospitals in entirely different circumstances may cause the efficiently managed hospital to go broke because it is attempting to play in a situation where community forces have stacked its deck. Equal rate structures imply equal community medical needs and support of hospitals. This is patently not the real world.

PAYMENTS CANNOT BE STANDARDIZED

Cost payment systems are bad, but the notion of changing from a cost-based to prospective payment mechanism, as presently understood, to escape the disincentives of a cost system is a myth.

The ultimate rationale of any price is justified by the costs incurred to produce goods or services. A market price is determined after considering its costs of production and marketing. If the price does not exceed its cost, no enterprise in any industry can produce a particular product or service.

Hospital care is not divisible. If a service is essential, it must be provided. A phasing-out of some services can be achieved if there is another alternative reasonably available, but where no alternative institutional option can be exercised, the only choice is to continue to operate an unprofitable service.

Any payment method must therefore have a direct relationship to the costs of operating a particular hospital. This does not mean that all existing systems need to be scrapped. It does mean that standard rates for all hospitals are unworkable. If a hospital is to be at risk for its pricing decisions, then postaudit adjustments for profits are completely illogical within an external rate review system.

The fundamental point about payment is that it is a process, and there can be no mechanistic approach to rate setting because of the many interrelated variables that affect hospital efficiency.

When management consultants judge the efficiency of hospitals, they work from a series of institutional performance indicators, and adjust the efficiency rating from its norm, either up or down, because of the unusual circumstances. Through experience, the extent of the adjustment required to reflect earnest, competent administrative effort can be judged.

USING PROSPECTIVE PAYMENT

Before any form of payment system can succeed, a large battery of performance indicators must be assembled and the conditions defined for approving variances for each indicator. Given the present state of knowledge about hospital operation, no other method can cope with hospital efficiency issues. All other schemes will eventually lead to gross inequities. Equitable treatment of hospitals is a necessity if efficiently operated hospitals within their individual circumstances are to maintain financial health, and this is the most sensible of goals for any payment program. Inequitable systems pose the long-run threat that efficient, well-managed hospitals with unique sets of unfavorable circumstances may be forced into bankruptcy.

The use of well-defined performance indicators and approved variances will not completely separate the efficient from the inefficient institutions. Assessment of quality of care levels is also an essential element to be measured and considered. Medical audit programs may ultimately fill this gap. They are now internally developed and monitored in hospitals, and must be externalized into a set of standardized parameters of medical care.

Such an event will be a long time in coming and will involve several basic issues in the philosophy of medical care.

The increasing scrutiny of quality of care has raised operating costs because new, detailed control measures, which require additional institutional procedures, are introduced as a response. Any modification that attempts categorization of hospitals will be inequitable. The initial failure will be the downgrading of medical quality in high-cost but efficient hospitals, and this will ultimately result in substantial deterioration. A long-run failure will develop because hospitals will sooner or later actively oppose the continuation of inequitable treatment by a payment system that is not based on performance indicators.

An individualized institutional payment system will require a large investment of research funds to develop meaningful performance indicators and quality assessment profiles. Several years of serious effort will be required.

Unfortunately, the imperatives of the American political process will probably ignore the need for this research. The round of legislative proposals for a national health insurance program with prospective payment requirements are global in their assumptions of practicality. It will most likely take the threatened collapse of several hospitals with national reputations before the reality of careful profile development is recognized as an imperative for an effective program.

A meat-ax approach by government should be intensively opposed by all nongovernment hospitals. If the opposition does not succeed, then hospitals can look ahead to a piecemeal program of financial propping-up of individual institutions through the use of special grants. Ultimately, the hospital field will come to see that government aid on a random, special-need basis brings about government control of hospitals on a piecemeal basis. By then the final curtain will have been lowered, and the struggle will have ended without a shot being fired in anger.

These thoughts are not a plea for a return to the good old days of uncontrolled expansion and autonomous institutional rate setting. In essence, what has been proposed is a method for identifying efficient and inefficient institutions, even those in adverse circumstances, through the development of appropriate performance indicators; for recognizing and controlling hospital expansion and development by relating reasonable need and financial responsibility; and for establishing a way to reward superior financial performance and to place poor performance at risk.

The four essential characteristics of any payment system are:

1. an established rate structure that has been reviewed by an outside authority and approved on the basis of acceptable standards of effi-

cient operations that use performance indicators and case mix as the fundamental inputs;

2. the establishment of a reasonable relationship between total debt and annual capital expenditures by size of institution, so that PL 92–603, Section 1122 reviews are not more frequently required for larger hospitals;

3. a review of the results of hospital care by an external agency to determine that the quality of medical care meets minimally acceptable standards;

4. that where external reviews exist there are no postaudit adjustments that eliminate cost factors or limit net surplus.

The goal of any system of paying hospitals for services to government program beneficiaries must be the maintenance of fiscally healthy institutions that provide readily accessible care of a quality nature at a desired level of service in a reasonably efficient manner. It is in the public interest that hospitals never compromise this goal.

Part VIII

Modern Technology

Chapter 35

Changing Patterns in Medical Care

Efforts to improve efficiency and contain hospital costs do not directly affect the major problems of medical care. The culprit that is forcing more and more dollars to flow into hospitals is neither inefficiency nor poor management, but rather a rising demand for hospital services tied to an inflation over which health care institutions have no control. Hospitals are caught between changing patterns in medical care and national economic practices.

THRUST TO DO BETTER

For the past 50 years, hospitals have been busy trying to keep pace with medical needs for more equipment, more specialized personnel, and more space for diagnostic procedures. Without consciously attempting to do so, the role of the community hospital has been permanently altered in responding to the needs of physicians. Increasingly, the hospital has become technology oriented. Social and religious motives of the past that led to the development of the voluntary hospital system have been pushed aside by the rush into specialization and intensive programs of care with their increasing emphasis on quality assurance. The modern hospital has moved from the primary ingredient of bedside nursing care to a diagnostic and treatment organization manned by specialist physicians and specialized nursing and technical personnel, all geared to finding answers for the causes of human malfunctions and then repairing them as expeditiously as possible.

The thrust for doing better has led to substituting technology for the consoling efforts of a friendly and caring nurse, who could offer little else a half century ago. Yet, the basic motivation of those who choose health careers has remained unchanged. The result has been to regard illness as an evil to overcome, to fight with all available medical weapons, and, when these prove inadequate, to find new and better weapons that can do the tasks. This blending of social ethic, enhanced professional education, and improved technology has led to a constant thrust to improve the results being obtained; to be able to perform operations that 20 years ago were considered too dangerous, to make a more rapid and safe diagnosis with noninvasive techniques, to return persons to health more quickly, and to prolong life. These are the intellectual rewards to the health professional.

The economic side of the equation—the cost to the patient, the cost to the employer, or the cost to the taxpayer—has not been an issue of concern in the past to physicians. Medical meetings used to be exclusively devoted to clinical subjects and discussions of new techniques and procedures. Even today, these are usually the only items on the agendas of physician meetings. Only within the last few years have medical agendas occasionally been broadened to include malpractice insurance and unusually long lengths of patient stays. Little else of an economic nature is typically discussed by physicians, except for the protectionist activities of each specialty group.

ECONOMIC QUESTIONS

With increasing frequency, representatives of the public are raising medical economic questions they want considered. What matters if a person can be rehabilitated from a heart attack when life savings are wiped out? The real question then is whether the costs of coping with disease have reached a point where they are disproportionate in achieving the last one percent of improvement that is possible. Has the point been reached where a fresh look is required?

Hospitals and those who pay the bills are concerned about economic questions, but neither side can come up with an acceptable alternative to the present situation. The government's approach has been to impose controls limiting the dollars it is putting into health care. This strategy does not address basic issues. Hospitals continue to strive for higher standards of patient care with the rationale that their mission is to alleviate and cure illness. The government talks money, the hospital talks patient care, and neither addresses itself to the concerns of the other party. Behind this posturing lies a dismal truth: no one knows what course of action should be followed to contain rising medical care costs.

The road ahead is not clear. During the past decade, there has been a milling around, hoping against hope, that somehow a way would develop that would break the impasse, but nothing has happened. Instead, government has tightened controls while hospitals continue to broaden their diagnostic and treatment capabilities. Both are equally right, but both are equally wrong.

Ambulatory Care

Probably most people would agree that if patients can be satisfactorily treated on an ambulatory basis, this is an economical way to provide the care. Until recently, hospitals have been noticeably reluctant to address this approach, even though hospitals have been into ambulatory care for decades in their laboratory, x-ray, physical therapy, and emergency care, and in university settings and outpatient clinics.

In the private practice arena, hospitals have not been in competition with physicians, even in communities that have experienced severe shortages of physicians. Hospitals have gone along with the medical profession's insistence that the recruitment of new physicians in a community is not a concern of hospitals; it has been, and still is, the sole province of the medical profession. The medical profession believes that when a new physician applies for hospital privileges, this is primarily a matter of concern to medicine, and hospitals should stay out of the matter.

Without realizing the implications of this position, hospital boards of trustees have gone along with this viewpoint. Trustees who also are active in business often see physicians as entrepreneurs trying to protect themselves from the encroachment of government; so when physicians say they are in private practice, the trustee's natural reaction has been to agree, which is a vote for nonparticipation by the hospital in recruiting new consumers for their services.

If hospitals are to escape the influences of the past, they must begin to change their ways and be willing to influence the quality and specialization of new physician manpower. This is a relevant consideration for hospital governing boards: to be concerned about the kinds and numbers of specialists and family practitioners in their communities. If the public is going to use ambulatory care as an alternative to hospitalization, then there has to be enough of the right types of physicians available to provide primary care. When there is an insufficient supply of the right kinds of specialists, a hospital must decide whether or not it should do the recruiting and provide new specialized facilities, and the extent to which it should guarantee or underwrite the incomes of the physicians recruited. If a hospital does not accept this responsibility, there will not be a rapid shift to ambulatory care. In most communities, it is unlikely that the medical profession, by itself, will undertake this responsibility because of personal economic considerations.

Whether or not the patient should be diagnosed and treated on an outpatient basis or on an inpatient basis has, up to now, often been decided by insurance coverages and the effect of the medical procedures upon the patient. Lately, the malpractice situation has tilted more frequently toward an inpatient admission situation. If in doubt, physicians usually hospitalize a patient.

In addition, if physician efficiency is increased by hospitalization because of the coordination and convenience of specialized instrumentation and trained personnel, then physicians usually prefer hospitalization.

Neither malpractice nor physician efficiency, however, brings on economic considerations of the person paying for a service. If, however, a person asks about the outcomes of diagnosis and treatment, and whether or not it would change, then medical economics comes into play and the equation changes. If a patient will recover to the same degree and at the same rate as an outpatient, rather than as an inpatient, then the obvious choice should be for the least costly method of providing medical care. Relatively few studies have addressed the health delivery system from a viewpoint of the outcome of illness. It is an area worthy of considerable exploration.

Prevention of Illness

There is an increasing belief that the way to limit health care expenditures is to concentrate on keeping persons healthy, rather than on returning them to health after they have incurred an illness. Hospitals, by their very nature, are repair oriented and are filled with patients whose health is already impaired. Up to now hospitals have neither had a significant role in the prevention of illness nor has there been a concerted effort among physicians to prevent illness. Physicians are disease problem solvers who are concerned with discovering and treating medical breakdowns. They, like hospitals, react to what is discovered and do not have a primary concern with preventive medical practices.

As the landscape of health care is scanned, those most actively concerned about keeping people well and out of both the physician's office and the hospital are the third party payers. To the extent they can decrease office visits and admissions, lowered utilization will improve their financial condition. To date, they have lacked a strong willingness to try innovative programs that might lead to these results. Blue Cross has chosen to support the HMO concept, perspective rates, utilization review, and controls on capital expenditures of hospitals as the way to limit the outflow of its dollars to institutions. This, of course, has not been successful, as can be attested by the fact that 50 out of 71 Blue Cross plans lost a total of $455 million in 1975.

The time has now arrived for third party insurers to consider seriously other methods of cost control. A worthwhile set of ideas might be drawn from the automobile insurance arena, where excess premium rates are charged for drivers with accidents or moving violations, or, conversely, by granting credits on premiums for drivers with long safe driving records.

A prepayment plan might offer a variety of premium rates. For persons who have had a heart attack or a stroke, there might be a surcharge on the basic premium rate, unless subscribers could present evidence that:

- They are on a regular exercise program.

- Their weight is controlled.

- They have attended a course for patients with heart disease dealing with ways of changing life style to live successfully with a disability.

Annual certification might be required in order to demonstrate continued adherence to the program. Upon receipt of an attesting statement, the premium would be lowered to a standard rate.

In the event that subscribers are healthy, they might be given credit for proper diet, exercise, nonsmoking, and other positive health indicators, thus having the benefit of a reduced premium. Where the employer now bears the full cost of the premium, it might be required that a subscriber receive the difference between a regular premium and a reduced premium, or, conversely, be required to pay the difference between a regular premium and a surcharge that might be levied for poor health maintenance practices. Such a program would be prevention at the point it would most likely be effective. The role of the hospital would be to provide training programs that would be needed for each specific disease entity.

Health Maintenance Organizations

An alternative to the present system are health maintenance organizations. Since they have been widely publicized as greatly reducing hospital admissions and thereby costs, a comprehensive appraisal should be made of their impact. In comparing fee for service with prepaid care, several considerations point toward continuation of fee for service.

CHANGES IN NURSING

Nursing care, like physician services, has also undergone considerable change in the last decade. No longer does a nurse stand up when a physician enters the nursing station. The disappearance of this symbolic gesture reflects changes that have taken place. In terms of time, physicians spend perhaps ten minutes on a nursing floor seeing patients, reading charts, and writing orders. The other 23 hours and 50 minutes of the day, the nursing staff observes and cares for patients. Today physicians, in large part, do not render care to their patients; rather, they direct the care a patient receives. Because physicians spend so little time with a patient, they must depend on nursing observations about changes in the condition of the patient. This has brought about changes in nursing and nursing attitudes.

Modern floor nurses expect to be involved in decision making about patients. They see themselves as participants in this process, no longer subordinates who unquestioningly carry out physicians' orders. This has led to the development of the concept of primary care nurses, who are responsible for the laying on of hands with patients. They function in a manner akin to that of a first sergeant in the army, accepting direction from the company commander, but with considerable freedom as to how to achieve the desired results. This change in the nursing role is sometimes upsetting to older physicians who are accustomed to unquestioned acquiescence from nursing personnel. Buttressed by court opinions on the responsibility of the hospital for patient care, nurses now report to their superiors in the organizational hierarchy any actions or decisions of physicians they consider detrimental to the welfare of the patient.

This shift in the relationship of the nurse to the physician has occurred because of an increasing technological approach to patient care in hospitals. Fifty years ago, a hospital was a building that contained patient beds and a few small marginally effective ancillary services. Today a hospital is primarily a group of ancillary services with beds attached. The increased use of ancillary services is growing at a rate about three times the rate of bed activities. No longer do physicians observe a patient, listen to various tonal sounds, and review a small number of laboratory and x-ray reports. They now order large batteries of tests and procedures, call in other specialists, and transfer the patient to specialized units for intensive care. Where they once started all intravenous therapy on a patient, this function is now performed by the nursing IV team. As technology has routinized physician's activities in the hospital, it has also freed up time. They no longer need to sit and observe a patient undergoing acute physiological changes, but can simply write an order transferring the patient to a unit with appropriate monitoring equipment under the direction of a nurse skilled in their use. Medical technology has increased both the breadth and depth of knowledge with the resultant shift of many activities from physician to nurse, which in turn has significantly modified traditional roles.

THE CHANGING ROLE OF PHYSICIANS

Through the last half century, as a hospital has evolved into a technology-based industry, the public has not understood how the role of the physician in this setting has changed. In their mind's eye, hospitals and physicians are regarded as one, with the physician dictating and controlling all activities associated with a hospital. This myth is so deeply implanted in society that the government acts on this traditional understanding in setting new rules and regulations for controlling hospitals. With increasing frequency since 1966, Congress and HHS have initiated controls that penalize hospitals for physician activities. As surrogate customers, physicians exert a great deal of influence on hospital operations. In multihospital communities, most physicians behave as customers, often threatening to shift their inpatient practice from one hospital to another unless their demands for specialized equipment and facilities are met. In effect, they shop on behalf of their patients and personal needs as expeditiously as possible.

To the hospital, physicians are consumers that need to be catered to if the institution is to hold or expand its share of the local market. A hospital cannot deal with impunity toward physicians. They are separate and apart from the hospital, even though they are also part of the hospital. This relationship is not understood by the public or government officials, who assume that hospitals control physicians' activities in the hospital. In actual practice, a hospital does not even control the number of physicians on its staff. It merely sees that physicians who apply for staff membership are reviewed by their peers to ensure that they will perform their professional duties with a reasonable degree of proficiency.

Once a physician is admitted to staff privileges, a hospital has little effective control, except in monitoring professional standards. Individual practitioners determine which patients they will admit, at what time, and which laboratory, x-ray, and other diagnostic and treatment procedures are needed by their patients. They do this without sensing any institutional constraints. As independent entrepreneurs, physicians decide what time of the day they will arrive at a hospital to see their patients, when they will go on vacation, and how hard they will work. As a group, physicians believe that as long as they practice medicine at an expected level of competency, the institution may not exert any other authority over their performance. This attitude is basic to the current hospital-physician relationship and has prevailed since the turn of the century.

CONTROLS

With the introduction of Medicare and Medicaid, the attention of government officials has turned toward controlling the amounts of monies spent on hospital care for recipients of their programs. This approach culminated in the Economic Stabilization Program of 1972–1974 and has been subsequently reintroduced in the form of proposed caps on increases in hospital revenues. Such proposals are premised on a belief that hospitals have authority to control the ways in which physicians use hospital resources in treating their patients. When penalties are imposed, they apply only to hospitals, not to physicians. Thus, even though the collective acts of a medical staff may force hospital charges to be higher than approved revenue caps, penalties are not placed on physicians. Thus, professional patient care decisions remain unrestricted and unmodified.

In essence, the demand for hospital services continues to rise and requires third party payers to seek rate increases in premiums regularly. To stay in the market, the third party response to slow the rise in costs has been to restrict payments to hospitals by a continual redefining of allowable costs, all aimed at reducing or limiting the outflow of premium dollars. Yet, control of demand depends on physician decision making since physicians determine admissions to hospitals and the ordering of services to be provided. Hospitals do not participate in either type of decision; they are only facilitating agents and, therefore, have no role in controlling demand for their services. Yet, hospitals are singled out by government programs and third party payers as the cause of uncontrolled escalating costs and are the focus of regulations.

Controls will not succeed because they are applied at the wrong point in the health care system. In order to affect demand, the physician-patient relationship must become the focal point of control. This can take one of several forms.

Some students of reimbursement believe that medical care demand will remain uncontrolled unless the patient pays part of the cost of hospitalization. They argue that many of the existing prepayment plans pick up first dollar costs as part of the benefits and impose no economic decision making on patients. Thus, a physician does not have to deal with economic pressure applied by patients who might request medical services on an outpatient basis if available and appropriate to their needs.

A suggestion often made for cost containment purposes is to control the number of physicians by type of specialty in a given area. Under this approach, the number of physicians is predetermined for each specialty in a given geographic area. Physicians are then permitted to bid for a franchise in their specialty. When awarded, their patients can be admitted to the hospital and receive full benefits under a prepayment plan. Those physicians who elect not to participate would then largely be restricted to an office practice since their patients would not qualify for third party coverage for hospital admission. Franchise grants would probably be made by the local health systems agency.

Another suggested plan would be retroactive in its application. Physicians would be free to use their own best clinical judgment with regard to the hospitalization of patients, but in the event the hospitalization fell outside the limits that are determined as acceptable by utilization review or PSRO criteria, physicians' fees would be penalized by the same percentage as that incurred by the hospital.

All of these approaches are aimed at curbing demand for hospital services and are pointed at the place where medical decisions are made—the physician-patient relationship—and not at the hospital, which has no control over demand for its services.

HOME CARE

In a different frame of reference, the concept of resorting to home care frequently receives attention. From this perspective, advocates of home care see it as a way of shortening the length of stay of the patient or as an alternative to hospitalization.

This has led to the development of ambulatory surgical centers where the patient has a one-day stay for a minor procedure, and all of the subsequent days of care are handled in the home. Studies that have been conducted on this approach indicate that approximately 30 percent of a typical hospital surgical volume can be transferred to this program.

If obstetrics is considered, the question might be raised about home deliveries, since obstetricians indicate that 85 out of 100 births are uneventful. The issue, however, relates not to the 85 percent, but to the 15 percent who encounter difficulties at birth. Since physicians cannot be assured ahead of time that they are handling all of the 85 percent, neither they nor family members are usually willing to run a 15 percent risk; therefore, nearly all births occur in hospitals, which will continue to be the site of nearly all deliveries in this country.

Traditionally, home care has been a service provided by hospitals to those who need assistance in the home; if home care is not available, the program requires that a patient move to an extended care facility. Even though home care programs have been around for many years, they are not growing in number. Of the more than 7,000 hospitals in the United States, only 270 operate these services. It seems unlikely that the future will see a change in this pattern, even though the need for such a program is probably high, particularly for elderly persons. Hospitals recognize that home care is not a substitute for hospitalization. Home care is seen by physicians as an alternative to admission to a nursing home, but not as an alternative to admission to a general hospital. Physicians tend to view home care as a service more closely akin to nursing home care rather than hospital care and, therefore, not of real advantage as an alternative to hospitalization.

CHANGE IN PUBLIC PERCEPTIONS

In recent years, as changes have occurred in hospitals, there has been a corresponding change in public perceptions. Largely through government actions, public attitudes have begun to jell about reorganizing the health delivery system. The concept that a hospital is a private corporation is being modified into that of a public utility.

Physicians have also begun to feel these winds of change. Though they still strongly believe that they are an independent profession and entrepreneurial, they are cautiously beginning to wonder when they will become controlled rather than controlling decision makers in medical care.

This change in physician thinking reflects changes in public attitudes. Today, physicians no longer introduce themselves at social gatherings as Dr. Jones. They are far more likely to say, "I'm Jim Jones," a subtle but meaningful distinction reflecting awareness of the attitude shifts now underway. What they subconsciously recognize is that a physician is now only another cog in the wheel of medical care delivery and not its sole agent controlling all elements and functions.

The present day insistence of government on avoiding unnecessary duplication of hospital services and equipment has led to an emphasis on a community's medical needs rather than on its institution's past achievements as a basis for justifying an expansion of services. Consequently, hospitals can no longer concentrate only on acute illness services to the exclusion of all other health needs, but are being required by HSAs to be meaningful participants in the development of comprehensive health care centers.

Those in the health field have, for years, believed that quality of medical care is untouchable. However, today the public may no longer share this belief. The public may be undergoing a real and permanent shift in medical attitudes, so that they are now more concerned with cost rather than quality. If this is so, hospital trustees are obliged to be sure that the focus of effort is directed to the demand side of the medical care equation and not on cost containment, which will cripple the health care industry to the point where it can no longer adequately perform its role. Certainly trustees can assist hospitals in achieving improved productivity; however, to believe this is the greatest problem confronting hospitals ignores the more important and fundamental causes leading to the public's present concerns.

The pursuit of medical excellence in quality of care can no longer be the sole goal of a hospital. It now appears that trustees must squarely face this question: "What does the American public expect of its health delivery system?" Will the goal be a revitalization of the hospital's long-standing concerns about quality of care, or will it become one of cost control even at the expense of quality? The battle has just begun, and the outcome will not be known for several years. Whichever route is eventually chosen, the results will have a profound and lasting impact on a system that has been laboriously created by dedicated trustees, hospital personnel, and physicians.

Chapter 36

Perspectives on Ambulatory Care

INTRODUCTION

While ambulatory medical care may seem to be a new concern to the health field, it is one of the oldest forms of health care. Many students in training programs may first remember a field trip to a dispensary. It was as depressing an experience as visiting the back wards of an insane asylum. Since those days, hospital costs have gone up to proportions that were never anticipated.

In the late 1960s, when rapid cost increases occurred along with a substantial reduction in primary care physicians, a patient's complex medical problem was divided up among a host of physician specialists. This led many observers and participants of the medical care system to wonder anew about the possibilities of redeveloping ambulatory care programs.

In the past ten years, a variety of approaches have been worked out. Medical centers have tried to straighten out the chaos in their outpatient clinics, the federal government has accepted the belief that ambulatory care is the cost containment wave of the future, and general hospitals have initiated ambulatory care programs to cope with medical problems of patients that overlap several areas of medical specialization.

EXAMINING THE POTENTIAL FOR AMBULATORY CARE

When hospital administrators begin to organize their thoughts about ambulatory care, they probably start by wondering how medical care in a physician's private office might be changed. As they quietly probe members of the medical staff as to what does go on, or during an office visit of their own, they may carefully observe just how the place operates. Soon they

381

begin to see new potentials for rearranging the delivery of ambulatory medical care services.

Administrators may learn that the medical diagnostic and treatment equipment available in a physician's office is in reality quite limited and reflects the physician's special interests in medicine. They find an office with a full supply of syringes, some drugs, and examining rooms perhaps with some special equipment. In a group practice there might be a centralized medical records room, a laboratory, pharmacy, and x-ray. In a large group practice, there may be a cystoscopy and outpatient operating room.

In further talks with medical staff members, they often discover physicians are interested in hospital outpatient clinics so the medically indigent are kept away from their private patients. Some specialists may be interested in starting their own ambulatory program, such as a neurological diagnostic center, because of income potential, or in having the hospital set up a program to provide expensive equipment and technician assistance because they want to avoid the necessary investment and risk involved.

As administrators get into the heart of the matter they figure out that the difference between the old and the new concept of ambulatory care is the proposed scope of service, sponsorship of the program, and, in the case of HMOs, the financing mechanism.

In the past, potentially profitable ambulatory care programs were solely the property of physicians and woe to the hospital administrator who began to talk as if the hospital were more than an economic nonentity. The development of HMOs legitimized the sponsorship of medical care by nonphysician entities, though much resistance might be encountered.

The inquiring chief executive officer has two major questions to decide if the hospital is to sponsor some type of ambulatory care. One is location, either on the hospital grounds or at some distant location. The other is the role and mission of an ambulatory program. Should it be developed to provide primary medical care, or should it be focused on specialty clinics serving needs not met by private practicing physicians? This has appeal where several different specialties are required to diagnose and treat a particular medical problem, such as pain, diabetes, sickle cell, headaches, or back injuries.

COST ADVANTAGES

Specialty clinics are a response to filling a serious unmet need that exists but cannot be met in a totally physician directed organization. On the other hand, ambulatory surgery centers have developed as an economic opportunity, providing lower direct cost to patients by eliminating overhead and a battery of routine tests usually required for inpatient admissions.

When hospital literature is reviewed for studies that clearly establish ambulatory care programs' cost advantages, none are to be found. There are many studies and *a priori* statements that demonstrate that, through the elimination of the routine daily service charge, a cost reduction is possible if ambulatory visits replace inpatient care. It all depends on how costs are counted.

In the September 1976 issue of *Inquiry,* Richard A. Elnicki reports a cost analysis of substituting outpatient for inpatient care in Florida and comes to the conclusion that outpatient care is a more expensive affair than inpatient care if more than four outpatient visits are required, because of lost wages and travel expense.[1] For one visit, the cost is estimated at 25 percent lower than the first inpatient day. In general Elnicki concludes that cost savings from substituting outpatient for inpatient care are minmimal at best.

In studies of ambulatory surgical centers, cost differences between a freestanding center and a program located in a hospital are found to occur. Hospitals use average costs in their accounting distribution, rather than marginal costs. In addition, the routine standing screening procedures required in a hospital facility raise total costs.

If cost reduction is the rationale for increasing ambulatory care programs, it is a will-of-the-wisp hope. If continuity of care, preventive medicine, patient convenience, and access are the goals, then ambulatory care is a useful concept and will probably increase both the total amount of health care rendered, its quality, and with it the total health care bill.

PHYSICIAN CONCERNS

There are several potential organizational restraints operating in hospitals that affect ambulatory care programs. When a hospital offers such a program it will usually be seen by physicians as an economic threat. Most physicians become concerned whenever additional providers arrive in their marketplace, even though they always talk about being overworked and having more patients to care for than they can possibly handle. In a similar vein many communities have experienced overt as well as subversive physician activities when a new ambulatory service is planned by nonmedical groups outside of a hospital. If medical staff appointments are needed by physicians in freestanding clinics, difficulty often arises in obtaining medical staff membership.

Fifteen years ago, membership in the local medical society was often a prerequisite for any type of medical practice in a community. Today, lack of this membership no longer bars practice in the community.

A classical point of view in a medical staff dominated by private practice physicians is that salary arrangements inhibit physician productivity, while fee-for-service reimbursement encourages maximum effort. This may be so, but only in circumstances where diagnosis and treatment procedures are straightforward, the fee structure is already defined, and complex, unusual diagnostic and therapeutic procedures are avoided. For ambulatory care programs this means that readily identifiable procedures that are not complex, have standard fees already established, and do not involve several physician specialists will fit the fee-for-service model of primary care programs and ambulatory surgery centers. In complex diagnostic areas, such as headache or pain clinics where several specialists may be required for one patient, their participation is not so clearly identifiable, thus making salary arrangements more useful.

When a fee-for-service arrangement is proposed, there are many hospital situations where physicians will balk at initiating an ambulatory care program because of hospital sponsorship. Physicians tend to see it as unethical for a hospital, even though they have not reached out to fill the medical service gap. Too often their response is that all people in the service area are receiving needed medical care. Ignored is patient convenience, continuity of care, and the fact that community studies conclusively demonstrate unmet medical need and demand.

The key to success in an ambulatory care program is to have an adequate number of physicians providing quality service. In inner-city areas the attractiveness of traditional forms of medical practice to new primary care physicians has steadily diminished, and the number of primary care physicians has declined. Until new elements of attractiveness are provided, such a trend will not be reversed. The establishment of an ambulatory care program adds nothing to this situation, unless the program appeals to young graduates in medicine.

Realism is essential in developing a program to attract new physicians to a community. There are at least two ways an ambulatory care program can appeal to physicians. The first is for the program to provide an opportunity for physicians to develop a specific panel of patients. This means that physicians retain the right to either accept or reject patients for their panel. Since some physicians do not desire to treat certain types of illness, they eventually will leave a practice if forced to provide care in which they are not interested. Staff physicians with the right acceptance can identify more closely with their patients and will have an increased concern for the patients' well-being.

The second way is for ambulatory care physicians to have an opportunity to practice on a fee-for-service basis whenever possible. New physicians are encouraged to settle in a community if they are provided incentives for above average productivity and a guaranteed fee for service. This arrangement places a floor under their income, but does not restrict their total earnings if they exceed the budgeted number of visits for the guarantee.

Because incomes of established physicians in private practice are frequently significantly higher than in ambulatory care programs, physicians recruited may leave after a short tenure if they cannot approach income levels that are available through independent practice.

Direction and supervision of physicians in an ambulatory care program when sponsored by a nonphysician-owned entity is often a sensitive issue and should be handled by a medical director. Whether the physician is fulltime, parttime, or consulting should be based on a recommendation by a medical director, approved by a majority of the fulltime physicians, and appointed by the governing body. All appointments, both fulltime and parttime, should be made by a written contract in which specific authority, responsibility, and accountability are defined. A desirable contract should include:

- the physician's responsibility for maintaining a practice schedule that has been approved by the medical director;
- participation in limited weekend, evening, and on-call service as determined by the medical director;
- the maintenance of a medical staff appointment at a local hospital;
- the responsibility for providing competent medical care to patients on his or her service;
- participation in the work of physician committees of the ambulatory care program as assigned;
- a grant of a power of attorney to the ambulatory care program for billing and collection of patient fees;
- responsibility for visiting hospitalized patients daily, or as frequently as desirable, from his service;
- recognition of the authority of the ambulatory care program for establishing a physician's fee structure;
- referral of patients to the consulting staff of the ambulatory program when additional specialized medical care is required.

The contractual responsibilities of the ambulatory care program should include:

- a definition of the method of payment and productivity level required;
- provision of the same fringe benefits as other employees of the program;
- provision for an annual contract that may be amended with 90-days notice after the first year;
- payment for malpractice insurance at the customary current limits of liability;
- authorization for the purchase of additional fringe benefits through a reduction in the minimum income guarantee of a compensating amount at the direction of the physician;
- the payment of professional and staff dues;
- provision annually for four weeks vacation;
- provision of two weeks of professional leave annually, with expenses paid by the program, for approved educational activities;
- annual review of the physician's medical and administrative performance and providing him with a written evaluation;
- authorization of the physician to accept or reject patients assigned to his service.

The contract provisions outlined apply to both a primary care program and to specialty clinics.

IMPLEMENTING AN AMBULATORY CARE PROGRAM

In the past, delivery of ambulatory care services has usually been a loosely organized program geared to the convenience of physicians and program staff. In the future a major job of ambulatory care must be implementing an organizational structure consistent with health care delivery patterns acceptable to community expectations, which is personalized care.

Scheduling System

A key element to accomplishing this goal is the scheduling system used by the program. Traditionally, a block appointment system has been used, where several patients are given appointments at the same time, usually at the beginning of the morning or afternoon hours. This type of scheduling system unduly penalizes the patient who must wait an inordinate period of time to see a physician and also creates periods of lower productivity for physicians and program staff during the late morning and afternoon hours.

A preferred method of scheduling for patient convenience is an appointment system. Typically about 80 percent of patient appointments are kept and can be adjusted as operating experience determines a specific rate for a given program.

Development of Teams

Another characteristic of an ambulatory care program should be the development of teams directed by physicians and supported by other personnel. Organizationally, an ambulatory care program should stand as an independently functioning unit within a hospital. Its medical director should be the administrative head of the program. This person is responsible for developing policies and procedures within the scope of authority of his position as established by the hospital administration.

Program directors should be responsible for daily operations. Their duties should include developing and maintaining the following functions:

- job description
- wage and salary control
- position control
- procedure manuals
- personnel policies consistent with hospital policy
- credit and billing procedures within the overall hospital financial system
- marketing activities
- short-term planning—annual
- inventory control

Operations

The operations of an ambulatory program should be grouped into three functional areas: nursing staff, business function, and professional staff.

Each area should be directed by a working supervisor. For example, the nursing staff should be directed by a designated chief nurse, who in addition to clinical responsibilities, also provides the necessary decision making to keep the nursing staff functioning efficiently and effectively. The two other areas should also have persons appointed to provide the necessary coordination and decision making needed for their activities.

The typical physician's office employs two ancillary personnel per physician. Guidelines for an integrated urban health strategy issued in December 1976 by the Health Services Administration of the then Department of Health, Education, and Welfare (HEW) call for a three-to-one ratio as a ceiling in primary health care delivery systems, which is also typical for organized group practices.[2] However, these ratios only have significance if the program is defined.

A primary care program needs to be more than competition for a private practicing physician's office if it is to meet the needs of the public in a modern way. Medical care delivery is a system with many components and functions. A major problem today with its traditional form of organization is that a patient in need of a variety of diagnostic procedures, tests, and consultations must drive all over town to obtain the necessary service, often during several different days. It is an inconvenient, time-wasting experience.

An organized ambulatory care program should make one-stop medical care a reality. This means that two-to-one or three-to-one ratios are meaningless. For example, a comprehensive primary care program should include functions for an organized approach to patient reception and scheduling, a medical records system, billing, and secretarial services in its business office. Its professional services, other than physicians, ought to include health education, pharmacy, laboratory, x-ray, electro-diagnostics, and social service. The nursing staff should use both registered nurses and nurse practitioners grouped into teams with the physician staff.

A nurse practitioner can expand the productivity of a physician by about two-thirds. The AMA *Profile of American Medicine* reported the number of visits, per week, to general practitioners as 186.3.[3] With a nurse practitioner, this capacity could be expanded to 310 visits per week, the available hours of service lengthened, and the unit cost of providing diagnostic and treatment capability significantly reduced.

To supplement the three divisions of the program, other arrangements are needed for comprehensive care. Formal referrals should be made through an organized system for dental, optometry, and podiatry services when required. Even though these practitioners are on an independent, but affiliated basis, it is desirable to have them located in the same building.

At a later stage of development, consideration may be given to incorporating these services into the ambulatory program.

Since other medical care specialists beyond the primary care physicians will be needed to provide additional diagnosis, treatment, and hospital services, a referral panel should be established.

Laboratory services for complete blood counts, blood sugars, pregnancy testing, and urinalysis should be available at the primary care program, as well as any other laboratory test that has a high volume and low capital cost. Arrangements should be made for an electrocardiogram and pulmonary function studies.

A referral capacity should also be developed for indigent patients to determine government support and provide medical care payments. Other arrangements are needed for mental health, drug addiction, and alcoholism treatment.

Location

The location of an ambulatory care program is another important factor. A usual rule of thumb is that the patient should travel 20 minutes or three miles for primary medical care. There should be easy parking and public transportation to the site.

Marketing

Simply establishing an ambulatory program, even under conditions of significant medical demand, will not generate patients. The public must know that a program has been started, its method of operation, and the services available. Potential patients must be aware of the program and be persuaded of its merits. The program will need more than "walk-in" patients. Therefore, it must develop an effective program of communication and promotion.

Traditionally, medical services have been circumspect in their promotional activities. However, in the last several years, HMOs, health insurance carriers, Blue Cross, Blue Shield, and Planned Parenthood have used promotional techniques to make the public aware of their products and services.

A properly planned effort to promote an ambulatory care program is a positive opportunity rather than a necessary evil. For effective promotion, the ambulatory care program must use an integrated communications concept. The developmental planning for an effective marketing program requires specialized communication knowledge and skills to reach the target population. This kind of marketing involves:

- who should be the spokesmen;

- what meanings and concepts should be conveyed;

- what communicating channels are most effective in delivering specific meanings to the target population;

- which parts of the target population should receive specific information.

A specific program must identify for the public their need for medical care and how the services of the program can efficiently and effectively satisfy their needs. Many media and communicating problems must be solved in the context of community characteristics in order to develop an effective marketing mix to promote an ambulatory care program.

Because the operating expenses of a new medical venture are high and can only be offset by quickly developing a patient clientele, it is important that, prior to its opening, a well-planned promotional program generates a willingness to try the medical services being offered.

A parallel requirement to a marketing effort is a satisfactory initial operation of the ambulatory care program. Patients must be promptly scheduled and seen. Staff personnel must be pleasant, concerned, and competent, and the facilities must be attractive. In essence, an ambulatory care program is entering into a competitive market situation, even though there is a potential unmet medical demand. It must be a desirable place for receiving medical services that is recognized for quality and convenience.

SUMMARY

Most of the ideas discussed have been focused on the characteristics of a general medical care ambulatory program. This kind of program is more comprehensive than the usual type of specialty clinic a hospital develops within its institutional boundaries. A hospital clinic may be anything from a designated time to see a particular kind of patient in the emergency room, such as a venereal disease clinic, to an elaborate clinic operation with 50 or 60 staff members and its own facilities.

In selecting a general type of ambulatory care program it is assumed that this is an area of great interest to most general hospitals. It is a response to the need for primary care physicians. The demand for medical care is probably greatest at this point. This has been recognized by the rapidly developing area of family practitioner residencies. Hopefully, these graduates will remain in the community.

Probably the major determinant of whether a hospital moves into ambulatory care programs is the attitude of the medical staff. Even though it has the potential of providing quality, comprehensive care in a new way, an ambulatory care program will receive physician support only from specialists who view it as a referral source. Other members of the medical staff in general practice, internal medicine, pediatrics, and obstetrics usually examine such a proposal in clinical terms, and then quietly take a position based on the economic factors that affect them.

Ambulatory care will come of age on the hospital scene in the next decade. As John F. Kennedy said in his 1961 inaugural address, "Let us begin."

NOTES

1. Richard A. Elnicki, "Substitution of Outpatient for Inpatient Hospital Care: A Cost Analysis," *Inquiry*, September 1976, pp. 245-259.
2. December 1976. Health Services Administration.
3. American Medical Association, *Profile of American Medicine.*

Chapter 37

Planning a Primary Care System Using Computerized Models

Those directly involved in the creation of a primary care system for the disadvantaged must respond to a multitude of initiates fostered by governmental and philanthropic organizations that offer financial support or that otherwise can affect the operation of a health care system. On one hand, there are many programs intended to improve the access and availability of health care to neglected populations. Some of these are community health centers, HMOs, quality assurance programs, physician assistants (PAs) and nurse practitioners (NPs), family practice residencies, and health networks. On the other hand, the adoption of any "innovation" must be tempered by the practical need to maintain an economically viable care system that can serve health needs of the population with a permanent, stable operation. Thus a manager or planner with an operational primary care system is faced with a paradox of immense practical importance, namely to exploit opportunities for program and operational improvement of the health center but to do so in a systematic, organized way that keeps economics of the operation in proper perspective.

One approach used by the Medical Center of Gary, Inc. (MCG), Gary, Indiana, utilized a set of computerized models. This permitted a strategic but detailed analysis of changes to the program and operation of the health center. Their use has created a systematic process for planning an evolving urban primary care system that serves the Gary population.

THE GARY HEALTH SYSTEM

Gary has experienced an outmigration to the suburbs of health care providers, which has left it with less than one-third the national ratio of

---

Reprinted with changes, from *Health Care Management Review* with permission of Aspen Systems Corporation, © 1978.

primary care physicians to population. In conjunction with the exodus of providers, four new hospitals have been constructed in the suburbs surrounding Gary. This has added strain on both the primary and secondary health care systems that had served the city. With the suburban hospitals involved in aggressive expansion programs, the Gary patient "market," particularly those with private insurance, has become subject to much competitive pressure. The urban Gary health care system has found itself progressively less able to compete in this struggle with dwindling resources.

Without adequate numbers of primary care providers, the existing primary care system is overcrowded. Those patients who are able to seek services elsewhere do so, leaving the Gary system overburdened with patients whose payment for services is automatically discounted or nonexistent. The Gary hospitals then have a smaller referral base, which is also biased against ability to pay. Furthermore, it is not that Gary is unable to support a quality health care system adequately, but the services in the city are now being duplicated in the suburbs.

Thus Gary reflects many of the national health care issues: rapidly rising costs, maldistribution of providers, duplication of hospital facilities and urban-suburban competition. A similar set of conditions exists across the country in hundreds of localities. The particular organizations involved may be different, the personalities certainly are different, but the general environment in which the health care system is functioning is similar.

To counteract these trends, the MCG has laid the groundwork for the development of an ambulatory primary care group practice in Gary for several years. The MCG jointly administers a family nurse practitioner program with the division of nursing at Indiana University Northwest. They also manage the Model Cities Family Health Center, which serves 1,500 Gary families primarily on a fee-for-service basis.

DEVELOPMENT OF THE AMBULATORY CARE MODEL

The MCG provides primary care and supports the provision of general health services. The proper evolution of the services offered by MCG is the central planning problem. It is a complex one because of the interaction between the needs and the provision of care.

To assist in quantitatively accounting for these interactions, a primary care model was developed. The development began two years ago in an effort to secure foundation and federal money to cover the start-up costs of an ambulatory primary group practice. The model's major purpose was to provide a systematic mechanism for relating demands to services and then computing the costs of service. Accordingly, three interrelated modules were developed to: (1) estimate potential demand; (2) determine staff requirements; and (3) provide a *pro forma* cash budget.

The Primary Care Potential Demand Module

The northern two thirds of Gary, with a population of 140,000 people, served as the target area. This population and its area became the focus for a population-based approach.[1] The demand module was developed to determine the potential demand at the medical center. Figure 37-1 summarizes the general approach.

First, potential demand of the target population was corrected for both social and economic factors. It was assumed that only 75 percent of the black population and 50 percent of the white population would use primary care providers within the city. An explicit function relating utilization to family income was developed but discarded, since it proved to be an inadequate description of demand.

Second, potential demand for each census tract within the target area was corrected for the geographic accessibility between the particular census tracts and the site of the ambulatory primary care facility. For Gary, in regard to potential demand due to distance to the facility, no reduction in demand was assumed for persons living in a three-mile radius of the facility. A straight line reduction in potential demand equaled zero at a distance of seven miles from the facility. This distance function was developed for the particular circumstances in Gary and may not be applicable to other situations. More complicated distance functions were rejected because they lacked justification.[2]

Finally, remaining potential demand numbers were further reduced to reflect the existing medical care system. Some 22 fulltime equivalent (FTE) primary care physicians practice within the target area, and their yearly patient load was computed using overall physician productivity measures.[3]

The local service utilization pattern was used to determine the potential demand in visits per year for the population left in each of eight age-sex cohorts for each of eight services. The output of the demand module showing these results is found in Table 37-1. The choice of the eight age-sex cohorts is based on the logical subdivision by age and sex according to children (less than 15), young adults including women of the childbearing ages (15 to 44), adults (45 to 65) and older persons (greater than 65). The illness, or service type, was derived from discussions with the medical staff. Furthermore, these categories are not uncommon in the planning literature.[4]

Figure 37-1 Design of Demand Module

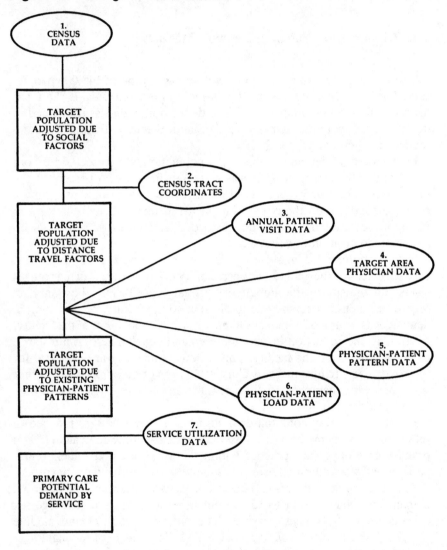

Table 37-1 Number of Patient Visits per Year by Age/Sex Cohort and Illness Type

	Cohort	1 Male 0-14	2 Female 0-14	3 Male 15-44	4 Female 15-44	5 Male 45-64	6 Female 45-64	7 Male 65+	8 Female 65+	Total
Acute	1	7,033.54	8,566.76	7,431.57	4,611.33	4,438.34	3,390.50	984.68	616.23	37,072.94
Chronic routine	2	2,344.51	2,855.59	2,972.63	4,611.33	3,328.75	3,390.50	1,969.36	1,232.46	22,705.13
Chronic follow-up	3	2,344.51	2,855.59	1,486.31	2,305.66	2,219.17	2,260.33	1,477.02	924.34	15,872.93
Health maintenance (Λ 15)	4	18,756.10	22,844.70	—	—	—	—	—	—	41,680.00
Health maintenance (Σ 15)	5	—	—	7,431.57	4,611.33	6,657.51	3,390.50	1,969.36	616.23	24,676.50
Nurse visits	6	9,378.05	11,422.35	5,945.26	9,222.65	3,328.75	3,390.50	2,461.70	1,540.57	46,689.00
Trauma	7	7,033.54	8,566.76	4,458.94	6,916.99	2,219.17	2,260.33	984.68	616.23	33,056.64
OB/GYN	8	—	—	—	13,833.98	—	4,520.67	—	616.23	18,970.88
Total		46,890.24	57,111.74	29,726.28	46,113.27	22,191.70	22,603.33	9,846.80	6,162.29	240,645.65

The Primary Care Potential Demand Module takes the following seven inputs and produces a table listing the potential primary care demand by service for each of eight population cohorts. (See Figure 37-1):

1. census data
2. census tract coordinates
3. annual patient visit data
4. target area physician data
5. physician-patient pattern data
6. physician-patient load data
7. service utilization data

The Primary Care Providers Staffing Module

The potential demand was put into the staffing module, which produced a projected staffing pattern. This module uses a linear programming approach to allocate optimally primary medical services to meet the predicted primary care demand, a method used by others.[5-7] Details concerning the model development are contained in Whitford.[8]

In the Gary setting, eight different categories of manpower are considered fundamental to the primary care mission:

1. general or family practice physicians (GP)
2. pediatricians (PED)
3. obstetrician/gynecologists (OB/GYN)
4. internists (INT)
5. family health practitioners (FHP)
6. pediatric health practitioners (PHP)
7. OB/GYN health practitioners (OB-GYN HP)
8. licensed practical nurses (LPN)

Health practitioners HPs can either be NPs or PAs. The FHP can work with either the general practice or the internal medicine patient. The use of health practitioners rather than RNs reflects the bias of the Gary practice setting. With only slight alteration in the input data, RNs could be used.

The same eight service classifications used by the demand module are used in the staffing module. The demand for each of these services in the form of annual office visits was produced by the demand module. (See Table 37-1.)

The staffing module also uses a construct called service techniques. A service technique is a combination of health care providers who are capable of satisfying a specific set of services. Again in conjunction with medical and administrative personnel, eight service techniques were identified and used in the staffing module:

1. GP/LPN
2. PED/LPN
3. OB-GYN/LPN
4. GP/FHP/LPN
5. GP/FHP/LPN
6. PED/FHP/LPN
7. OB-GYN/OB-GYN FHP/LPN
8. INT/FHP/LPN

The staffing module is capable of determining staffing patterns to meet the specified demand under one of the following three objectives:

1. The supply of primary care services is greater than or equal to demand, and physician, health practitioner, and LPN costs are minimized.
2. The supply is greater than or equal to demand, and physician usage is minimized.
3. The supply is maximized under limited physician, health practitioner, and LPN employment.

Given one of the above objectives, four data sets must be supplied:

1. a table of annual manpower costs for each type of manpower
2. annual demand for each type of service from the demand module
3. maximum staffing of each type available
4. a table of times in which each team of providers (each service technique) can provide a particular service; for example, GP/LPN can provide service for illness type acute in 12 minutes for the GP and 6 minutes for the LPN

Two types of output are obtained. The first, which is found in Table 37-2, is the allocation of provider teams (known by the service techniques) to supply the specified demands allocated by specific services. Also total annual medical personnel costs are given. The second output, which is found in Table 37-3, provides the final staffing pattern according to the category of personnel. When the demand data for Gary were input, it was determined that an additional 40 primary care providers along with 80

Table 37-2 Staffing Module, Personnel Allocation

Illness/Service Type	Number of Demanded Visits
Acute	
PED/LPN	12,616
PED/HP/LPN	24,456
Chronic Routine (PED/HP/LPN)	22,704
Chronic Flare-up (INT/HP/LPN)	15,872
Health Maintenance	
Children (PED/HP/LPN)	41,600
Adults (GP/HP/LPN)	24,676
Nurse Visits (PED/LPN)	46,688
Trauma	
GP/LPN	25,036
PED/LPN	8,020
OB/GYN (GP/HP/LPN)	18,972
Total	240,640

Table 37-3 Staffing Module, Staffing Pattern

Speciality	Number of Personnel Required
Physician (GP)	18.84
Physician (PED)	18.20
Physician (OB/GYN)	—
Physician (INT)	2.88
Health Practitioner (GP)	37.68
Health Practitioner (PED)	36.48
Health Practitioner (OB-GYN)	—
Health Practitioner (INT)	5.76
LPN	59.52

health practitioners would be needed to meet fully the potential demand existing in Gary.

Although the staffing module was limited by its inputs and the strict assumptions that must be made in using such a technique, it does provide several benefits. It forces the planner to examine closely the assumptions and data on which staffing judgments are made. It permits a convenient mechanism to all data supplied and quickly evaluates the effect of changes. Finally, it creates in some sense an "ideal" staffing pattern; the judgment of the planner is still essential, but the model provides additional information on which to base judgment.

The *Pro Forma* Cash Budget Module

The model had been developed to include the demand prediction and staffing design when HEW announced guidelines for the Urban Health Initiative Program under Section 330 of the Public Health Service Act. With the estimates of potential demand and staffing need from the demand module and the staffing module, projections were made for the utilization and staffing of an ambulatory primary care center in Gary that would qualify under the Urban Health Initiative Program. In order to establish whether such an ambulatory primary care center could attain self-sufficiency in Gary, a *pro forma* cash budget was needed. The budget module was therefore developed to translate utilization and staffing projections over a three-year period into *pro forma* revenue and expense budgets.

The budget module was designed to be time dependent. Service utilization projections, and direct and indirect costs are input for 24 time periods. *Pro forma* cash flow revenue and expense budgets are generated by the budget module for these same periods. These time periods could be 24 months in a two-year time span, 24 quarters in a six-year time span, or any other logical combination of periods and total time span.

The output of the budget module gives the line item revenues and expenses, the net revenue (loss) for each time period, and the cumulative net revenue (loss) as seen in Table 37-4. From the final *pro forma* cash budget, the manager can make direct determinations of payback, the time period during which the net investment in startup costs is recouped, and the net investment. More sophisticated calculations leading to return on investment, net present value, or yield can be derived from the output data.

The budget module does not include rates of inflation of either costs or revenues. If the circumstances are such that the relationships between the rate of inflation of costs and the expenses will vary over time, this will have to be accounted for in the input data or corrected in the output.

The relevant financial output factors are highly dependent on the patient utilization projections. Working from the total unmet potential demand produced by the demand module, the manager, over a period of time, develops a projection or a series of projections of the actual patient utilization. The input of the budget module does not require estimates of the type of services required; this is taken care of in matching the type of staffing to the type of demand. The input of the budget module must, however, break out the patient visits for each time period into four cate-

Table 37-4 Output from Final *Pro Forma* Cash Budget (Time Periods in Quarters)

	Time Period											
	1	2	3	4	5	6	7	8	9	10	11	12
Start-up costs	84,000	—	—	—	105,000	—	—	—	—	—	—	—
Direct health expenses	17,673	60,543	88,377	104,761	181,508	188,394	195,279	230,793	250,086	253,529	256,972	260,414
Supp. service expenses	—	—	—	—	9,125	8,775	8,925	8,975	9,475	8,975	9,075	8,975
Administrative expenses	30,788	59,695	59,695	59,695	82,830	82,830	82,830	82,830	88,330	88,330	88,330	88,330
Net expenses	132,461	120,238	148,072	164,456	378,463	279,999	287,034	322,598	347,891	350,834	354,377	357,719
Net income	—	27,225	68,063	116,589	184,674	241,496	298,319	340,936	365,635	393,761	421,886	450,012
Net cash flow	(132,461)	(93,013)	(80,009)	(47,867)	(193,789)	(38,502)	11,285	18,338	17,744	42,927	67,510	92,293
Cumulative net cash flow	(132,461)	(225,474)	(305,483)	(353,350)	(547,139)	(585,642)	(574,357)	(556,019)	(538,275)	(495,349)	(427,839)	(335,546)

gories. In the Gary area these are initial office visits, repeat office visits, initial hospital visits, and repeat hospital visits.

The output of the staffing module that provides the type of personnel and the amount of time needed by those personnel to fulfill the potential demand for each service type is an excellent tool to structure charges to reflect costs. In Indiana, however, and in many other states, charges for ambulatory services as reimbursed by Medicaid and Medicare are not directly related to costs. Only four categories of charges for the revenue budget were selected. The eight services used in both the demand module and the staffing module can be divided into these four categories, or further adjustments in the model can be made.

The following sets of data are required to produce the Revenue *Pro Forma* Cash Flow Budget:

- billed revenue rates for services

- utilization rates for ancillary services

- per primary care visit

- percentage of revenue lost due to indigents

- percentage of revenue lost due to discounts

- projected distribution of patient visits by period

The input data for the Expense *Pro Forma* Cash Flow Budget are structured in such a way to assist the manager in cost accounting. Total costs dependent on production units—that is, visits—are computed by the budget module based on unit cost factors provided as input. Staff costs are based on the hiring schedule and the salary, both provided as input. The time independent total salary cost calculated by the staffing module is related to the salary costs per period used by the budget module, but they are not directly comparable.

The costs are divided into categories of direct health care expenses, supplemental health care expenses and administration expenses. For each category, four sets of data are needed: (1) a table of salary expenses for each individual by time period; (2) costs directly related to staffing; (3) unit costs related to the number of office visits; and (4) fixed costs.

No account for a delay in cash receipts due to late payment is made by the model. The manager can introduce such a factor by artificially adding an appropriate delay in the patient utilization projection, which will delay all revenue but also delay unit costs.

THE GARY MODEL PROVED USEFUL

The Gary model proved particularly useful in negotiations with HEW Region V staff and Project Review Committee. As questions were raised, different utilization projections, cost factors, salary ratios, and utilization rates were put into the budget module to obtain *pro forma* budgets. The effect of different inputs on the bottom line could be quickly measured.

In August 1977, the ambulatory primary care program in Gary was funded under the Urban Health Initiative Program. The projections showed that by the end of the third year of operations, 80,000 patient visits per year would be serviced by eight primary care physicians and 16 health practitioners. The total startup cost is estimated to be $585,000. The ambulatory primary care group practice is projected to show a quarterly profit during its seventh quarter of operation.

The utility of any development is in its use. It would be misleading to state that the model as developed for the Gary health scene is a panacea for the planning problems faced. It is not. It is, however, a tool that has been useful in several ways. It has created a disciplined approach to the collection of data and the statement of assumptions regarding the planning for the ambulatory care group practice. It has become a convenient tool for easily changing data and assumptions, and evaluating the results. It has provided confidence to investors who might finance the start-up of any group practice. Finally, it has created an atmosphere for the coordinated discussion of determining demand, providing supply, and computing economics. All these features lead to better planning and should lead to better decisions.

Much has been written about the impact of technology on medicine. The process of evaluating both the benefits derived from technological improvements and the cost of such improvements is topical. Much has also been written about the potential impact of technology on health care delivery. The primary care group practice model described earlier takes established modeling technology and applies it straightforwardly to the problem of setting up and monitoring a primary care practice. No doubt widespread use of these and similar tools can assist the health care manager or planner as the problems of health care delivery grow in complexity.

NOTES

1. M.A. Baum, "A Model for the Examination of Urban Primary Care Health Care Delivery Systems with Special Emphasis on the Poor" (Washington, D.C.: The American University, 1971). Ph.D. dissertation.

2. L.J. Shuman, C.P. Hardwick, and G.A. Huber, "Location of Ambulatory Care Centers in a Metropolitan Area," *Health Services Research* 8, no. 2 (Summer 1973): 121–38.

3. American Medical Association, *AMA Profile of American Medicine, 1976–1977* (Chicago, Ill.: AMA).

4. A. Donabedian, *Aspects of Medical Care Administration: Specifying Requirements for Health Care* (Cambridge, Mass: Harvard University Press, 1973).

5. P.T. Ittig, *Planning Ambulatory Health Care Delivery Systems* (Ithaca, N.Y.: Center for Urban Development Research, Cornell University, 1974).

6. K.R. Smith et al., "Analytic Framework and Measurement Strategy for Investigating Optimal Staffing in Medical Practice," *Operations Research* 24, no. 5 (September-October 1976):815–41.

7. C.P. Schneider and K.E. Kilpatrick, "An Optimum Manpower Utilization Model for Health Maintenance Organizations," *Operations Research* 23, no. 5 (September-October 1976):869–89.

8. J.P. Whitford, "Primal Medical Care Model," (West Lafayette, Ind.: Purdue University School of Industrial Engineering, 1977). Master's project.

Part IX

Planning the Future

Chapter 38

Puzzlement for Hospital Planners

DUPLICATION OF SERVICES

If there was ever an enigma for hospital planners to unravel, the problem of institutions doubling and redoubling services is likely to become a classic in the field. The rallying cry for planners and cost controllers is for hospitals to stop duplicating services. What does this mean?

Government regulated planning is fast developing into a powerhouse of authority and control. Hospital administrators need to organize their thoughts and arguments to discuss and deal with appropriate definitions and their implications if a cliché is to be prevented from leading hospital planners into unwise decisions.

Planners have amassed greater authority than their abilities to cope with the emotions aroused by the specter of wasted scarce resources. Until the need for total balanced hospital operation is recognized as an organizational imperative, the dangers will remain. Present day planners are also reacting rather than acting to understand the complexities of hospital operation.

It is deceptively simple to state that hospitals should stop duplicating existing services because it wastes scarce resources. With more than nine percent of the GNP of the United States, or more than $200 billion, spent annually on all forms of health care, it is easy to find support for this statement. Unfortunately, what this statement means has not been defined in its operational implications.

The issue is not as simple as it sounds. To decide whether or not a duplicated hospital service is wise or unwise involves a series of considerations, some financial, other psychological, and still others of institutional survival.

The cliché, "stop duplicating institutional services," usually refers to preventing the development and operation of a hospital service or department in another hospital, when a less expensive alternative is to use an existing hospital service to its maximum capacity. Cobalt therapy, open heart units, and obstetrical services are examples used to plead the case.

Specialized hospital services or departments will become lower unit cost operations because of additional economies of scale if their use is maximized. This concept depends, however, on the basic technological process, the available knowledge, the capital investment required, the number of skilled people on hand, and the ability to control the market.

How much greater efficiency is there in a ten-man barber shop than in a one-man operation? The basic technological process is always the same, one man and a pair of scissors. All that can be done is to spread the overhead of the operation. Compare this with a large capacity computer company that operates in a batch process mode handling premium notices for a dozen life insurance companies. To add one additional company will generate almost total profit; to lose one company will not significantly reduce costs. To hospitals, the benefits of either nonduplication or sharing services is someplace between these two extremes.

The problem of duplicating services has both an internal and an external aspect for an individual hospital. Internally, it means an unnecessary expansion of facilities or services. Externally, a second hospital creates excess capacity by organizing the same service, which is not needed. Consequently, on internal doubling of services, planners talk about excess institutional capacity, and externally they refer to it as duplication of services.

SHARING SERVICES

The other side of the coin for nonduplication of services is shared services. When a person wishes to avoid duplicating a service, a provision must be made to make the blocked service available to patients hospitalized in the institution. In other words, the potential total range of medical care and support services must be available to all patients, whether they are in a 50-bed rural hospital or a 500-bed medical center. It does not imply that all potentially useful programs should be on hand in small hospitals, but rather that a plan has been organized that operates smoothly and reliably to transfer patients to a facility that offers the service.

In the national medical care system, many shared services are available, or in a reverse sense, steps have been taken in communities to prevent duplication. These services include blood bank centers, computers, intensive care newborn nurseries, intensive care units, coronary care units, burn units, trauma centers, renal dialysis services, transplant services, tissue-typing centers, emergency rooms, operating suites, outpatient clinics, pharmacy departments, housekeeping and laundry services, dietary kitchens, parking, rehabilitation services, obstetrical care, psychiatric units, neurosurgery, neurology, proctology, plastic surgery, ophthalmology, pediatrics, metabolic diseases, health education for patients, hospital staff education, medical education, abortion clinics, radiation therapy, laboratory, pathology, radioisotopes, anesthesia, open heart stations, printing, maintenance, billing and collection, and administrative services.

The only essential hospital function is nursing care service, and even in this specialized area, efforts at nonduplication occur.

WHAT IS A HOSPITAL?

The ultimate question left after mentioning the range of hospital services that have been limited or shared is, "What is a hospital?" Apparently its only essential function is nursing.

For about 20 years this question has been deliberated. It was first defined in the late 1940s in Hill-Burton legislation when a definition became essential for licensing. Subsequently, in the mid-1960s, the same kind of problem was faced when federal legislation dealt with nursing homes, skilled nursing home care, and extended care. With the present emphasis on legislating health care planning, it has arisen again, this time in the context of subunits of hospitals. The old definitions are no longer useful.

If legislated planning is to prevent unwise duplication of hospital services, a new definition of hospitals is needed. A careful look must be taken at existing theories of administration if rational, workable guidelines are to be developed. Since all hospitals today exist as a corporate form of organization, the theories of corporate structures should be used to locate meaningful benchmarks.

DECIDING ON SPECIFIC PROGRAMS

Seven Elements of Concern

Although the accepted planning process now in vogue is well thought out, it does not reflect the total scope of issues with which hospital administrators are concerned. The individual hospital corporation must analyze seven major issues when it considers whether or not to start, phase out, or expand any particular program.

Reasonable people within an organization frequently disagree over the importance of each element in decision making on a specific program. The reason for differing opinions is that personal judgment is involved in determining when to duplicate services. The information needed for this decision is a mixture of value judgments and hard data. In the last analysis, the elements reflect the overall costs of operating a hospital, though some have either a secondary or tertiary relationship to costs.

Operating Cost

The seven elements of concern apply equally to internal and external expansions. Of the seven elements, two are direct cost considerations. The first is the operating costs of a hospital service. These are the expenses incurred by hiring personnel, buying supplies, and retraining people, and the overhead costs, such as housekeeping, telephones, maintenance, insurance, and services needed from other hospital departments. Offsetting operating expenses is the amount of revenue that will be generated by the service to pay for the additional costs. This equation then must be analyzed in terms of the productivity level that can be attained, and an estimate must be made of optimal efficiency. If this is ignored, the charges for the service may be too high and unfair to patients. Just because there may be a sufficient number of patients who will pay twice a reasonable charge for a service is no reason to ask them to do so when it is operating at 50 percent efficiency. Too often the question of equity is ignored or disregarded by hospital people promoting a project or by physicians striving to develop a particular medical capability.

Capital Investment

The second cost element is capital investment. To start a new service, special rooms and equipment may be required. Modern medical procedures often require several hundred thousand dollars in building expansion or remodeling, as well as in expensive instruments. This is a one-time cost that must be made to initiate a new service, so it is capitalized, or, in accounting terms, the cost is allocated over the anticipated life of the service. Generally speaking, a new service in a hospital has a capital cost of 2½ to 3 times the operating cost.

Technological Process

The third and fourth elements of technological and organizational processes have a secondary relationship to hospital costs. They are real, but are buried in the issue of overhead costs; they may either be insignificant or of major importance, depending on the size and complexity of the new service.

A third element, which reflects the variety of things that are mixed into an organization called a hospital, is technological process. The mechanics or technology of preparing and delivering a meal to a patient is altogether different than giving medication, a radioactive isotope procedure, or a linear accelerator treatment. In many services, the technological procedure is so complex that heavy demands for cooperation and servicing are experienced by many other hospital departments.

In other cases the procedure is so simple that there is a negligible effect. The impact of the technological process is particularly serious when it involves major mechanical services in a hospital, such as electrical, air-handling, sterility, and specialized patient services. Many times the technology of a service must also be related to the availability of outside support services from other corporations. This is often judged on the reliability of the instruments. A major part of any technology consideration is its rate of obsolescence.

Organizational Process

The fourth corporate element is organizational process. A hospital structure exists to control and direct the functions and services that it provides. When a new service is under consideration, there must be an analysis of its present control mechanism to assess its ability to incorporate a new program. How good are its training capacities, its recruiting abilities, the quality control procedures, the financial controls, and its resourcefulness in handling the unpredictable? For small, unspecialized programs, no difficulties are encountered. When large, technologically sophisticated services are to be operated, a long hard look at the organizational process is required.

Unfortunately, planning agencies rarely have the courage or ability to assess the administrative capacity of a hospital when facing the issue of duplicating services. Yet, the ultimate success or failure of a new service hinges on this. Sooner or later planning agencies will have to begin to make judgments about the competence of administrative staffs in hospitals. When this step is taken, hospitals will experience planning agencies as adversaries rather than as friendly and helpful.

Time Perspective

The last three elements are tertiary in their cost relationships but are of equal significance. The fifth element is time perspective. If an individual knew that in four years there would be a need for two new units of a particular service in two hospitals, would it be better to start both at once on a smaller basis or to phase them in sequentially?

Often, public interest reaches a peak on a particular project, and it cannot be rekindled in the future. Is it wise to capitalize on this interest and start two units, or is it better to risk a lack of future concern and an inability to amass the necessary resources to start a second unit? Another way of looking at this issue is to consider risking a major commitment of hospital resources in one large project or spreading the financial risk by starting two smaller units so that, even if it fails, both institutions will survive.

Human Behavior

The sixth element is human behavior, particularly that of the physician. Status, ego satisfaction, technical capability, and amenability to external pressures must be considered. If a hospital does not move ahead and develop a new program from time to time, some of the more competent and concerned physicians may shift their loyalties to another hospital and thereby depreciate the quality of care in their present hospital.

Also, within the present organizational structure there may be such a high degree of empire building and isolation from overall hospital concerns that any new service that impinges on present activities will be undermined by incumbent dictators.

A decision to do or not to do something in an organization is a two-way street. Those who desire to make a change must accept it as well as to those who will be affected by the change. This fact is often overlooked by planners busily preparing a new design for tomorrow's modern medical care.

Acceptability in the Marketplace

A corollary that operates with the human behavior element is the seventh element, the acceptability of a new service in the marketplace. A hospital service must be desired and used by patients and physicians. One of the most researched areas in planning is the problem of patients and physicians, particularly patient convenience. Acceptability also means whether or not Blue Cross, Blue Shield, commercial insurance carriers, and government programs will pay for new services. Some desirable programs of care are often excluded from payment under these contracts. For example, there are severe limits to reimbursement for health education services and for service to medicare and medicaid patients when planning approval has not been given for a new service.

Applying the Elements

Determining when duplicated hospital services should be prevented or allowed is a complex judgment in terms of these seven elements. No standardized formula can be applied evenhandedly to reach a decision. Within the limits of existing knowledge, the best that can be done is to apply these criteria to a situation as dispassionately and as analytically as possible.

Planning literature frequently uses open heart stations, cobalt bombs, and laundries as examples of wasteful duplications. There are obvious examples of abuse, but these have been overemphasized, and little credit has been given for the voluntary restraint of hospitals in other service areas.

With a lack of sophistication and experience in present day planning staffs, it is unlikely that a reasonable capacity now exists for handling decisions of this complexity. To grant authority to planning agencies for controlling hospital initiative and avoiding duplication of services is to risk stifling progress in medical care.

To understand the potential for damage, all a person has to do is review government hospital systems. Innovation in the technology of medicine and in hospital administration is not a hallmark for them. Most new developments have arisen in medical systems where greater flexibility has been available.

The most common observation about the cause of duplicating services is that physicians influence trustees and hospitals to create unneeded programs of care. This is true to a limited degree. Trustees, administrators, and community members also encourage unneeded programs.

With the list of opportunities for avoiding duplication of services already listed, it is obvious that this criticism is overworked. An administrator wants to satisfy an important and useful clinician, but also wants the hospital to survive and prosper as an institution, which means the expansion of both the range and depth of services.

What needs to be recognized is that the government bureaucracy fears coming to grips head on with the medical profession. To confront the freedom of private enterprise openly is to risk shaking one of America's fundamental tenets and to arouse emotional responses rather than reasoned responses.

Knowing this, bureaucrats mask the goal of controlling medicine by using a tangential approach; they develop control mechanisms for hospitals that they know will impinge on physicians. An example of this tactic is restricting the number of cystoscopy rooms in a hospital. When the hospital is prevented from expanding to meet the needs of urologists, the ultimate effect is felt by the specialists who need more operating time. Sooner or later, urologists will leave the community to work in a nearby hospital that has expanded to meet their needs.

Another problem with the bureaucrats' strategy is that it creates a situation of conflict in a hospital, and the wrong people are held accountable by physicians. For any defined population there are criteria to determine the number and type of specialties needed. It is more sensible to confront the issue head on than to start a process of obfuscation. Unfortunately, the political impact of organized medicine is so powerful that the new designers of medical care systems choose not to deal with them.

Another alternative to hitting the medical lobby directly is to encourage the consumer advocate. This is an attempt to get someone else to do a job that the bureaucrats dread.

The operation of medical care in this country involves the manipulation of a system that is highly complex. Simple answers to sophisticated problems provide only irresponsible responses. The best intended consumer advocate cannot overcome ignorance by the best of intentions.

This does not imply that there is no role for consumer representatives. Planning agencies must present choices to public representatives to force consideration of the value of one patient's life as compared to the alleviation of pain or impaired functioning of a much greater number of people.

Such choices are extremely difficult, but the persons making them today are the hospital administrator and the physician. In all probability, this practice will continue.

Without courage in planning activities, mindless duplication of services will continue. Until much more thoughtful consideration is given to the kinds of issues raised, hospital operation will remain a puzzle to hospital planners, and needless doublings will occur.

Chapter 39

Progress in Planning

HEALTH PLANNING LEGISLATION

Hill-Burton

Shortly after the close of World War II, hospital planning emerged as a requirement of the 1946 Hill-Burton legislation. Until recently, hospital planning was highly informal, unsophisticated, and conducted on a voluntary basis. Much of what passed for hospital planning was catch-up planning, where the local hospital built beds as fast as it could raise the money to keep up with the increasing population that was moving into its primary service area. There was no concern with overbedding or retiring long-term debt with empty hospital beds.

Comprehensive Health Planning

With the advent of P.L. 89-749 and Comprehensive Health Planning (CHP) in 1969, a more comprehensive approach to health care planning developed. The planning process remained basically voluntary, however, decision-making bodies were formed at local and state levels and were composed of consumers and community representatives.

From 1969 to 1970, these CHP agencies were responsible for reviewing and commenting on proposed health care programs. They had no authority to approve or disapprove these programs, however, and their activities were limited primarily to federally supported projects. In many cases, CHP agencies' plans and priorities were inconsistent with other federally sponsored programs, such as the Regional Medical Programs. Around 1970, state legislatures began to enact certification of need laws to establish a process of mandatory review and approval for all health related programs regardless of sponsorship.

Social Security Amendments of 1972

Requirements specified in Section 221 of P.L. 92-603, the Social Security Amendments of 1972, empowered the secretary of HEW to withhold or reduce reimbursement to hospitals under Medicare and Medicaid if capital expenditures were inconsistent with area health needs as defined by the designated planning agencies. Section 234 of P.L. 92-603 required health facilities to receive planning agency review of any anticipated capital expenditure in excess of $100,000. Furthermore, the hospital's capital expenditure plan had to be projected for at least three years.

National Health Planning and Resources Development Act

To hospitals, P.L. 92-603 imposed increasing responsibility to sophisticate and document planning efforts never before required. As if this legislation were not enough for hospitals, Congress passed P.L. 93-641, the National Health Planning and Resources Development Act of 1975. This law gave greater authority to the planning agencies, imposed cost controls, potentially reorganized planning areas, and, to some, paved the way for national health insurance. The law sought to accomplish its goals in four major ways. First, it required a state-by-state implementation of certificate of need programs. Next, it replaced or extensively revised Hill-Burton, Regional Medical Programs, and Comprehensive Health Planning with a uniform, layered planning and development system extending from the national to local levels. Third, it established a method for evaluating the appropriateness of existing health care services and facilities. Finally, it proposed creating a national accounting system for monitoring the volume and costs of services provided by health care facilities.

Hospital responsibilities in planning under P.L. 93-641 are extensive and hold that federal officials have the authority to intervene in the health delivery system. When enacted, Eugene J. Rubel, HEW's Bureau of Health Planning and Resources Development director, stated: "We (the federal government) are now very definitely intervening in the private practice of medicine and in the organization and operation of health care institutions and the primary reason is dollars."[1]

Reflecting on the recent history of health care planning in the United States, it has been an era of perpetual change, which is likely to continue. Hospitals who fail to recognize the dynamics of health planning legislation and the changed nature of health care planning are going to have an increasingly difficult time.

OTHER FORCES

A number of forces other than health planning legislation have been at work, but all focus on the hospital's front door. They include:

- a continuing rise in construction costs

- increasingly complex and costly medical equipment

- increasingly higher interest rates

- a greater proportion of hospital revenue from cost reimbursement sources

- prospective rating programs

- a larger number of average gross square feet (GSF) per bed

- greater acceptance of comprehensive health planning

- greater intervention at the federal and state levels

- greater emphasis on ambulatory care

- a more mobile population, as well as a growing one

- a rising expectation among the public for more adequate health care delivery systems, resulting from increased public awareness of health care costs

All of these pressures have changed planning requirements for the future.

Well known to all have been the rising costs of construction. Between 1960 and 1967, construction costs rose approximately 3 percent per year, but between 1967 and 1971, construction costs escalated at an average annual rate of over 10 percent. Within the last three to four years, construction costs have increased at a rate of 12 to 14 percent or a total of approximately 40 percent during the period. Many metroplitan areas have reported hospital construction costs in the neighborhood of $100 to $120 per GSF. These costs are approximately double those for typical school and office space construction in the same region because of the complex requirements of a hospital building.

Not only has the cost per GSF been escalating, but the average number of GSF per bed has also been increasing. As hospitals have added new

programs that have enhanced the comprehensiveness of the services offered, proportionately less of the total space has been devoted to beds and
to direct nursing care activities. Stated another way, most of the growth
realized in the last few years has occurred in the ancillary departments,
such as emergency room, laboratory, and x-ray. A half century ago, nursing
units made up over 50 percent of all of the available floor space in a hospital.
Today, nursing units represent approximately 20 percent of the total gross
square footage of a hospital. Where hospitals averaged 600 to 650 GSF
per bed in the past, the typical community hospital is now being built in
the range of 1,000 to 1,200 GSF.

The impact of these increases on the voluntary not-for-profit hospital
has led to two trends:

1. Old, obsolete hospitals will be closed because of their inability to
   cope with the capital funding problems of rebuilding.
2. New hospitals in new communities will not be built because of the
   high initial costs involved in a freestanding venture, but may be built
   if part of a multihospital system.

An historical perspective, shown in Table 39-1, reveals that the financial
implications of a major capital program are clear.

Given these conditions, existing hospitals will have to broaden their
horizons and take on responsibility for building and operating additional
hospitals in a local multihospital system. Gifts and community fund raising
will be unable to provide the basic capital fund requirements to build new
freestanding hospitals.

Table 39-1 Historical Perspective of Financial Implications

Factor	1965	1975	1980
Average GSF per bed	600	900	1,100
Average construction cost per GSF	$45	$70	120
Minimum size project	100 beds	200 beds	200 beds
Construction cost	$2,700,000	$12,600,000	26,400,000
Project cost (est.)	$3,518,100	16,512,300	35,600,000
Fund-raising factor	1,500,000	1,500,000	1,500,000
To be financed	$2,018,100	$15,012,300	$34,100,000
At 70% of project cost	1,412,670	10,508,610	23,870,000
Hospital's obligation	$ 596,430	$ 4,503,690	$10,230,000

The increased amount of dollars needed to be financed and what the hospital must contribute become an effective barrier to undertaking the project.

Many states have enabling legislation allowing a bonding authority to be established for not-for-profit hospitals, but with high interest rates and underwriters requiring proof of a positive earnings history, with a minimum debt service coverage of 1.5 times, this is a difficult, if not impossible goal for many hospitals.

In recent years, the investor-owned chains have expanded into areas needing beds. Often these hospitals are located in rural or growing suburban areas. The investor-owned chains have moved into areas that the not-for-profit voluntary hospitals have believed undesirable or were not foresighted enough to venture into developing communities. Even if a particular hospital had the foresight, the financing of such a project may have been impossible. There has been a trend for large metropolitan hospitals to build satellite hospitals in growing suburban areas. The purpose for such a move is twofold: (1) The home base hospital seeks referring satellite hospitals, thus, guaranteeing protection of its service area and financial viability; or (2) the satellite hospital may ultimately be the home base hospital when the home base hospital is vacated.

The financial implications of either an investor chain or not-for-profit voluntary hospital expanding into developing areas are significant. Assuming that both will build a 200-bed hospital, the financial differences shown in Table 39-2 become evident. The not-for-profit voluntary hospital must finance $13,068,000 more than the investor-owned chain. The difference may be even greater, since the investor-owned company can elect to do part of its financing by issuing additional shares of stock and thereby, have equity money in the project. These differences could prove to be the devastating factor in developing such a project.

Table 39-2 Financial Differences Between Proprietary and Not-for-Profit Voluntary Expansion

Factor	Proprietary	Not-for-Profit Voluntary
Average GSF per bed	900	1,200
Average construction cost per GSF	$ 100	$ 120
Size of project	200 beds	200 beds
Construction cost	$18,000,000	$28,800,000
Project cost (est.)	$24,282,000	$38,851,000
Fund-raising factor	—	$ 1,500,000
To be financed	$24,282,000	$37,350,000

NOTE

1. Eugene J. Rubel, Statement to the Press, January 1975.

Chapter 40

Health Planning and Regulation by 2010, A.D.

The difference in opinions about the planning and regulation of health care that exists in the United States is well described by Eugene Field's *The Duel* in the opening verse:

The gingham dog and the calico cat
Side by side on the table sat;
'Twas half-past twelve, and (what do you think!)
Nor one nor T'other had slept a wink!
The old Dutch clock and the Chinese plate
Appeared to know as sure as fate
There was going to be a terrible spat.[1]

Between today and 2010, tumult and confusion will characterize events. There will be multiple clashes of personalities, institutions and government, ethics and financing, and decentralization versus centralization as two contrary views are sorted out. One basic opinion holds that economic and behavioral science theory is sufficiently mature to provide guidance for solving the most complex problems in health care delivery. The other opinion holds that the pragmatism and initiative of local people, exercised within broad review and control limits, will ultimately develop a more useful, responsive health care system.

As these two broad themes bob and weave against each other through the next three decades, their wider implications will be argued within the concepts of freedom.

The true believer in institutional initiative will point to past achievements within earlier freedoms to plan and operate an expanding health care system. However, the loss of these freedoms, through planning and regulation, will occur in three different ways.

First, all institutions must be not only equal to, but the same as, every other institution. This equality can be achieved only by reducing institutional freedom to a common, standardized level.

Second, institutional freedom is threatened by inflation. Inflation destroys a hospital's capital and diverts its diminished income from clinical to support service expenditures.

Third, the role of the hospital must be altered to serve as an agent for securing change in health care and to become a provider for social services, as well as health care services.

These three dimensions will be the major forces used to justify the drive for dominance of the federal government in health care. Missing will be the fact that the best results in health care occur when its management is left to people who know something about it.

If the societal forces now at work and likely to remain in force are correctly perceived, then there are two issues to project within these parameters: the characteristics of planning and regulation in 2010; and their effect on the scope, shape, and mode of operation of health care delivery.

The only error-proof predictions are that there will be change and there will be a difference. Thinking in probability terms, a three percent annual error in prediction means a miss by more than 100 percent in 30 years. Therefore, it is quite easy to be committed to the idea that the best that might be hoped for three decades hence, is to find that one's thoughts were still aiming in the right direction.

In itself such a hope is no mean achievement. The best of footings for 30-year predictions is the historical observation that, once societal forces have changed from low, sweeping waves to their being compressed and having increased choppiness. The length of time a societal force persists has been significantly diminished. This means that the faint breeze now blowing may become a raging cyclone 30 years from today.

The health care system is a part of society and will take on new shapes and forms as the fundamental institutions of the government accommodate new understandings of the roles and functions.

Planning and regulation of the health care system in the twenty-first century will reflect what happens to the roles of the judiciary, executive, and legislative branches of government, and the future role of state government. It will also reflect what occurs in energy generation, monetary policy, foreign affairs, and new medical knowledge.

Developments in each area will heavily affect health care. Collectively, they may either reinforce or cancel out each other. Despite the popular view that events are predictable and that a person's course is steadily upward toward a better life, the Dark Ages remain a reminder that fortunes can recede for centuries.

To the degree that people are in control of the future, that institutions of government reflect pursuit of the public good, and humanity among people progresses, the years ahead can be approached.

THE FUTURE OF PLANNING

The progressive logic of events is more predictable than its timing. The present issues in planning have set the stage for the next series of changes. Out of cost containment efforts and ineffectiveness of health systems agencies will arise expanded authorities for regional planning, with greater authority over future capital decisions of institutions and individual providers.

In the process, technical capabilities of HSAs will slowly improve. Centralized data on the therapeutic results of treating common diseases and meaningful manpower statistics will be developed. Sophisticated forecasting techniques will gradually be applied to health care issues.

A period of intense data collection and manipulation will occur. By the last decade of the forecasting span, refinement of this new data will be pointing toward the simplification of the data base, with a sense of relief that at last stable and reliable key statistics have been identified and proved acceptable for forecasting need, demand, and resource allocation, and for making planning decisions.

It is now many years since the report of the Commission on Hospital Care was issued and laid the foundation for the Hill-Burton Survey and Construction Act. Their report is still more advanced in planning techniques than the ones currently in use. If the years ahead move as slowly as those of the past, rationalization in planning will still be an unaccomplished objective.

Two possible organizational events may enhance the effectiveness of planning. The signs of one, increasing the accountability of the planning agency for the quality and cost-effectiveness of its decisions, are already present. Much of the planning being done at this time is on the basis of what ought to be, in terms of some unproved model of a regionalized health care system that is colored by unattainable objectives introduced by consumer elements in the decision process. Within the next three decades, consumerism, the *second* event, will be removed from the local level and raised to, and limited by, broad policy-making decisions at the state or federal level. The local planning level will then become technically oriented and limited to approving programs that are consistent with national health policy and are cost-effective.

This shift in organizational authority will be forced by providers as they seek accountability from planning agencies through the courts. Sooner or later such actions will stimulate a realization that consumer politics and naive decisions are interfering with excellence in planning.

In summary, the year 2010 will find planning operating within a defined and prioritized set of policy decisions set at the federal level; an accurate and useful data base; collapse of local governance in planning; sophisticated planning methodologies; and the freedom of institutions to propose and planning agencies to dispose of proposed programs and services.

Capital funds of institutions will not be pooled, but obsolete and un-needed facilities will not be modernized, and will slowly disappear as health care facilities.

THE FUTURE OF REGULATION

Regulation in health care will follow a separate course of events. Financial and operational regulation will be substantially different than now experienced.

Within the next decade, the present heavy reliance on regulatory activities will be accepted as counterproductive. The existing practice of issuing a steady, never-diminishing stream of promulgation of new regulations will overload the system and reach a point of absurdity.

A New Form of Control

Federalization of the hospital system will be considered and rejected on a political basis, and gradually detailed administrative regulations will be modified. Out of this process will rise a new form of control. It will be focused on clinical programs and services. It is not unlikely that the composition of a hospital medical staff, by specialty, will be determined at the planning agency level.

This authority will be exercised on the rationale of balancing hospital services against community needs and the optimal use of medical manpower. As existing medical knowledge is refined, accountability for patient outcomes will be more squarely placed on physicians.

While institutional regulation will moderate and will be specific in nature, clinical regulation will increase. This shift will provide the impetus to accelerate the growth of large group medical practices. Patient choice of physician will be replaced by patient choice of physician group.

Financing of medical care is unpredictable because of the possibility of a national health program. Even though the common wisdom is that a national health program is inevitable, this is more political speculation than political reality. The overriding fact is that the federal budget is unbalanced and is likely to remain so. As long as this is so, only an irresponsible Congress would enact such legislation.

Unless there is a basic restructuring of Congress, the political process will remain expansionist, and annual federal deficits will be a continuing fact of life. If the political system is modified and a restructuring of Congress occurs, then national health insurance will become a probability.

Rate Review Will Be Universal

Regulation will continue and increase for hospital and physician reimbursement. No truly prospective reimbursement system will develop, but rate review of hospital and physician charges will become universal. Planning and financial regulation will not become vested in one agency, but authorization for recovery of capital investments will remain a planning agency function, despite current fears that P.L. 93-641 will become the authority for developing a supra-agency for planning, financing, and operational control.

While these predictions may now appear as unrealistically conservative, the overriding societal forces now arising are a growing mistrust of government and an understanding that their area of operational competence is not unlimited.

CHANGES THAT WILL TAKE PLACE

With the outline of future planning and regulation drawn, what will be the changes that will take place in the providers of medical care?

Larger Corporate Groupings

As long as there is any opportunity for provider responses beyond existing control mechanisms, they will take place. The most clear-cut change that will occur is the massing of larger corporate groupings of physicians and of hospitals.

The driving force for provider changes will be a continuing concern about the cost of medical care. Federal pressure will remain on hospitals and physicians, including limitations on medical practice income. The provider response will be to develop more hospital-based practices and group practices, including a substantial use of nurse practitioners at the primary care level. There will be a significant increase in the formal organization of medical practice.

Expanded Administrative Role

As a corollary, the division between clinical and administrative medicine will become quite distinct, with departmental leadership in the medical staff clearly a function of the hospital administration. Quality assurance and appropriate use of hospital resources for diagnosis and treatment will be under constant scrutiny. There will be little room in Washington for the point of view that increased regulation does not improve cost performance in the medical care system. Cost shifting, rather than cost savings, will still be a regulatory issue in the twenty-first century. It is doubtful that the cost issue in medical care will be confronted in any sensible way during this period.

Mergers and Consolidations

Hospitals will respond to cost control pressures by continuing to merge and consolidate services. Because free enterprise concepts are deeply rooted in American society, the investor-owned national chains will continue to expand, and a corollary chaining in religious hospitals and large nonprofit community hospitals will also take place.

By 2010, the number of hospital corporations will probably be around the one thousand mark. The total number of hospital units will also decrease, as obsolete rural hospitals are not replaced, and larger hospitals at a greater distance will be expanded to meet the rural demand for medical care. Along with this shift will come a comprehensive ambulance network and the development of articulated primary care centers from a distant medical center.

Increase in Elderly Population

Another factor that will create a demand for the expansion of acute care beds at the secondary and tertiary level is a steady increase in the elderly population. The United States will face what Sweden is now facing in two more decades. On the other hand, if there are medical knowledge breakthroughs not now anticipated, such as one comparable to antibiotics, the expected need for expanding hospital services may not occur.

Roles and Missions

Hospitals will routinely develop role and mission statements that define that part of the health care marketplace they wish to serve and the reasons they plan to do so. One of the persistent scrambles between hospitals and planning agencies will be the issue of appropriate institutional roles and missions. This will probably be a serious point of contention between the two organizations, with no authority granted to the planning agencies to do much about how an institution defines its marketplace.

Along these lines, one of the major issues in the years ahead will be the extent to which federal planners try to expand institutional social services, with hospitals preferring to maintain a medical care posture. The struggle will be determined on the basis of funding, with hospitals believing that the federal government's desire to transfer social services to their area of concern is because of a need to use health care dollars for social services not fully funded on a direct support basis.

Reimbursement Mechanisms

The argument about appropriate reimbursement mechanisms will remain a topic of major interest. The payment mechanism will be called prospective, but restrictions in its application will leave the mechanism short of being a truly prospective payment system. Some form of rate approval will be centralized in a federal agency.

Watching over these coming changes will be their appropriate functions. The day of the insurance broker, local merchant, and community lawyer and banker will fade in the hospital boardroom as chaining of institutions grows. The corporate board of directors concept will gradually evolve and local boards of trustees will become advisory in nature.

SUMMARY

As the calendar turns to 2010, the present system of planning and regulation will have disappeared. Planning will be implemented to carry out a defined national health policy, and local planning agencies will be technical arms for processing local data and plans into a national scheme for health care.

Regulation will remain separated from planning activities and will have two major elements: (1) the financing of medical care; and (2) the evaluation and control of clinical activities within rather specifically defined areas of interest.

In this coming period of twisting and turning, as planning and regulation bite into existing hospital and medical practices, the result will be as described in the final verse of *The Duel:*

Next morning where the two had sat
They found no trace of dog or cat;

And some folk think unto this day
That burglars stole that pair away!
But the truth about the cat and pup
Is this: they ate each other up!
Now what do you really think of that![2]

NOTES

1. Eugene Field, *The Poems of Eugene Field* (New York: Charles Scribner's Sons, 1911), p. 1.
2. Ibid.

Chapter 41

Convertibility of Hospital Facilities

Until the federal government created the magic numbers of 4.0 beds per 1,000 population and an average occupancy rate of 80 percent, the hospitals in this country did not have much interest in facilities conversion. But that changed abruptly in the fall of 1978 when it was decreed that henceforth, each HSA would be judged against these numbers by those who provide its annual financing at HHS. For those employed by HSAs, it became self-evident that the numbers were not debatable. The concern over the bed supply in each HSA area became lost in the bureaucratic struggle to conform. Conforming now has a higher priority than using good sense, as focusing on the following two aspects will demonstrate: (a) the inability to recycle a highly specialized single purpose building to another activity; and (b) what happens when parts of a hospital building are no longer used for acute beds.

INABILITY TO CONVERT HOSPITAL BUILDINGS

The first can be summed up as follows. A building that has been constructed as a general hospital cannot, in most situations, be used for anything but the purpose for which it was built.

If it should come to pass that a hospital is closed and razed so that the raw land can be put to some other use, passersby are likely to question the wisdom of tearing down a building that, in their opinion, looks sturdy and appears to have some useful life left. Knowing this may happen, a

---

Reprinted with changes with permission from *Hospital Progress*, October 1979, © 1979 by The Catholic Health Association.

governing board is usually reluctant to agree to such a course of action. The dramatic effect of a massive iron ball smashing against bricks and glass is something that cannot be hidden from the community. It is impressive to watch that ball swinging back and forth, destroying everything with which it comes in contact.

Unseen are the reasons that lie behind this action. Long before the headache ball goes to work, the conclusion had to be reached that the facility was obsolete, outdated, and not able to be sold, and that the costs of conversion and bringing the building up to code requirements exceeded the revenue-generating capabilities. Even after such information is carefully compiled and the decision made that the building must go, there is still a reluctance to do it.

Alternative Uses

What are the alternative uses? The list is neither long nor satisfying nor often accepted as being true. The alternatives range from none to physician office building, extended care facility, residential home, or as office space for community agencies. Realistically, it should probably start and stop with none.

Physician Office Building

The idea of converting a hospital or a major part of one to a physician office building is one of the more popular notions. If physicians resist and refuse to move in, they often are regarded as not being loyal to the hospital. The fact that the space is laid out wrong, that traffic patterns do not make sense, and that the office is located in the innards of a hospital lacking an identity of its own is often overlooked or minimized. If people are objective about this use, it is obvious that any physician who would office in such space lacks good judgment about what is needed for a successful office practice.

Extended Care Facility

The next most likely suggestion is to turn the hospital into an extended care facility or, if it is a partial conversion, to use some of the nursing units for this purpose. The need for additional nursing home beds can usually be demonstrated, particularly in communities that have static populations or slow growth rates. But since need is not the same as demand, difficulties are experienced when it is recognized that the filling of these beds depends on finding enough patients willing to pay the cost from their own resources, since Medicare reimbursement is inadequate. The crucial element in this kind of conversion is fiscal viability. If the hospital has excess beds and is running a low average occupancy rate, the chances are good that it has a marginal financial picture, which is made worse by moving into extended care because reimbursement is often below operating costs.

Other problems of a serious nature exist in this kind of conversion. A related financial problem is the allocation of indirect costs to patient cost centers. In freestanding extended care facilities, the indirect expenses apportioned to the patient day cost are lower than those in a general hospital. When the general hospital continues to operate with these subacute beds as part of it, the basis of a never-ending argument with the third party payers is created. Even though the indirects are higher, they are legitimate inclusions in cost reimbursement in spite of the fact that they represent a disproportionately higher expenditure per day of care. Since the monies available for subacute care are more limited than for acute care, the resistance from third party payers to paying a higher cost per day to the hospital for this kind of care than they would have to pay to a freestanding facility designed for this purpose is understandable.

In addition, there are space configuration problems and patient factors that need to be considered. An acute nursing unit lacks the needed space required for out-of-bed activities of elderly patients and is overequipped with bedside mechanical services. Extended care patients need to get together since the institution has, in reality, become their home. Units are built with this in mind so that when an acute facility is converted, a capital expenditure must be made even to meet minimal standards for this type of care. This presents a particularly difficult hurdle because it requires investing current dollars in an older building, not only to modify the structure to house the contemplated program, but to bring the structure up to the latest code requirements as well. This is risk taking with considerable front-end money needed before the new program can become operational.

Residence for the Elderly

Another alternative that may be considered is to convert a nursing unit to a residence for elderly persons. This is more apt to be proposed in church-related hospitals than in nonaffiliated ones. This kind of conversion is even more difficult to accomplish since privacy is lacking, the amenities are not present, and the dining and recreational areas are missing. Psychologically, this kind of activity housed in a general hospital has adverse effects on the residents who view the location in a negative way.

Social Agencies

Another possibility is to use surplus space to house social agencies of the community. If the program is medically related, it may be possible to make it work, such as for a tumor registry. However, if what is needed is office space, the design of a nursing unit is not satisfactory. When used as offices, it represents a compromise between an inadequate budget and a program that is not adequately funded; it is simply a way to balance a budget at the expense of the persons employed by the agency.

About the only successful type of conversion has been when a diploma program in nursing has been phased out by a hospital, and the school of nursing building has been used for administrative purposes and inservice training programs. Accounting, personnel, executive offices, and purchasing can usually be shifted into this building, freeing up space in the hospital that can be remodeled for other uses.

When a hospital has experienced a steady decline in admissions and patient days over several years and reaches the point that it must consider closing its doors, it may be suggested that the facility be turned over to an investor-owned hospital chain either as a sale or under a management contract. Typically, the reasons for the decline are not related to the lack of managerial skills, but stem from the location of the hospital and the changes that have taken place in the community that immediately surrounds the institution. The chances of making any sustained significant turnaround in the patient days and admissions are not very good. If a sale is considered, potential purchasers are going to base their bids on the cash spill-off that can be obtained, and not on depreciated or replacement value of the buildings. This often comes as a shock to those wanting to sell the facility because the bid may turn out to be 30 to 40 percent of the book value.

The difficulty of finding alternative uses for an entire hospital is recognized by investment houses, banks, and those who hold mortgages on them. In the event of default in meeting payment schedules, they are reluctant to force bankruptcy because they appreciate that a hospital is a hospital and has no market value for another purpose.

WHAT HAPPENS WHEN BEDS WITHIN AN INSTITUTION CLOSE DOWN?

It will probably come as a shock to HSAs when they realize that a successful program of deactivating beds is likely to increase the costs of hospital care rather than achieving a reduction. An example may illustrate why this is so.

An Example

Assume that a hospital is operating at a 62 percent occupancy rate and receives a notice that its licensed bed complement is to be reduced by a number that is the equivalent of one nursing unit. Assume, also, that after much internal discussion, the decision is reached to comply. How to make the mandated cut now becomes the issue. Two alternatives exist: (a) to close a few beds on each unit; or (b) to close one entire nursing unit. Good management sense will dictate the latter, and the hospital will then have a mothballed unit. At this point, the problem shifts to the financial arena and becomes one of allowable costs under the cost reimbursement formulas that affect the hospital. What was a direct expense has been shifted to an indirect one and, since the bed complement has been reduced, the indirects rise. If the hospital is in a state that has adopted a cost review commission program, the institution may find itself in a different category where the established ceilings had not taken into account this kind of problem, with the result that the hospital exceeds the ceiling.

Recognizing the inequity but also having learned from previous experience the difficulty of attempting to gain an exemption, the hospital will probably look for ways of putting the space back to some use that will be socially worthwhile but also profitable. If one can be uncovered and the mothballed unit is put back into service, new revenues will be generated for a program not previously offered by the hospital. These revenues represent new monies flowing into the hospital and become additional dollars being spent on health care.

On the other hand, if a use cannot be found and the unit remains idle, the cost of maintaining and depreciating it becomes an ongoing part of the indirect expense, which is now higher and results in a higher cost per patient day. In either case—the adding of a new program or the mothballing of the unit—the result is the same: more monies flowing into the hospital, one due to the introduction of a new program and the other due to the eccentricities of cost reimbursement as a method of paying hospitals.

If an alternative use is found, some capital expenditures may be required to make the space suitable for the new purpose. Again, costs rise since these capitalized items will be depreciated in current dollars and, if a loan was secured, the interest expense will also be included as an allowable cost.

The only avenue that leads to a reduction in a community's expenditures for hospital care is when a total hospital is closed and taken out of operation. Patients who would have been at the closed hospital now receive their care at other institutions in the area. This raises the other institution's occupancy rates and enables them to spread their indirect cost over a larger number of patient days. Yet, experience to date suggests a strong reluctance on the part of HSAs to attempt to push hospitals into closing in overbedded communities. The approach has been to nibble away at all of the hospitals as the only route that is politically feasible. The closing of beds increases costs; the closing of hospitals decreases expenditures. The closing of beds is politically feasible; the closing of hospitals is not.

Trade-offs

In order to increase the average occupancy rates on specialized units, the planning logic is to attempt to get hospitals to make trade-offs among themselves, such as hospital A giving up obstetrics to hospital B and, in turn, B gives up pediatrics or psychiatry or orthopedics or something to A. Trade-off of clinical services is a one-time activity in a game in which there are very few chips and many undesirable side effects that are overlooked or disregarded.

When obstetrical units are involved, the question of which unit to close may hinge on satisfactorily resolving the sterilization and abortion issue. When economic considerations overlap moral concerns, the wisdom of Solomon may be required to break the stalemates that develop. There is also the ripple effect that goes hand-in-hand with obstetrics. Since obstetrics is practiced by specialists who are also trained in gynecology, the loss of the former results in a loss in female surgery of between 50 to 80 percent of gynecology admissions. Where a hospital gives up obstetrics, it will certainly see a decline in gynecology and often may see a decrease in pediatrics as well. The outcome may well jeopardize the fiscal solvency of the institution and, in addition, may be disruptive to referral patterns of physicians and interfere with patient convenience. The issue of trade-offs is a complex one that goes far beyond the maintenance of an adopted standard occupancy rate for every hospital.

THE IMPACT OF FEDERAL GUIDELINES

In thinking about facilities and their conversion to other uses, some consideration needs to be given to the forces at work in the field that have led to this becoming of primary interest to hospitals. Two factors appear to be significant: (1) the HHS guidelines on numbers of beds per 1,000 population and occupancy rates; and (2) that hospitals may now be a mature industry that for the foreseeable future is going to have excess capacity. If the latter is the major reason, then the facilities conversions that take place will be due to what is occurring in the marketplace and will automatically correct themselves without government intervention.

If, on the other hand, the moving force behind conversions is due to the federally adoped guidelines, then an understanding of the impact of them is important. As promulgated, they call for HSA areas to reduce to 4.0 beds per 1,000 population if they are now above that number. If they are currently below the 4.0 for the area as a whole, they are expected to remain at that level. In either case, the area occupancy rate is expected to be 80 percent. If these conditions are met, the number of acute beds in service will decrease from the present 956,284 to 860,271, a proposed loss of 96,013 beds or 10 percent. Should these standards be obtained, the net effective bed rate will actually be much lower than the 4.0. In 1980 it was 3.79 beds and in 1985, it will be 3.59 beds. During this same period, the population of the country has been projected to continue to grow from 227 million in 1980 to 239 million in 1985.

The result of decreasing beds while population continues to expand means that occupancy rates will rise dramatically over the next several years. If the government standards were immediately enforced, the national occupancy rate of hospitals would be 93.4 percent in 1985.

Since these rates are much too high for the system to respond effectively to the public's need for hospitalization, the variable that has to be affected is the number of patient days per 1,000 population. By applying the government guidelines, the utilization rate has to decrease by 176 patient days per 1,000 population as shown in Table 41-1.

For the past 30 years, patient days per 1,000 population have steadily increased. The reversal in this trend can occur only if utilization review programs become effective or if HMOs significantly increase their enrollments to where they account for close to 17 percent of the population of the country, up from under the five percent now participating in them. By 1988, 41 million persons will have to belong in order to reach the 1,048 level. Even though HMOs are now experiencing this kind of growth, it must continue unabated until the late 1980s, with an annual increase in

Table 41-1 Acute General Beds, Occupancy and Patient Days Per 1,000 Population

Year	Average occupancy	Beds per 1,000 population	Patient days per 1,000 population
1978	73.6%	4.50	2,224
1980	80.0	3.79	1,106
1985	80.0	3.59	1,048 (−176)

enrollment of nearly 20 percent. To the extent that this does not occur, the average occupancy rate of hospitals will edge upward beyond the 80 percent occupancy rate.

Weighing the chances of reducing the total number of beds to the levels called for in the guidelines and the likelihood of reducing the utilization rates, it would seem that, on balance, hospitals will probably have a tight, but not unmanageable occupancy rate for the nation as a whole. But what will be true for the country will not be the situation in all communities. Areas that are rapidly growing will be experiencing bed shortages, even though they may have gone through periods of bed surplus in the mid-1970s. Many rural areas will continue to have low occupancy rates but will remain relatively immune from bed reductions because of political overtones. Inner-city hospitals will continue to phase out of existence because of inadequate reimbursement and a declining rate of admissions due to the number of physicians relocating to suburban offices. The tightness will occur in suburban areas of major cities and the sun belt region.

The result of each HSA attempting to apply the federal standards in its own service area is going to lead to criticism of the efforts of the agency. As occupancy rates creep upward, the hospitals in suburbia will receive an increasing number of complaints from members of the medical staff with regard to a tightness in admitting patients. When this comes about, administrative staffs of the hospitals are going to discover some desirable side effects they had not anticipated. The financial picture will improve, their ability to deal effectively with physicians will be enhanced, and productivity will rise. As the hospital executives in Syracuse, New York, have learned from this experience, the pluses far outweigh the negatives, and they would contend that utilization rates are lowered without adversely affecting the quality of patient care.

As it now stands, 69 percent (35) of the states are out of compliance on the beds per 1,000 population, and by 1985 this will be reduced to 56 percent (28) if beds are held constant and not permitted to increase. With regard to the 80 percent occupancy rate, 12 percent (6) are now in compliance. When the two criteria of both beds and average occupancy are applied to each state, only four—Connecticut, Rhode Island, Delaware, and Maryland—are substantially in compliance. Thus the adopted standards are now met by 8 percent of the states and will only be slightly greater by 1985. This does not represent a solid basis for government regulation as of the present time, but will change as population continues to increase. Some changes in the application of the guidelines would be helpful. These are:

1. Adopt 4.0 beds per 1,000 population as a national goal, not a goal for each HSA. By 1985, this will be met if no net beds are added to the delivery system due to the continuing increase in population. To the extent that HMOs have enrolled substantial numbers of persons, the percentage occupancy will be slightly lower.
2. Let each state adopt its own norm based on historical utilization patterns, but at a level that is based on a statewide occupancy rate that forces efficiency in hospitals.

Exceptions will need to be made, not only for unusual conditions in any one HSA, but for an entire state. The first place where this is apt to occur is the state of Minnesota. If the existing guidelines are imposed in that state, the 23,529 acute beds now in service will have to be reduced to 15,700, a drop of 7,829. This will be difficult to accomplish since on any given day there are now 16,753 patients in those beds, 1,053 more patients than beds. This same kind of problem will also be occurring in North Dakota, West Virginia, and the District of Columbia.

STRAIGHTFORWARD STRATEGY

The strategy of the hospital field is straightforward in dealing with facilities conversion. As a mature industry, a number of institutions are going to find themselves with excess capacity. On their own initiative they will seek to use such space for needed health programs that are revenue producing. Where these cannot be found, they will mothball whole nursing units rather than close a few beds on each unit. When pushed by HSAs to conform to federal guidelines, hospitals may initially be hard pressed to conform, but, by the mid-1980s, there will be a growing ability to meet the guidelines. In some suburban places there will be lines, whereas in inner-city hospitals they will still be struggling with low occupancy problems. In general, there will be a growing appreciation that a tight bed situation is not only manageable but desirable from an operational standpoint.

The balancing of the total supply of beds against the demand for those beds can never reach a zero sum in an HSA, a state, or the country as a whole unless the health delivery system is totally controlled by a centralized scheme, which would have to include dictating where each physician practiced. Short of that kind of program, the bed supply will remain in flux. By permitting some flexibility but holding it within the predetermined occupancy levels, another benefit will be obtained, a redistribution of physicians. Since physicians need to be able to admit patients, those just coming to a community will have to use those hospitals where they can get beds for their patients when needed. The adopted guidelines are unlikely to be met initially, except in a few states. By holding the lid on additional beds, the growth in population will gradually see the effect of the guidelines. As long as HSAs do not move precipitously to enforce them, the overall results will be beneficial. As of now, while the hospital field is concerned with the delicensing and facility conversions, they should take a wait and see attitude.

In summary, the following observations seem pertinent:

- Hospitals are single purpose structures that cannot, in most situations, be converted to other uses.

- HSAs are unlikely to be successful in closing entire hospitals and, therefore, will reduce the bed complements of all institutions in the areas that do not meet the occupancy guidelines.

- Reductions in bed complements will increase hospital unit costs.

- The only effective way to reduce costs is to close entire hospitals.

- Hospitals will discover positive benefits when operating in a tight bed situation.

- Hospitals should adopt a go-slow posture on facility conversions as a response to federal guidelines since population increases will bring about a need for them.

Chapter 42

The Quiet Revolution

Over the next decade the health delivery system will undergo radical change; change that is not now being given much consideration by either physicians or hospital executives. It will occur quietly and without fanfare, but when viewed ten years from now it will be identifiable as a revolution that has taken place, much to the surprise of many who lived through the turbulent years of the seventies, when hospitals and government were locked in a struggle that seemed to be never-ending. There will be problems, of course, but they will not be the ones that now dominate the daily diet of hospital administrative life. Long gone will be the bruising battles with HSAs and state rate review commissions. Concerns with bureaucratic meddling and tinkering with the system will be replaced with thoughts about improving productivity, the application of pricing services based on marginal cost concepts, and the realities of living in a free marketplace.

A LOOK AT THE PAST

Looking back over the past century, Odin Anderson has identified the major thrusts of the hospital field. He characterized the period from 1870 to 1930 as one in which all of the developed nations were concerned with growth and expansion of hospitals.[1] In the United States the number of hospitals grew from 450 to over 5,000. From 1930 to 1965, they all had a common problem: installing financing mechanisms for purchasing hospital care. From 1965 on, they had a mutual interest in controlling costs. This last phase was fueled by the rapid expansion of residency training that took place immediately following the end of World War II.

The growth in specialists and subspecialists led to a metamorphosis in hospitals. They had been patient care institutions offering limited diagnostic and therapeutic services, but they turned into large technologically-oriented enterprises that cost increasing sums of money to operate. As a result, the public came to believe that they were out of control.

THE PRESENT DESIRE FOR CHANGE

This is where hospitals are today. The point has been passed where doing a better public relations job of explaining these costs will be all that is needed to soothe the tempers of a disbelieving public. The answers of the past are no longer workable.

The evidence for change is piling up. There is a growing recognition that cost containment may be required to stem the rise in hospital costs; that both labor and management are now serious about restraining additional dollars from going into higher premiums for health coverage; that cost reimbursement is not a satisfactory method for reimbursing hospitals; that inefficiency is not penalized and efficiency is not rewarded under present financing mechanisms; that competition is noneconomic between hospitals; and that the present system is disjointed and uncoordinated. There is also a growing recognition that life styles need to be altered if better health for all is to become possible. As the list lengthens, those calling for change grow in numbers.

Significantly, government has now been joined by labor and management in desiring a change in the health field. This has been brought about as an outcome of collective bargaining. Over the years negotiations between management and labor on health are benefits centered on the items to be included without any real knowledge of the amount of dollars that were involved. After the fact, it was discovered that the costs were often much higher than had been anticipated, but the door was closed to reopening the matter at the next round of negotiations because benefits had been agreed to as a service inclusion in the health package without dollars being attached.

Because the benefits are often comprehensive, the only practical solution is for the corporation to maintain its commitment to the range of services by absorbing the annual hike in premium rate. The increased cost then becomes a bargaining point of the corporation representatives, who correctly point out that they have added dollars to the fringe benefit package and want it recognized by the union representatives. From their side of the table, the union may be unwilling to do this because it represents a benefit that is already in the package, and they probably feel that their membership will not acknowledge it as a new or additional benefit. By now both groups are looking for ways around this troublesome issue and recognize their mutual interests are served if they can contain hospital costs.

As the number of premium dollars has escalated in corporate budgets, there is a growing interest in using them to secure bids to provide health care so that competition can be introduced to the benefit of the large block purchaser of health care. For better or worse, the mutual interests of management and labor are joined with those of government in bringing about a major change in the way they do business with the health industry.

AVENUES FOR CHANGE

Assuming that change will occur because of the deep interest of management, labor, and government in bringing it about, the question that must be addressed is what avenue is most likely to be followed. Five options can be identified:

1. Continue the status quo.
2. Continue to increase regulation.
3. Introduce meaningful economic competition.
4. Alter physician behavior.
5. Alter consumer behavior.

The first two hold little promise for the future, as the events of the past clearly indicate. The status quo route of minding the store, of doing things in the way they have been done, will see only a continuation of present trends in costs and public attitudes. In a recent study, the authors' firm projected an operating cost per patient day of $190 in 1978, reaching $435 in 1986. Seventeen assumptions were made about various components of the hospital's operating expenses, including an inflation factor of eight percent per year. The result shows that the hospital field may be approaching the point where it is reaching the end of a road.[2]

The same holds true for the second alternative of continuing to increase government regulation. Both Scott Fleming and Alain Enthoven have pointed out that centralizing the control of 350,000 physicians and 7,000 hospitals ultimately leads to absurdity as attested by the number of law-suits now pending against HHS.[3]

Behind the government posture on controlling costs lies the belief that hospitals are inefficient and mismanaged. Unfortunately it is difficult to refute this opinion as long as cost reimbursement dominates the payment mechanism. To pay a hospital an additional dollar of revenue for each additional dollar of expense as it is incurred seems to the public mind as a way to encourage inefficiency. Hospital people deny this generalization and legitimately point out that the Economic Stabilization Program of the early 1970s far more seriously penalized the efficient institutions than it did the inefficient ones. They correctly point out that the fat became leaner, and the lean nearly starved to death. Notwithstanding this experience, the public disbelieves and will continue to do so until cost reimbursement is abandoned.

Public dissatisfaction is heightened when confronted with the costs of an emergency room visit, the problem of securing regular medical attention when moving from one community to another, the lack of sufficient numbers of primary care physicians, and the array of medical bills to be paid for a major illness; all of these are laying the groundwork for change.

The last three alternatives provide the hope for the future and are linked together. Moving away from payments that are cost reimbursed is not easy to accomplish, yet is essential to establishing meaningful competition. The barriers are substantial. To date, competition between hospitals has been noneconomic and has centered on providing more services of better quality, but not price. The present contracts between hospitals and Blue Cross will have to be modified. In most of them is a provision that the carrier is entitled to pay the hospital "costs or charges, whichever is lower." This effectively precludes differential pricing, and its effect is to require a hospital to offer its services to Blue Cross at the same price it offers it to some other group. This forces the hospital to apply an average cost or average price to all of its services, preventing it from using a marginal cost concept. Under such a Blue Cross contract where the hospital derives a substantial percentage of its revenues from this source, the hospital would be effectively deterred from seeking to bid competitively for small volumes because, were it successful, it would have to make the same rates available to Blue Cross.

In those states having rate review commissions a similar problem is found. For instance, in New York, the commission insists that all carriers be charged an identical amount for each unit of service, irrespective of the numbers of units involved. Such a policy by state rate review agencies is a barrier to competition.

BARRIERS TO CHANGE

Internal to the hospital are entrenched viewpoints that represent barriers to change. Medical staffs of community hospitals can be characterized as being overwhelmingly in favor of fee for service and free choice of physician. The establishment of a free marketplace runs counter to these ideas since it necessitates patients selecting both physicians and hospitals from approved lists with whom contractual relationships have been developed and spells out the range of service provided and the charges that have been agreed to by the two parties. If, as part of bringing about economic competition, the hospital finds that it must negotiate for physician services and fees, the medical staff is apt to resist. Whenever possible, physicians attempt to keep the hospital as an economic neutral with regard to their services. Anesthesiologists prefer separate billing, as do many radiologists and pathologists. Other specialists, such as cardiologists, emergency room physicians, neonatologists, and physiatrists, usually feel the same way. Given a choice they prefer that the hospital have no role in determining the charges for their professional services. To shift from these concepts is to move away from the status quo.

If hospitals attempt to do so, they can anticipate that physicians will consider their actions as a violation of the corporate practice of medicine. These state statutes limit the practice of medicine to natural persons. Overlooked in this line of reasoning is that there are already a number of physicians employed by hospital corporations in university medical centers, state mental institutions, community hospital emergency rooms, industrial medicine, chronic institutions, and in the rapidly developing health maintenance organizations. To avoid confrontation on this front, it is desirable to repeal these laws.

Even part of the planning act, PL 93-641, has built-in barriers to effective competition. Three of the ten guidelines used in evaluating a hospital's application for a certificate of need relate to cooperative planning. Under them a hospital is expected to develop its plan, share the information with other institutions in the same service area, and secure their agreement in cooperating with them. This same kind of cooperation is being forced by various state rate review commissions, who examine hospital budgets to be sure that their rate structures are similar for the same kinds of services. Not only is there no penalty for exchanging price and cost information between institutions, it is a desirable activity. If this occurred in other industries, it would be illegal, since it would be regarded as collusion or restraint of trade. The Department of Justice views hospitals as it does other forms of enterprise. It sees its responsibility as one of encouraging competition, not of encouraging cooperation and sharing arrangements.

If economic competition is to become the road that is followed, then the hospital field needs to work with Congress to remove the barriers that are now in place in PL 93-641. Price fixing and cooperation is as undesirable among hospitals as it is in American industry. To force either or both of these on hospitals is not in the public interest.

To date hospital executives have been unwilling to take public stands against these three guidelines, though privately they admit that the guidelines are a farce because they do not square with the real world and the competition that exists. Given a choice between the position of HHS or the Department of Justice, a poll would probably show that hospital executives favor the stand of the Justice Department, since it would free them to use their managerial talents to the maximum, rather than having to use their manipulative skills.

One of the most difficult barriers to overcome will be to move hospital governing boards away from the status quo. Trustees listen thoughtfully to medical staffs, and if they sense that the physicians associated with a hospital do not want to make any changes, they are likely to take the same position. They are not likely to alienate the prevailing viewpoints of the medical staff.

This bias suggests that the hospital—particularly the community, nonprofit institution—will react to changes in the marketplace, but will not attempt to shape the marketplace to protect the service area of the hospital.

THE ADVANTAGES OF A FREE MARKETPLACE

Before addressing the ways in which the health delivery system can be restructured to bring about changes in physician and consumer behavior through economic competition, a look at the advantages of a free marketplace may be useful. Price competition, as such, is missing from the hospital scene due to hospitalization insurance. Patients neither know nor are concerned about the size of their hospital bills and in many cases are not even concerned about the monthly premium since it is paid by an employer. A large percentage of those who use hospitals are shielded from both a cost and a price impact. Under economic marketplace conditions, however, the hospital and the physician would be placed at risk, since the purchaser would be contracting for large blocks of service on behalf of individuals, and the best price would likely be the determining factor on the placement of it.

This is quite different than it has been in the past, where dollars were not even considered. When a hospital found itself losing market share, its response was likely to be to increase its operating costs and charges for its services. This resulted from beginning new diagnostic or treatment services and renovations to plant and equipment, all for the purpose of attracting new physicians to the medical staff. In some situations a physician recruiting program was included that guaranteed incomes and underwrote the costs of physician office space.

The lack of economic competition is evident when hospitals are compared by size ranges. The smallest hospitals always have the lowest costs, and the largest hospitals the highest because they have the most comprehensive range of services, which makes them more desirable from the standpoint of the physician. Thus, higher cost becomes associated with better quality of care, and low cost with an inferior level.

When competition enters the picture, cost becomes a factor and will lead to improved efficiency since those who remain inefficient will discover that they are pricing their services too high to be competitive. Bidding will result in hospitals sharpening their pencils and resorting to the application of marginal costing in determining their bids.

When a free marketplace condition is obtained, hospitals will become reluctant to cooperate with other hospitals or to exchange pertinent financial information. Like other forms of enterprise, they will come to appreciate that the pricing of hospital services is proprietary information.

ECONOMIC COMPETITION

Gaining acceptance of the idea of a free marketplace for hospital and physician services will be difficult, not only because it is a shift from the status quo, but because it also moves the risk taking from the third party carrier to the hospital and the physician. Cost reimbursement to hospitals, and reasonable and customary fees to physicians embody no financial risks to either of them. By introducing competitive factors, the leverage shifts, and both hospitals and physicians find that managerial acumen is a valuable asset to possess.

The shifting of risk, which now rests with the third party carriers, can be accomplished through the adoption of a capitation method for paying for health care services. By putting out bids and having them accepted, the cost of paying for hospital and physician services largely becomes a fixed cost to the prepayment agency and a variable cost to the providers, depending on how many units of service are used during the contract period.

In the past entering into such a contract made little sense to either physicians or hospitals since both were paid for each unit of service furnished to a patient. There was no need for providers to put their services up for bid; the marketplace only required that a third party be billed for services rendered.

Rapid Growth of HMOs

Over the last year, however, a new phenomenon has begun to develop that will bring about significant changes in the next decade. The early steps in the formation of HMOs climaxed with the passage of the federal act in 1973. Even though such organizations had been in existence since World War II, their influence was primarily restricted to the West with the Kaiser-Permanente Plan, to New York City with Health Insurance Program (HIP), and to Washington, D.C. with *GHA*. In those circles this act was viewed as a way of triggering widespread development of this kind of payment system. For some reason the expected did not occur until 1977 when enrollments in HMOs moved sharply upward.

The present statistics now suggest rapid growth is in the offing. An Inter Study Survey found in 1978 that there were 199 HMOs, up from 165 the previous year. Enrollments stood at 7,354,000 in 1978, up 13.9 percent from the previous year.[4] (See exhibit 42-1). In the Federation of American Hospitals journal the following six facts about capitation plans were reported:

1. The number of hospital days per 1,000 members in plans is 488.
2. In HMOs with more than 100,000 members, the average is 408.
3. The median family premium is $89 per month, and the range is from $75 to $95.
4. In HMOs operating ten years or more, the premium is $81 per month.

Exhibit 42-1 Inter Study Survey, August 1978

	1977	1978
Number of HMOs	165	199
Change from prior year	−5.7%	20.6%
Total enrollment	6,330,676	7,354,121
Percent of total	5.2%	13.9%
Group practice and network models		
Number of HMOs	120	141
Percent of total	73%	71%
Number of members	5,894,174	6,714,811
Percent of total	93%	91.3%
IPA models		
Number of HMOs	40	58
Percent of total	24%	29%
Number of members	413,852	639,310
Percent of total	7%	9.5%
Number of new HMOs (1 year)	16	29
Average size of plan	38,368	37,713
Percent of members in HMOs larger than 100,000	71%	69%

Source: Jon B. Christianson, *Do HMOs Stimulate Beneficial Competition?* (Excelsior, Minn.: Inter Study, 1978).

5. There are 1.14 fulltime equivalent physicians per 1,000 members in all plans.
6. The rate of physician utilization is 3.8 total physician visits per member per year.[5]

These numbers are attracting the serious attention of purchasers of health care services. Though the individual can never bring about these kinds of results, the big block purchasers can achieve it on the individual's behalf by dealing with capitation plans. The elements of such a plan call for the formation of a corporation that will enroll subscribers, either individually or through a group, and in turn contract with hospitals and physicians for large volumes of service at a fixed cost to the corporation. Both free choice of physician and hospital are restricted to the parties of the contract, except for highly specialized services.

Looking ahead for the next ten years and realizing that government, labor, and management are now all in the same camp with respect to containing hospital costs by fostering growth in capitation plans, the stage is now set for its rapid development. An annual growth in membership of 20 percent per year from 8 million in early 1979 will result in 1988 in 41,300,000 persons being covered. It seems likely that this will take place.

As these plans grow in numbers and increase in size, they will loom larger in importance. In those sections of the country where their growth is the most rapid, the managerial abilities of the hospital administrative staff will be a crucial factor on the viability of the institution trying to survive in a highly competitive economic situation. Efficiency and control of costs will become of much greater significance than is now the case. Three trends will be recognized:

1. As enrollments in capitation plans grow in a given community, there will be a proportionate growth in interest among hospitals in achieving increased efficiency.
2. As capitation plans grow, the reasonable and customary fees concept will proportionately decline in importance as a method of paying for physician services.
3. In those communities where the majority of physician and hospital care is delivered through capitation plans, the role of the HSA will be markedly different than its present one.

The Role of HSAs

Instead of attempting to put as many roadblocks as possible in front of hospitals wishing to make capital expenditures, the HSA will, of necessity, move from this negative type stance to a more positive one where it will become an agent to encourage competition. In those communities where hospitals are deeply involved in competition, the HSAs will have no meaningful role in monitoring their capital expenditures since marketplace forces will automatically come into play. Once several capitation plans exist in the same service area, the need for the HSA disappears. If a hospital wishes to expand, renovate, remodel, or re-equip, the decisions are made by determining if it can still remain competitive in bidding on new contracts offered by the capitation plan. If a hospital decides that the capital improvement program it has in mind will put it at a competitive disadvantage it cannot overcome, it will forego the expenditure.

The HSAs role will be to advocate adherence to established standards of performance and quality of constuction of facilities. In many ways the HSAs will probably adopt a role similar to that performed by the Federal Aeronautics Agency, which establishes and monitors standards of aircraft performance. Under economic competition it will be unnecessary for an HSA to concern itself with the number of beds per 1,000 population, average occupancy rates, numbers of CAT scanners in the service area, or other such ratios or numbers.

Government Role in Development of HMOs

If hospitals elect to join with labor and management in bringing about meaningful economic competition, they need to take a hard look at the role of government in the development of HMOs. The 1973 act had a number of provisions that proved to be detrimental to HMOs rapid expansion. The scope of services turned out to be so comprehensive that the monthly premium charged the subscriber proved to be too costly to be saleable in the open market.

Rather than seek federal grants to establish HMOs, those groups considering the formation of one would be wise to avoid federal involvement as it is now prescribed. A new plan cannot afford to cater to low socioeconomic groups either, since to do so may make the HMO unattractive to middle income families who will view it as a program for the poor. To be saleable a capitation plan has to provide a range of services dictated by a monthly premium level that is competitive against all other offerings and has to be appealing to middle income families, similar to the pattern followed by Blue Cross in the early 1930s when that program was established by the teachers in Dallas, Texas. Wide social acceptability among the public is as necessary now to the marketing of capitation plans as it was to Blue Cross 45 years ago.

Because of the availability of federal grant money, there is a strong temptation to apply for a grant when establishing an HMO because of the heavy up-front costs that occur in the first two or three years. Grants appear to minimize the risk taking, which may turn out not to be the case. The restrictions and requirements that are built into the use of this money may lead to a Catch-22 situation, where the range of benefits that must be offered by a federally qualified plan are so broad that the cost of providing them exceeds the price that can be charged in the marketplace. Grant money is used to subsidize the gap between revenues and expenses. This is rationalized on the basis that as more persons are enrolled and as the management information system becomes more refined and stabilized the gap will be closed. What may happen is that months will pass without recognizing the basic problem, a benefits package that is too costly for the premium charged to subscribers. Then when the federal grant expires, the realities of the competitive marketplace may come into play, and the capitation plan will have to face its true costs and revenues.

Revolving Loan Fund

If economic competition is to become a moving force in the health field, the present HMO act should be replaced with a revolving loan fund. A number of advantages would result with this type of support for capitation plans. Its greatest strength would be that the forces at work in the marketplace would not be tampered with, but the plans would remain responsive to the conditions as they exist in any given community; whereas, a grant postpones coming to grips with economic consequences. Under a loan, the plan would have to address the question of repayment as part of its decision to seek such funds. It forces a realistic look at the benefit package, a hard-nosed appraisal of the actuarial estimates used, and a thorough understanding of the competition in the marketplace as to what can be charged for monthly premiums. A loan fund recognizes the heavy start-up costs and facilitates the establishment of capitation plans, while at the same time requiring the discipline needed to survive in a free market.

THE RACE TO CONTROL CAPITATION PLANS

Since less than five percent of the population of this country is now enrolled in capitation plans, there are going to be many more formed in the next few years. Those who can be expected to do so include Blue Cross, commercial insurance companies, groups of physicians, investor-owned hospital corporations, community hospitals, and industrial corporations.

Examples of each are already on the scene. Blue Cross is involved in 66 HMOs; commercial carriers are experimenting in selected areas along with some of the investor-owned groups; physicians are forming Independent Practitioner Associations (IPAs) in California, Colorado, and Massachusetts; large nonprofit hospitals in metropolitan centers like Chicago are gaining experience; and industry is carefully observing the HMO of the R. J. Reynolds Tobacco Company in Winston-Salem, North Carolina. The results to date are mixed, but are interesting as enrollments begin climbing at a rapid rate.

With all of this increasing interest, hospitals are going to have to move decisively in this development, or they will abdicate their pivotal role in the health delivery system.

As capitation plans grow and multiply, hospitals will come to appreciate they have both much to protect and much to offer to the changing health scene. Over the past 50 years hospitals have become a technologically-oriented industry that is both labor and capital intensive. These high cost specialized resources need to be used as productively as possible and must remain alert to changes in their marketplace and their share of it. The best way to do this is to control or influence as much as possible what goes on in that arena. They will face competition from these other groups who will be as interested in forming capitation plans as well. A variety of arguments will be used to keep hospitals from taking the initiative. The most difficult one to cope with for the hospital will be from the medical staff. Physicians will probably favor the formation of an IPA that will sponsor a capitation plan and will be opposed to the hospital moving into this position. They will probably pressure governing boards to prevent it.

With the growing concern of industry in capitation, industries can be expected to use the leverage provided by the size of the dollars spent on health care premiums to assure maximum results. Once started, physicians will quickly appreciate that this can also economically threaten them and that the size of their practices may be reduced as the plan enrollment increases in the local community. Once this is recognized the climate will shift, and hospitals can take the leadership in forming capitation plans and may even have support from the medical staff. When physicians feel threatened, the hospital may be viewed by them as offering the best alternative among those that are available, even though under former circumstances this would have been considered undesirable.

Those hospitals that fail to take the leadership in the capitation movement will, in time, find themselves competing along the traditional avenues for a smaller and smaller share of the market. There will be exceptions to this trend, but in general it will hold. Only those hospitals in communities where capitation plans are not available will escape, along with highly specialized services in medical centers where the service is one-of-a-kind.

The race to control capitation plans has just begun in earnest, and the importance of the plans on the health delivery system has just begun to be recognized. They bring a new set of problems that are different than those now faced by hospitals. In doing so, however, they provide an avenue for reconciling public attitudes and hospital viewpoints through a previously untried approach, a free marketplace where economic competition becomes the determinant of who survives and who does not. The thoughtful application of economics to the hospital scene will not only strengthen the ability of this industry to respond to the public, but can be woven together with ways for altering physician and consumer behavior through economic incentives or disincentives.

A PATHWAY TO THE FOREFRONT

Having looked at the coming decade, a positive program has to be developed, or else the increasing regulations and procedures being ground out daily in Washington are going to bring the health delivery system to a dead stop. To avoid this, plans must be developed and implemented. These can be built around the following conclusions:

- Hospitals now engage in noneconomic competition but need to operate in a free marketplace.

- Cost reimbursement as a method of paying hospitals has to be replaced with a pricing system of generating revenues.

- Hospitals need to operate in an environment that rewards those institutions with managerial expertise; conversely, those hospitals that operate inefficiently have to be automatically economically penalized by the forces at work in the marketplace.

- Management and labor are now serious about the need to find appropriate alternate health delivery systems.

- Hospitals should take the lead in bringing about a rapid expansion of capitation plans as the best method of encouraging economic competition.

- In order to gain public acceptance and financial success, capitation plans should avoid accepting federal grants because of their onerous restrictions, and should initially aim at enrolling middle income families and not bring in those from low socioeconomic groups until public acceptance is assured.

- Hospitals should recognize that physicians will want to keep them as economic neutrals with respect to their own economic interests and that this area must be dealt with in a tactful manner.

- The need for health systems agencies will decline at an inverse rate to the growth in subscribers in capitation plans.

Within these broad conclusions that will foster the quiet revolution of the coming decade, several specific recommendations will prove helpful in speeding up the changes that are going to take place:

1. Abandon the 1973 federal act that created health maintenance organizations.
2. Establish a federal loan program on a revolving fund basis that may be tapped for the development of new capitation plans.
3. Encourage hospitals to take the lead in the formation of capitation plans by mandating preferential treatment by HSAs.
4. Eliminate state laws on the corporate practice of medicine.
5. Seek federal legislation to bring hospitals under the provisions of antitrust laws.
6. Eliminate the requirements in third party reimbursement contracts and state rate review commissions that prevent the application of marginal cost pricing of hospital services.
7. Develop working coalitions with local industry groups to foster the rapid expansion of capitation plans as the best method of encouraging economic competition.

These seven steps are not a panacea that will solve the problems of the future for the hospital field and its relationship with the public. It only represents a beginning effort in finding a new pathway that will establish hospitals in the forefront of the quiet revolution that is now just underway.

These steps depart from the traditions that built the health care system of this country, but in a broader sense the road just outlined will lead hospitals into the mainstream of American life where the ability to compete successfully in a free marketplace determines the winners and the losers. It is worth the effort.

Exhibit 42-2 Blue Cross Association Enrollments in HMOs

Year	Number of HMOs	Number enrolled	Increase in enrollment
1975	36	1,100,000	—
1976	50	1,300,000	200,000
1977	62	1,437,000	137,000
1978	66	1,500,000	63,000

Source: Telephone conversation with Arlene Fong, Blue Cross Association, Chicago, Ill.

Exhibit 42-3 ANCHOR—Chicago HMO*

Year	Number enrolled	Increase in enrollment
12/31/76	13,595	—
12/31/77	17,771	3,376
10/31/78**	23,295	5,524

* Five offices in Chicago area.
** Ten months only.
Source: Telephone conversation with Judy Liplut, ANCHOR, Chicago, Ill.

Exhibit 42-4 COCARE—Chicago HMO

Year	Number Enrolled	Increase in enrollment
6/1/77	3	—
6/30/78	10,000	9,997
10/1/78	15,000	5,000

Source: Telephone conversation with personnel at COCARE, Chicago, Ill.

Exhibit 42-5 Minneapolis—St. Paul HMOs

Year	Number of HMOs	Number enrolled	Increase in enrollment
1971	1	35,996	—
1973	3	54,945	17,949
1974	5	70,116	15,171
1975	6	83,908	13,792
1976	7	104,410	20,502
1977	7	143,068	38,658
1978	7	189,585	46,517

Source: Survey by TriBrook Group, Inc., 1979.

Exhibit 42-6 NORTHCARE—Chicago HMO

Year	Number enrolled	Increase in enrollment
1/1/76	5,982	—
1/1/77	7,803	1,821
10/1/77	9,623	1,820
1/1/78	11,271	1,648
10/1/78*	14,079	2,808

* Nine months only.
Source: Telephone conversation with Jenny Burnagin, NORTHCARE, Chicago, Ill.

NOTES

1. Odin Anderson, "Comparative Health Delivery Systems" (Lecture delivered to TriBrook Group, Inc., February 24, 1978).

2. Personal communication.

3. Scott Fleming, "A Perspective From An Organized System." A monograph prepared as a discussion paper for the HOPE Committee on Health Policy, Project HOPE, the People-To-People Health Foundation, Inc., n.d.; Alain C. Enthoven, A Rational Economic Design For National Health Insurance April 28, 1978, Michael M. Davis Lecture Center for Health Administration Studies, University of Chicago.

4. Federation of American Hospitals, *Review*, 11, No. 4 (June 1978): 32.

5. Ibid.

Chapter 43

Playing the Numbers Game with HSAs

Requirements, documentation, and statistics are inevitably going to become a way of life in securing approval for hospital projects. Trade-offs, smoke-filled backrooms, and other subtle forms of political persuasion will remain but will become of secondary importance. Both will be necessary to steer an application to a successful conclusion, but the proportion of each is going to change. Numbers have become the name of the game.

PROBLEMS DEALING WITH AN AGENCY

A Horror Story

Just because hospitals are going to have to do a good job of supplying factual information does not mean that the planning agencies have a solid data base available for use. In many cases, the hospital is going to have to supply its own. There are four keys to dealing with an agency: documentation, patience, a cooperative attitude, and political savvy. Before describing the mix of these that is desirable, a horror story may put into perspective the problems that may be encountered.

Even though hospitals are going to have to reach new heights in the sophistication of information submitted in certificate of need applications, the decisions of HSAs to approve or disapprove are often based on political considerations that have little to do with the factual data that demonstrates need. In this example, the agency board was too large, with 41 members. The majority of them had little knowledge or prior contact with the health care delivery system except as patients. In addition, the staff members of the agency lacked the necessary capabilities. Most of them had accepted as their first priority the conducting of a patient origin study. The board had concurred that this was a compelling need, but two years later it still had not been commenced.

Though the federal law creating comprehensive planning agencies and its successor, the health service agency, are specific on the time periods for each step in the review process, these are often not adhered to in the course of events. In this case, the hospital expected the approval process to require six months from the date submitted. Nine months later the hospital had neither an approval nor a denial of its application. Considering that construction costs were rising at the rate of 0.8 percent per month, this was costing the hospital $80,000 per month on its $10 million capital program.

When this application was first submitted, the project review committee decided not to act on it until they disposed of a pending application from another hospital that wished to build a satellite institution in the same service area. Not wanting to make an unpopular public decision, the agency had instructed the representatives of the existing hospital to get together with those from the hospital wanting the satellite to see if they could not agree on a program that would result in only one hospital. These instructions had been somewhat perplexing to the governing board of the hospital already in operation for two years since they had a new facility. Believing that cooperation was needed, they held seven meetings with the other hospital over a period of three months, until it became obvious to the staff of the planning agency that neither would budge from their initial position. By then, the hospital wanting to build the satellite had received approval on its application, but could not secure a zoning variation from the county commissioners for the height of its proposed building.

When the existing hospital came back before the project review committee, three trustees, two administrative persons, a hospital consultant, a hospital architect, and two medical staff members came to the meeting prepared to discuss the expansion plans. As requested, they arrived at the hearing at 5:30 P.M. only to find seven applications were to be considered at that meeting. Because the staff of the agency considered the existing hospital's application a particularly difficult problem, it was shifted from first to last on the agenda. When finally ushered into the hearing, the time was 11:30 P.M. The hospital representatives, thinking they were in for a long grueling session, were surprised to be asked only two questions by agency board members, both of which clearly indicated the application had not been read. At 11:45 P.M., they were excused so the board could deliberate. The next day the hospital administrator was informed that the application was being deferred for one month since a newly arrived staff member had been assigned to the application and would be contacting the hospital within a few days with a list of further information needed to complete the application. This was a bombshell to the hospital board since they had paid out over $75,000 to their consultant and architect to ensure complete documentation. They had also been complimented at the hearing by the chairman, who indicated their application was the most thorough one he had ever seen in his four years on the agency board.

A week later, the consultant and the administrator met with the new staff member and reviewed the request for additional information. It turned out that 95 percent of it was contained in the original submission, and the new staff member had not carefully read the material. The missing documentation dealt with developing a table showing the educational levels in the community, major industries in town, and sources for securing additional nursing personnel.

At the next hearing of the review committee, the agency staff recommended approval. This time the hearing lasted 20 minutes, and three questions were asked. The one question that stumped the administrators was: "If we approve this project and it is to be financed by long-term debt, how are the poor people going to pay for hospital care?"

To their surprise, the hospital representatives learned the next day that their application was again deferred, and they were requested to meet once more with representatives of the other hospital to discuss building only one hospital. When it was pointed out to the agency staff that such a meeting was no longer between equals since the other hospital now had an approved project and they did not, the agency staff agreed but insisted on the meeting on the basis that they would run the risk of jeopardizing their pending application. Once again the meeting was held. The administrator of the other hospital proposed that he would support the pending application before the project review committee, but in return he wanted support before the county commissioners on his appeal for a zoning variation. He was turned down.

At the next meeting of the project review committee, the application was approved and in turn all the levels up the line concurred. Total elapsed time from start to finish was 13 months. Out-of-pocket costs to consultant and architect were $77,000, plus escalation in project due to lost time over and above prescribed time limits, $560,000.

What Happened?

In thinking about what happened in this case and comparing it with others, the striking aspect about all of them is that few applications seem to move smoothly through the approval process, no matter how well documented or how much attention is paid to the political equation. It is clear that a hospital has to do its homework as a first step, or it is not apt to go beyond this point. This does not assure approval, but it does enhance the chances of reaching a successful result.

HOW TO DOCUMENT APPLICATIONS

Patient Origin

The first major step is the numbers game. The starting point is to determine the geographic area where the population looks to the hospital for its health care services. This may or may not be the same as the subplanning area established by the agency. If not, a potential problem may be turned into a hospital advantage. (See Table 43-1.)

In Table 43-1, the agency did not take into account subarea eight, which contributed 5.5 percent of the patients to the hospitals, and made no provision for beds for patients from out of the service area, which amounted to another 10.5 percent of the patients. These omissions can put in doubt the validity of the work of the agency staff.

Population Forecast

Having looked at patient origin, the hospital is then in a position to know what population to count and to project into the future to determine the basic service population it serves. The majority of the agencies do not have an approved population forecast, which puts the hospital at liberty to select one. In the community being considered, 17 different forecasts

Table 43-1 Patient Origin Data

Agency established area	Hospital patient origin study	
Subarea 1	4.6%	
2	5.7%	
3	7.6%	
4	5.8%	
5	0.7%	
6	37.4%	
7	22.2%	
Subtotal	84.0%	
8	5.5%	16%
9	10.5%	
Subtotal	16.0%	
Total	100.0%	

Source: Confidential Client Study, TriBrook Group, Inc., 1978.

were available, including those of the county planning department, school system, highway department, chamber of commerce, telephone company, power company, water resources board, and a host of others. The variations between them were significant. After considerable analysis, the hospital elected to use the county planning department figures because a comparison between what they had projected and what actually occurred over the past 20 years clearly showed them to have the greatest reliability. For hospital purposes, the population shown in Table 43-2 was adopted.

These figures correspond to the definition of the planning agency's area but not the beds needed for patients using the hospital from subarea eight and out of the area, which needs to be included at the point bed projections are made.

Market Share

Before that is developed, the question to be answered is, "What share of the market does the hospital have from this geographic area?" Since four hospitals serve the area, an analysis of hospital discharges from all four is essential in determining market share. This is reflected in Table 43-3.

While Hospital A is clearly the dominant institution in the area, the purpose of this exercise is to determine what percent of the population in each subarea looks to Hospital A for acute care. From that percent the share of the market can be determined. (See Table 43-4.)

The importance of knowing the number of persons to be served is to be able to have beds and services in place no sooner or no later than they are needed in the future and in the right amount.

At this point, it might appear that the bed determination is a straightforward use of statistics once the basic service population has been deter-

Table 43-2 Population Forecast

| Community | Actual | | Projected | |
	5 years ago	This year	5 years from now	10 years from now
1 & 5	10,552	16,380	17,275	18,261
2	31,007	38,949	43,645	48,341
3	5,444	5,963	5,762	5,561
4	28,599	29,176	29,176	29,925
6	63,615	69,338	73,592	77,846
7	37,864	45,452	51,135	56,818
Total	177,081	205,258	220,960	236,752

Source: Confidential Client Study, TriBrook Group, Inc., 1978.

Table 43-3 Analysis of Marketplace by Hospital

Hospital	Subareas of planning area					
	1 & 5	2	3	4	5	6
A	86.4%	33.2%	81.8%	49.5%	68.3%	84.8%
B	8.8%	4.8%	13.0%	11.6%	21.1%	8.2%
C	4.5%	21.0%	5.1%	35.5%	7.5%	6.5%
D	0.3%	41.0%	0.1%	3.4%	3.1%	0.5%
Total	100.0%	100.0%	100.0%	100.0%	100.0%	100.0%

Source: Confidential Client Study, TriBrook Group, Inc., 1978.

Table 43-4 Basic Service Population of Hospital A

Community	Percent of population using hospital A	Basic service population of A		
		Now	5 years out	10 years out
1 & 5	86.4	14,001	14,926	15,778
2	33.2	12,619	14,490	16,049
3	81.8	4,910	4,713	4,549
4	49.5	14,405	14,628	14,813
6	68.3	46,777	50,263	53,169
7	84.8	35,579	43,363	48,182
Total BSP		130,291	142,383	152,540
Actual population		205,258	220,960	236,752

Source: Confidential Client Study, TriBrook Group, Inc., 1978.

mined. This is not the case since there are a number of factors that are as much judgment as quantitative, leaving considerable room for debate with a planning agency. One of the toughest questions of this kind has to do with a changing share of the marketplace. In any projection, a deviation in a straight line trend extrapolation is always an educated guess. When the trend line reverses, for example, the determination becomes even less educated and more of a guess.

When a hospital has aggressive management, it can substantially increase its market share in a few years. Since the tools of planning are inadequate in coping with anything but a constant market share, judgment becomes the crucial element. Since neither agency boards nor staff members feel comfortable with these shifts, the hospital experiencing a market share change needs to keep good records on patient origins over several years and preferably over a ten-year span. The hospital is then in a position to portray this change when submitting its certificate of need.

Utilization

Having come to grips with market share, the question of how often people are going to use the hospital needs to be resolved. Since planning concerns the future, usually at five- and ten-year intervals, judgment again becomes the important determinant. The grossest method is to project all kinds of acute clinical admissions against all the available beds in the hospital. Nationally, this resulted in 1974 in 3.33 persons per 1,000 being in hospital beds at any given point in time. But this number can vary from less than 2 per thousand to more than 5 per thousand depending on the number of physicians in an area, the ways in which doctors use hospitals, and the availability of beds.

Because the mix of patients can vary by type of care required (medical/surgical, pediatrics, obstetrics, psychiatric), this overall number is not useful in determining the beds needed in a hospital, yet many of the planning agencies apply a state norm on an overall basis for determining beds that is not directly related to the bed and patient mix in the community or individual institution. Table 43-5 reflects a typical utilization by major clinical service.

By using clinical services, recognition is given to inhouse rigidities, such as the nonmixing of pediatrics with obstetrics. Since basic service population times utilization rate yields the number of full beds, the varying of the use rate affects the beds required. This has been recognized by HEW, which holds the use rate constant. In most states, a patient discharge study was conducted in late 1973 or early 1974 and is now being applied for determining beds needed through 1980 in each state. This is akin to the

Table 43-5 Historical Utilization Pattern of Hospital A

Service	Year	Utilization ratio
Medical/surgical	1970	2.13
	1973	1.93
	1975	1.96
Pediatrics	1970	0.20
	1973	0.18
	1975	0.19
Obstetrics	1970	0.15
	1973	0.11
	1975	0.10
Total all services	1970	2.50
	1973	2.23
	1975	2.25

Source: Confidential Client Study, TriBrook Group, Inc., 1978.

Civil Aeronautics Board acting on a request for additional routes by a major airline based on data and information that is six years old.

Unfortunately for hospitals, the consequences of this are likely to be of considerable importance in capital financing. In many instances the application of a constant utilization factor will result in a hospital becoming out of conformance with its state plan, even though its occupancy rate may average higher than 85 percent. Should this occur, the hospital may have difficulty with the capital money market if it is financing its expansion or replacement program from long-term debt. Being out of conformance with a state plan prevents securing a letter of conformance from a regional HHS office in case a Federal Housing Administration (FHA) loan is desired. If the debt instrument selected requires a rating from Moody's or Standard & Poor's, this may also be affected adversely as well as the sale of bonds itself, since the prospectus will have to state clearly the lack of conformance, which makes such an issue a marginal one to investors who, because of a lack of knowledge about the health field, rely on official statements for guidance.

The importance of utilization rates as an indicator of how hospitals are used cannot be overemphasized. It is a mixed bag of a number of factors at work that include:

- availability of enough physicians to care for the public
- physician patterns of using hospitals conditioned by their clinical training and malpractice concerns
- extent of third party coverage among the public
- availability of hospital beds in the community
- impact of utilization review

Projecting Future Occupancy Rates

Table 43-6 shows the numbers that need to be watched, analyzed, and projected.

This kind of data becomes most helpful as the baseline for deciding what is likely to occur in the future at five- and ten-year intervals. But a person needs to highlight relationships before moving forward. For instance, a series of questions needs to be asked, such as (using Washington[1] figures):

- Why is it the U.S. has 4.4 beds and Washington has only 3.6, a 24 percent difference in supply?

Table 43-6 Comparison of Various Utilization Factors—1974

Area	Geographic population	Beds	Dis-charges	Patient days	Util. rate	Average length of stay
			Per thousand geographic service population			
United States	209,689,100	4.40	156.7	1,217.0	3.33	7.7
California	20,601,000	3.9	146.1	974.9	2.67	6.71
Massachusetts	5,818,000	4.5	153.5	1,300.9	3.56	8.5
Maryland	4,151,300	3.1	107.9	901.8	2.47	8.4
Washington	3,448,100	3.36	149.2	835.7	2.29	5.6
Alabama	3,539,000	4.69	174.4	1,292.4	3.54	7.4
Florida	7,678,000	4.5	166.8	1,236.9	3.38	7.4
Michigan	9,044,000	4.2	149.6	1,227.9	3.36	8.2

Source: National Center for Health Statistics, *Vital and Health Statistics*, Series 13 (Washington, D.C.: National Center for Health Statistics, 1974).

- Even with 24 percent fewer beds, why is the state using only 68 percent of the beds compared to 76 percent nationally?

- What is the meaning of 835 days or 68 percent of the national rate of 1,217 patient days per 1,000 population?

- Why are there such wide variations in the average length of stay from one state to another?

It is these kinds of questions that require answers when the information relative to a particular hospital and community differs from the measurement applied by the planning agency. They center not only around utilization at the institutional level, but within clinical services and by kind of physician specialization. In a few years they will be determined by disease entity. Refinement after refinement will be added year after year in the decade ahead.

In addition, there will continue to be much debate over the average occupancy rate of 80 percent that a hospital needs to maintain. Small and rural hospitals simply cannot run at such a level. What are the implications for the future? Are they fewer rural hospitals, no small hospitals, and greater traveling time from home to hospital for the public?

Those persons associated with paying for hospital services have agreed that the answer lies in reducing the number of hospital beds in operation as the only realistic way of holding the line on rising hospital costs. Anything that contributes toward this is a step in the right direction.

In an attempt to limit the supply of hospital beds, the HSAs will require increasing documentation by the hospital. In the future, the 1122 submitted by a hospital can include Tables 43-7, 43-8, 43-9, and 43-10.

Table 43-7 Exhibit Often Required by HSAs

Census tract studies	Admissions per 1,000 population
Population movements	Patient days per 1,000 population
Dependency ratios	Beds per 1,000 population
Growth changes and projections	Bed need projection
Average income per family by age groupings	Average length of stay
Number of average wage earners per family	Definition of service area
Basic service population	

Table 43-8 Exhibit Often Required by HSAs

Occupational categories	Utilization rates by clinical service
Education levels attained	Mortality rates
Housing units	Morbidity by age-sex-ethnic
Patterns of traffic movements	Projected bed distribution
Driving times	Birth rates by age of mother
Labor market outlook	Stillbirths per 1,000 deliveries
Major industrial accidents	Premature births per 1,000 deliveries

Table 43-9 Exhibit Often Required by HSAs

Projected construction costs:	Health personnel surveys:
By function/GSFs	Professional
By building system	Paraprofessional
Estimated costs of operation:	Health resources inventory
Projected operating statement	Social resources inventory
Explanation of bad debts	Alternative health delivery systems
Financing method:	Linkages with other providers
Source of funds	Physician office locations
Letters of intent	OPD visits by service

Table 43-10 Exhibit Often Required by HSAs

Planning assumptions	Plans of other hospitals
Cultural—ethnic pockets	Trend of ER admissions
ER Rate per 1,000 population	Classification of ER cases by degree of illness and diagnosis
Ratio of inpatient admissions to ER visits	
Ambulance responses per 1,000 population	

In all, 54 exhibits may be called for by the HSA. If a hospital decides that it needs assistance from an architect and consultant in preparing its application, the out-of-pocket costs may range as is shown in Table 43-11.

APPLICATION STRATEGY

Thus, the cost for playing the game has become enormous. As the staffs of the HSAs become more knowledgeable, they will see an increasing need for data and completeness before acting on the application. To the extent they want to know more about the facilities and the financing, the higher the cost will go to the hospital. Since neither the staff nor the board members of the agency have reason to deal with consultants or architects from the standpoint of paying for these services, they are likely to be unaware of the costs associated with requesting additional information. How much information is enough may be ultimately limited only by their own concepts of adequacy of data.

Within a few years this will become a major bone of contention between hospitals and planning agencies. Both have a real stake in knowing as much about a project as is possible, but the burden of paying the cost for providing it rests with the applicant. This, in itself, is apt to put a brake on the number of applications submitted by individual institutions and to increase the scope of the project to be reviewed.

Instead of taking several projects a year to the planning agency for review, the hospital is likely to combine several of them into one application and make a concerted effort to secure approval. There is considerable logic in this approach when it is appreciated that the political realities require thoughtful consideration in the development of an appropriate strategy for walking the application through the approval process.

Table 43-11 Typical Professional Fees for Development of an 1122 for $10M Program

	Low	High
Role and program study	$40,000	$70,000
Project feasibility documentation:		
Revenue/expense forecasts	$10,000	$25,000
Fund-raising feasibility	$5,000	$10,000
Site master plan	$10,000	$26,000
Financing alternates analysis	$10,000	$20,000
Preliminary A and E participation	0	$155,000
1122 application preparation	5,000	25,000
Total through 1122 completion	$80,000	$331,000

To believe that adequate documentation and careful analysis of trends and statistics will speak for themselves is relying too much on agency staff and board members' willingness to wade through all of the information contained in a complete and thorough application. All this really does is create a climate that applicants know what they are doing, but in no way guarantees acceptance of their plans. It is the first step, but not the only one that needs to be taken. Planning an appropriate strategy is of equal importance, is time consuming, and may be frustrating.

Before the hearing on an application, there are seven steps that are necessary to assure the best possible hearing:

1. About three weeks before the meeting, free up the calendar and hold the majority of working time to concentrate on the succeeding steps.
2. Prepare a packet of simple, easy-to-read information about the project for each agency board member.
3. Before distributing the packets, try the material out on several persons who are relatively unfamiliar with the hospital.
4. Make revisions as needed.
5. Schedule individual appointments with all agency board members at their convenience as to time and location.
6. Review the packet information in about 30-minute, individual interviews during the week before the hearing. Answer all questions honestly and openly.
7. Schedule a half-day meeting with the staff of the agency, and review the total application in detail with them.

If these steps are followed through at the time of the meeting, the applicant will have a sense of the discussion that is likely to take place and can plan on bringing the appropriate representatives of the hospital to the hearing. Who is appropriate depends on an evaluation of what is needed. At the minimum, for a major project, the chief executive, the chairperson of the board, a well-respected member of the medical staff, the architect, and a consultant should be included. Others might include a local publisher, local politician, federal judge, or whoever fits the description of "bringing up the big guns." Applicants should decide who is to speak, make it short, and then respond to questions board members may have in mind. If the project involves a new clinical program, a knowledgeable physician should be part of the team making the presentation.

If a second meeting is required, the applicant should have a "skull" session over the strategy to be used for that meeting and not casually make the assumption the orchestration remains as was originally followed. This may be an opportunity to shift some emphasis or use other spokespersons who may be more effective.

THE FUTURE RELATIONSHIP BETWEEN THE HOSPITAL AND THE HSA

The road ahead is a rocky one. It will be a long time before the agencies are really geared up and able to do the job cut out for them. Hospitals will be encountering HSAs that do not have patient origin studies, approved population forecasts, or an ability to project bed needs in a community with changing market shares for the hospitals. Much patience and mutual understanding will be required between both participants. Even with this goodwill, the amount of time and dollars required will force hospitals to rethink the way in which they submit applications. They may be unwilling to put forth the effort to submit three or four applications a year. They will be more apt to bundle them together and make one major push per year.

Because of the emphasis on ambulatory care and the jaundiced eye increasingly cast upon additional beds, projects that are submitted for this purpose alone are going to experience difficulty in securing approvals. A better approach will be to put expansion beds in a package that includes other services and programs, renovations of existing space, or development of specialty beds to relieve pressure on the existing medical/surgical bed complement.

To date, planning agencies have not looked hard at the financial information submitted on an 1122. But as the agency staffs gain experience, the documentation is going to be much more detailed, and likely to require letters of intent and the general conditions of the financing package in the application. In fact, the financial data requirements could become so stiff as to be almost indistinguishable from a financial feasibility study. This could add between $450,000 and $150,000 to the cost of the 1122 application and drive the overall expense of submission to between $121,000 on the low side to a possible high of $445,000.

Finally, hospitals will have to meet the HSAs on the terms laid down by the HSAs. Where HSAs become too heavyhanded, there will be litigation to work out subsequent problems. Case law will inevitably be referred to as it grows and develops around the relationship between hospitals and the regulatory authorities.

Plato must have been a wise man. He foresaw difficulties of today in *The Republic:* "Democracy is a charming form of government, full of variety and disorder, and dispensing a sort of equality to equals and unequals alike."

NOTE

1. American Association of Hospital Consultants, *The Proposed National Health Planning Guidelines, An Analysis* (Arlington, Va.: American Association of Hospital Consultants, 1978.)

Chapter 44

How to Use the Planning Act Amendments

PROBLEMS PREPARING CERTIFICATE-OF-NEED APPLICATIONS

Since the passage of PL 93-641, the role of the consultant has shifted. Not only have the traditional activities continued, but the consultant has now moved into the position of being a "hired gun" for the hospital in putting together certificate-of-need (CON) applications. Out of these experiences has come an appreciation of what needs to be changed. The problems that were being encountered were found to be typical among most consulting firms and in the various states. A quick review of these may be helpful in appreciating the changes that have occurred.

Almost without exception, the time periods called for in the processing of a CON have been violated. In some cases this has become a serious matter if the timetable has slipped, because this affects either the size of the project or the financing. With inflation running more than one percent per month, a delay of three or more months could force a recasting of the project. This also requires pulling back the application and might lead to starting up the CON ladder all over again. On the other hand, leaving the application as is without modifying it would mean a less than totally honest presentation to the HSA or higher authority. This Catch-22 situation is being increasingly encountered by hospitals with large, complex capital projects.

One of the most frustrating experiences for hospital people is to prepare a CON application carefully; think through the project as carefully as possible; present the material; graphically, concisely, and clearly and come to the meeting only to find that little if any of the material has been read by the broad members. The frustration continues as the members proceed to discuss their concerns at length, which have been addressed in the written material in front of them, and then the chairperson, in the interest of time, does not permit any of the hospital's representatives the opportunity to discuss the problems. The frustration turns into rage if the hospital representatives conclude that the vote was lost because of a lack of familiarity with the information presented.

Almost as aggravating have been those meetings where a CON application seemed to be proceeding smoothly, only to run up against some board member who suggests the application should not be approved unless other conditions are agreed to by the applicant hospital. This has occurred so often that it has led to the Satterfield Amendment. The use of "either you do this or you do not get that" became difficult to deal with from the applicants' standpoints. They could not defend themselves, since they had no idea what might be suggested. In one sense, it became an unfair situation that was largely unrecognized by HSA members. When hit with an "either/or" situation, the hospital would automatically begin to calculate how much more delay they were going to encounter in the process, translate this time into money, and, more often than not, decide to comply.

The problem of securing a completed application does not appear to be solved. The amendments should have addressed this problem, but did not. When HSAs decide they have an obligation to deny as many applications as possible, the staff may be instructed to prevent this by repeatedly returning the application to the hospital for incompleteness. This is a time delaying tactic that is often successfully employed for several months.

CHANGES IN THE LAW

Changes in the law, of which there are about 36 of any degree of importance to a hospital, might be grouped into areas of concern that may well cause problems: those that appear to be advantageous to hospitals; those that might work against hospital interests; and those that appear to have little or no importance from the institution's standpoint.

Three New Health Goals

The troublemakers begin with three new health goals. The first requires each health services plan to detail personnel, facilities, and equipment, and to evaluate the degree of renovation required. It is not stretching the truth to state that there is not a staff of any HSA in the country that is competent to do this job. The disarming simplicity of the goal in no way reflects the complexity of this task. As a rule of thumb, about ten percent of the cost of a project is spent for architects, consultants, financial advisors, attorneys, construction managers, equipment planners, and so on, and this does not count the untold hours often spent by physicians and hospital personnel in preparing plans. This requirement will lead to HSAs looking for standardized rules of thumb to apply. Past experience would indicate that these are apt to become arbitrary and that in the future much time will have to be spent defending a well-thought-out project against the application of inappropriate criteria that is improperly applied.

The second new goal or priority is the identification and elimination of duplicate or unneeded services and facilities. This is a current issue in many HSAs and will become even more difficult in the next decade because of the third goal, the strengthening of competitive forces in the health services industry. This last goal is to be applauded because it will ultimately lead to a desirable restructuring of the health delivery system, but it will run headlong into the second new goal.

To explain this, assume a hospital has operated a physical therapy department for a number of years and one day finds that an HMO that was formed in the last two or three years and has now attained an enrollment of 50,000 or more has just established a similar department in its facility one block from the hospital. As part of a large remodeling and renovation project where a number of departments have to be relocated, the hospital finds its physical therapy space has to be relocated and includes this in its CON applications, dutifully noting that the HMO has just built duplicate facilities. The question then becomes moot as to whose ox is going to be gored. Clearly, the formation of the HMO is in keeping with the third priority, but does this mean that the hospital must abandon a service it has traditionally offered? Under the new amendments, the HSA is instructed to give priority to activities that strengthen competition. Resolving these two national priorities is sure to be the scene of much mischief in the years ahead.

Composition of HSA Governing Boards

The composition of governing boards of HSAs has its share of attention in the amendments. Labor organizations are encouraged to have a seat at the board table. Representatives of provider organizations are no longer required to live inside the boundaries of the HSA, and provider representation moves from one-third to one-half of the governing board membership. HMOs are recognized by suggesting that, if there is one or more in the HSA, they should be represented. Finally, a member of the governing board of a hospital is no longer counted as a provider, but may be regarded as a consumer. In a practical sense, none of these modifications are apt to be of much consequence in the work of an HSA, since the compelling guideline is that the decisions of the HSA must conform with the state plan. This becomes the controlling determinant of the decision-making process, not the composition of the board. Thoughtful persons serving on any agency or association board, even though committed to some other group, usually attempt to be supportive of their responsibilities as defined in the organization's objectives. It seems to be wishful thinking to believe that just because providers can now have a bare majority of an HSA board that this is going to change matters much.

Public Meetings

The fact that the amendments specify that meetings of HSAs must be public and that adequate notice must be given if requested means to a hospital that HSAs have a substantial argument in their favor if this provision is violated and they resort to the courts. As any person who has ever served on a public body knows, the casting of a vote in front of everybody is different than when it is cast in executive session. Hospitals are going to have to police HSAs in this regard since HSAs may tend to overlook this new requirement. When dealing with an HSA that likes to go into executive session and call meetings on short notice with no serious attempt to make meeting dates, times, and places known, the hospital should send a registered letter to the agency asking to be routinely kept advised of such matters.

Conflict of Interest Statements

Attorneys would say that the provision in these amendments requiring written disclosure by HSA board members of any conflicts of interest is not going to prevent these problems. However, if a hospital believes its CON application received an adverse decision because of it, the first thing the hospital should do is ascertain whether or not the agency has these written statements on file. If upon such an investigation it is determined they do not exist, the hospital is in a good position to go into court claiming that the agency was not following the procedural rules that are required, and the hospital stands a good chance of overturning the HSA decision. A question, however, may arise that should be addressed. At the state level, could the HSA reaffirm its position in the face of a court decision that held that a reversal of the HSA position was ordered on the basis of not following agency procedure? Or would the court decision only affect the action of the local HSA, still leaving free the action to be taken at the state level?

Performance Standards for HSAs

From the standpoint of the hospital, the amendments now set forth standards of performance to be adhered to by HSAs. This has been needed. Up to now, the performance requirements have been solely on the hospitals with respect to the CON process. One of the pluses now is the requirement that the Health Systems Plan be reviewed every three years, and revised as often as necessary. This will be of assistance, though it really does not go far enough. All too often agencies seriously lack data altogether, or if it exists the data may be so outdated that it is irrelevant. While the new amendments will help, much more detail should be specified at the next round of amendments to require such up-to-date information as a solid population projection, a patient discharge study annually, and a patient origin study from the institutions' standpoint. These are basic tools and benchmarks for the making of any informed judgments about beds and services and need to be required of HSAs.

Timing

One of the irritants in the hospital/HSA relationship has been timing. Procedures and criteria are often adopted following the submission of an application before it is on the agenda for action. This leaves open the question as to which criteria should be applied. Now they have to be "timely written," and there must be timely notifications. In addition, if the HSA requests information, it has to provide at least 15 days for compliance. This is going to cause scheduling problems in some cases within HSAs, where the minimum period of 15 days is going to extend the time frame to where it just passes the date of an HSA monthly board meeting. This will result in adding almost 1½ months to the processing of an application. As in the past, both institutions and agencies will collaborate in "winking" at this provision in the law. The important aspect is that the adopted ground rules for reviewing a hospital application cannot be changed after the agency signifies it has received a completed application.

Hearing Conduct

The hearing section of the amendments will be helpful in that it will serve to take much of the arbitrariness and capriciousness out of the conduct of a hearing. In doing so, the pattern that has emerged in California is likely to be adopted throughout the country. In that state, attorneys control the process in much the same way as a courtroom is controlled. Prior to hearings, lawyers often meet with hospital representatives for intensive sessions, reviewing questions they intend to ask and carefully structuring responses to be complete and factual. It is obvious to anyone watching or participating in this process that the adversary concept of law has now moved into the HSA arena.

At the state level of review it is important to note that the HSAs review is to be based solely on the adopted procedures and criteria, and the record created during the administrative proceedings. The HSA is forbidden to go outside the record. To support this concept, the local HSA is now required to have a record of its hearing on the matter. By requiring written records at both the local and state levels, an opportunity is thereby created for hospital representatives and their attorneys to review the records to determine if there were any procedural flaws. In the event any are discovered, the applicant hospital now has clear recourse to the court system.

If this section of the amendments is to be effective, hospitals are going to have to take the initiative in reviewing these records and going to court. The amendments also specifically require the state to adhere to its own published time schedule. This is a mixed blessing since the hospital will be faced with the question of deciding whether or not it wants to lose the time and encounter the expense that will be required if it decides to sue. This provision will probably not be used to the fullest extent possible because of these factors.

In the past, HSAs have tended to batch applications having to do with like services. The amendments now provide that these be considered on an areawide basis at least twice a year. It would have been preferable to have required consideration every six months, since the language that was used does not indicate these reviews have to be spaced evenly during the year.

Hospital Performance Standards

Prohibited from Lobbying

At the same time that performance standards were being required of HSAs, hospitals were not forgotten. Two are cited that need to be observed by institutions. First, they are prohibited from lobbying their CON with individual HSA members. Each hospital may wish to discuss with its attorney what constitutes lobbying. Past experience indicates that all too often HSA board members have not reviewed applications prior to a hearing. How a concerned hospital can now take the initiative in seeing that each individual HSA member is fully briefed and avoid the pitfall of lobbying is something that needs clarification.

Efficiency and Appropriateness

The other requirement now states that hospitals have to demonstrate efficiency and appropriateness even if the application is for replacing an existing service or facility. This suggests that the mere submission of a CON now puts the hospital at risk. If the HSA should determine that the service is not operating efficiently or that some other institution is considered to be more appropriate in providing the service, then the submitting hospital may discover, too late, that it has put that activity in jeopardy. To avoid this possibility, a hospital should carefully evaluate the other hospitals in the HSA service area, being sure to look beyond the hospital's primary service area to determine its exposure in this area.

Part C

Realistic Timetables

A new section of the amendments, Part C, which deals with the CON program, is now part of the planning law. Health maintenance organizations are exempt from this process if they meet the minimum requirements specified. In addition to the HMO exemption, there are two other provisions that may prove to be troublesome to hospitals. Hospitals are now required to establish realistic timetables for their projects or face withdrawal of certification. Timeframes are far more difficult to establish than is typically appreciated. After a CON is granted, two major hurdles can significantly affect a schedule. If a project needs to be brought before a local unit of government, the hospital may find that they have to appear before the zoning board, the environmental impact committee, the city beautification commission, the traffic commission, and the city council. Providing greater volumes of utility services may require meetings with these companies as well. Months may pass in the process of negotiating a way through this maze.

The other time delay involves capital financing when a bond has to be floated for the project. The amendments under Part C deal not only with timeframes, but costs as well. The hospital must specify the maximum amount of the capital expenditure. The wording does not define capital expenditure. Suppose it is advantageous for a hospital to roll over its existing long-term debt as part of its financing plan for this project. Is this part of its submission in the CON?

Since the money markets are volatile and often change from day to day and week to week, it is not possible to determine accurately either the costs associated with the bond issue or the timing of floating cost at the time of submission of an application. Because of this, the financing vehicle cannot be chosen too early. The best that can be done is to provide an estimate of the most likely financing mechanism and its associated costs. If the issue is undersubscribed at the time it is offered, still other problems are encountered. The vagaries associated with floating a bond issue require flexibility and wiggle-room that are not sufficiently appreciated by many HSA board members or their staffs. To put the total costs of a project at the maximum level or worst case possible is an open invitation to the charge of excessive cost. Dealing with this difficulty is apt to be a real trouble spot in the future.

Exemption Reapplication

In Part C a loophole has been covered. If an HMO establishes a service and that service or program is subsequently sold to a hospital, the exemption is not automatically transferable if sold or leased. Reapplication must be made for the exemption. This prevents a hospital from using an HMO as a conduit to get around the CON process. It does not, however, prevent the HMO from beginning a service that may directly compete as an unnecessary or duplicative activity, since the HMO does not have to qualify for a CON.

This kind of unrestricted competition has already occurred in Minneapolis, where eight HMOs enroll about 25 percent of the population in that community. Where HMOs either directly or indirectly control 75 percent of a hospital's admissions, the amendments provide that if the hospital files a CON, the HSA must approve it if it meets the needs of HMO subscribers or those who will potentially be enrolled. To a suspicious hospital operating in the traditional marketplace, this looks like a license to engage in unfair competition.

Looked at dispassionately, a hospital would be well advised to get in the middle of HMO development so that it can take advantage of these built-in protections for those who participate in economic competition. To continue to be regulated through the CON process while the competition is not puts hospitals at a disadvantage that was deliberately intended by the drafters of the amendments in order to hasten the interest of hospitals in HMOs. By including the provision that HMOs can count potential enrollments, they have further imbalanced the equation.

Physician Opposition

As yet, most physicians are unaware of the federal government's commitment to economic competition through alternative health delivery systems. They are still voting in county medical society meetings to support private practice and fee for service without any understanding of what has already passed into law. This set of mind will not be easy to cope with should a hospital move forward on the HMO front and actively participate in the formation of one. Hospital trustees and administrators can expect to meet considerable opposition from physicians.

Pass-Through Provision

The only pass-through that a hospital, subject to the CON process, is allowed is where they have code deficiencies, state licensure problems, or threatened loss of accreditation, provided that there is conformance to the state plan. If the hospital is in an overbedded area, this becomes the first consideration and voids the mandatory approval. However, if this is not the case, then the project must be approved, but its scope must be limited to the correction of the deficiencies.

This will be awkward for hospitals that intend to use this provision as the basis of an application. From a functional and operational standpoint, a hospital is a complex set of interrelationships in terms of building systems and traffic flows of people, patients, and material. To limit a project to cited deficiencies may necessitate overlooking needed remodeling or renovation that is more economical in the long run. This will force many hospitals to make a choice: to incorporate these additional renovations and run the risk of having the project turned down, or to exclude them, follow the guidelines, and know that they have created avoidable construction costs. To some, this will seem like a choice between blindly following the rules or opting to use sound judgment for that given situation.

Purchasing or Leasing Another Institution

In the event a hospital wishes to purchase or lease another institution, it will, in the future, be required to file notice of its intent 30 days prior to the occurrence. In order to comply with this requirement, a hospital will have to resort to the use of options in which the sale or lease is contingent only upon obtaining HSA concurrence. Since information that is sent to an HSA is a matter of public record, a hospital that notifies the HSA of such an intention runs the risk of having this proposed transaction known to its competitors and having them get into the act before the transaction is completed. To avoid this possibility, an option will have to be employed.

Additional Provisions

Under PL 96-79, physicians' offices are exempt from CON on the purchase of equipment. However, if a state is considering bringing physicians' offices in under this requirement, they have until September 30, 1982 to do so. Given the opposition that the medical profession has to regulation, it is doubtful that this provision will be exercised by many state legislatures.

Freestanding laboratories are also specifically exempted from the CON process. Although no definition of a freestanding laboratory is provided in the legislation, if a hospital created a subsidiary corporation where it held the majority control, this would not qualify for an exemption but would be regarded as an attempt to circumvent the CON process.

In some cases, hospitals have attempted to get around the $150,000 limitation by leasing equipment or by having it donated. This loophole has now been closed by requiring that the fair market value of the equipment be determined. If it exceeds the threshold level, it becomes a reviewable item for consideration by the HSA.

Another item is the new provision indicating that professional fees used in developing a project are now counted against the $150,000 level. This indicates that nearly all large, complex projects are going to have to be submitted twice to the local HSA, the first time at the point where they are considering engaging consultants and architects and then later when they have developed a definitive plan of action.

One of the difficulties encountered by hospitals in the past is where they received an approval through the CON and then had to submit to a rate review commission hearing only to be turned down. This should no longer be a stumbling block since the amendments now provide that those states with rate review commissions are required to coordinate their efforts with those of SMCC.

A new provision has been added that requires HSAs to collect data annually from each hospital on the 25 most frequently used hospital services, including the private and semiprivate room ratio. They are then required to make such information publicly available. Apparently a hospital has no choice about submitting the data since the agency can require compliance. However there is no indication as to how this is to be enforced.

The last major provision is a new grant program to assist and encourage the discontinuance of unneeded hospital services. It became effective April 1, 1980 and provides for grants to pay off long-term debt, to pay terminated employees, to retain employees, and to assist in reemployment. Applications for such grants must be made and follow the CON process up to the Secretary of HHS' office. At that point, the Secretary of Labor may get into the act as well. It will be interesting to see the extent to which this new program is utilized.

A MIXED BAG

The Planning Act Amendments represent a mixed bag of advantages and disadvantages. The two really significant points are the stipulations on procedural matters at hearings held by HSAs and the Satterfield anti-blackmail provision. These will be of great assistance in assuring hospitals that they can get a fair hearing on the issues they present in their applications. To be effective, however, hospitals may well have to take the initiative in seeing to it that they are used.

Chapter 45

Effective Planning and Reimbursement

Discussions about long-range planning for hospitals must seem to be exercises in futility for New York hospital trustees. The continual struggle to keep this year's budget balanced places greater emphasis on the present than the future. At times they must feel that there is no tomorrow with the uncertainties of reimbursement from Blue Cross, Medicare, and Medicaid.

The unpredictability of future reimbursement levels is sufficient reason to forget about developing a master plan. However, the best hope for institutional survival in periods of great uncertainty is planning activities. They may need to be more sophisticated and require more complex methods, but not to plan for a variety of contingencies is to invite future trouble.

LONG-RANGE PLANNING

Historically, the concept of long-range planning focused on facility construction and renovation. Programmatic planning was handled on an *ad hoc* basis. With the enactment of PL 92-603 and Section 1122 reviews for both construction and "substantial" charges in service, program planning became a necessity. A new element was added.

Change in Service

Today a long-range plan must include changes in the scope and type of services a hospital offers. When a board of trustees decides to close an obstetrical unit and convert it to general medical surgical patients, the regional HSA must approve the conversion of beds. No dollars are involved, and the $150,000 floor for 1122 is not applicable, yet there is a substantial change in service, so Section 1122 review is required.

The definition of substantial change in service has not been carefully defined by HHS regulations, and some zealous HSA staffs have adopted definitions that control even minor management decisions.

Prior to the time that PL 93-641 was enacted, many hospitals initiated, contracted, or expanded programs of care at will, without asking for an 1122 review, because they were reasonably sure that the agency staff would not learn about the change in service until long after it had taken place. With the new requirement that a hospital file a long-range master plan with the regional HSA, all changes are reported.

Reducing or Eliminating Services

In states where reimbursement regulations are in flux, Section 1122 reviews will frequently occur as hospitals shift their operations to cope with changing conditions. This means that their master plans must include both upside and downside conditions for the programmatic planning section.

Since long-range program planning has typically considered only the addition of new services, the uncertainties of reimbursement require inclusion of plans to reduce or eliminate services.

There are two ways to cut costs. One is to withdraw all hospital services from a particular class of patients, such as Medicaid enrollees, because the cost of providing this care exceeds the amount of payment for these services. This decision does not require an 1122 review, but will involve third party reimbursement negotiation.

The other method is to eliminate hospital services operating at a loss on either a program or department basis. The decision would require an 1122 review.

In the first instance the quality of care for the remaining patients stays the same, and no planning agency review is needed. In the second case, the quality of care will be decreased for all patients, but a greater number of people will be served, and HSA review is required.

Elements of a Master Plan

The usual elements in a master plan are not adequate to cope with fluctuating reimbursement. Typically, financial data center on cash flow projections with summary figures from operations to show how much of a net surplus is to be used for capital financing.

When the uncertainty of reimbursement is tied to a review requirement for substantial change in service, a hospital's master plan must have operations planning include both program changes, and revenue and expense estimates.

In the past a master long-range plan included a market analysis, projection of new programs requiring construction or renovation, building needs, and a financial feasibility. Under fluctuating reimbursement conditions, the scope of the master plan should be expanded to include a five-year budget projection with proposed shifts in operation when payments for hospital services are changed.

Most hospital administrations in the country are not at this level of development. Few integrate master plans and five-year budget projections. As other parts of the nation face a financial squeeze like New York's and implementation of PL 93-641, they will be forced to do so.

As an intermediate stage to cope with the vagueness of reimbursement, a master planning document should present a series of alternative projects based on a separate set of assumptions such as:

- to limit the purchase of new equipment to funds available in the equipment depreciation fund and building depreciation funds for renovation and minor facility expansion to implement the master plan;

- to maintain a three or six percent net surplus from operations for either implementing the long-range plan annually or for debt servicing for a loan to carry out the program;

- to conduct a fund-raising campaign;

- to use endowment income for debt service;

- a combination of these methods.

The use of each strategy has different financial and program implications as well as risks. The limits of each alternative change the scope and sequencing of a proposed plan.

Financing the Long-Range Plan

When an institution is using unrestricted endowment income, borrowing short term, and not fully funding depreciation to cover operating losses, the first priority is to achieve a breakeven operation.

Until a board of trustees faces this issue, it is trading future opportunities for survival. What it should do is ask the administration to develop a five-year revenue and expense budget for achieving a breakeven position, or a surplus from operations along with recommendations for eliminating program and departmental losses by cutting services or classes of patients.

These decisions are not administrative, but those of governance. They are difficult and not lightly taken. However, a trustee's failure to cope with operational losses and take the political heat for program reductions is to squander an institution's future.

Progress is a relative thing. If an institution is standing still while other hospitals are gradually spending resources for day-to-day operations, the other hospitals are relatively improving their position.

There is one other major alternative for financing a master long-range plan conversion of a voluntary nonprofit corporation into an investor-owned hospital. If it is assumed that cost-based reimbursement will continue, the financing advantage of a for-profit corporation is substantial.

For example, assume a 200-bed acute general hospital goes into operation today with a 100 percent mortgage for 30 years at a tax-free interest rate of 10 percent on $10 million that will fully depreciate on a 30-year basis. Also assume that 50 percent of the revenues are from cost-based reimbursement programs of Medicare and Medicaid, and that the federal government's rate of interest on equity is 10 percent.

This means that in the tenth year of operation the investor-owned hospital will have been paid about $900,000 more in reimbursement than a voluntary nonprofit hospital. Given the chance to sell stock, say with a 10 percent dividend, this means they can raise about $9 million in capital funds. Now, either the mortgage can be repaid or their plant once again can be expanded for additional revenue producing services; in other words, the financing for their long-range plan has been found.

In the present New York climate, the investor-owned idea is not workable. It is attractive in areas where hospitals still have an operating surplus. If New York hospitals ever overcome current reimbursement pressures, it is a useful concept.

In the meantime, hospital trustees should assure themselves that major government decision makers really do understand the fact that a hospital can only be successful medically, if it is first financially successful. Medical care services must be adequately financed, and underfinancing limits both the quality and scope of hospital care.

THE IMPORTANCE OF A LONG-RANGE MASTER PLAN

By interlacing long-range planning and operation realities into a master plan, the effect of increasingly restricted reimbursement can be vividly shown. Until both factors are jointly considered, trustees may not be aware of the significance of earlier decisions to divert the use of long-term funds into covering deficits.

An outcome of this type of operating, financing, and planning data is the elimination of wishful thinking by trustees that somehow things will change. A look five years ahead will point out the effect of declining market demand, growing plant obsolescence, aging medical staff, and increasing reimbursement restrictions in an inflationary economy. When its cumulative effect has been demonstrated, responsible trustees will earnestly seek to find alternative ways of preventing the predicted situation.

Affiliations, shared services, mergers, or consolidations between hospitals are more easily considered before a crisis, and the greater the number of alternatives that may be reasonably considered. Since institutional survival is important, a comprehensive master long-range plan is important.

No easy answers have been proposed to cope with uncertain reimbursement and long-range planning. However, the appropriate use of an institutional planning document will preserve and protect the best qualities of both private and public hospital care. Without it, trustees will not perceive the ultimate effect of uncertain reimbursement and continue the present practice of giving away piecemeal a community institution they respect.

Chapter 46

The Role of the Trustee, Physician, and Administrator

Up until yesterday, figuratively speaking, the planning function in a hospital was handled on a hit-or-miss basis. Whenever there was a prolonged use of corridor beds and a rising temperature in the medical staff, the board of trustees began to think about another fund drive and a dip into the Hill-Burton pool.

In those days, before hospital planning was placed under government regulation, boards of trustees relied upon a buildings and grounds committee, and a finance committee to map out the next step in the bigger and better approach to hospital care.

THE INSTITUTIONAL CHALLENGE

With the passage of PL 93-641 in 1973, which required a planning process in hospitals, this traditional approach to institutional planning became obsolete. The advent of certificate-of-need laws, 1122 reviews, and whatever else the old "B" agency required and the development of HSAs forced the recognition that planning was indeed a sophisticated, complex affair. Boards of trustees learned that the usual planning they had done through their committee structure was increasingly unable to deal effectively with the combined pressures imposed by community organizations; medical staff members; hospital administration; and local, state, and federal bureaucrats. Today, the institutional challenge is to organize all major elements of the planning process into a coherent whole to accomplish the goals established by the trustees.

Accomplishing Disparate Goals

This is no easy task. Each major element in the hospital setting has a set of goals and priorities that reflects its major interests and concerns,

489

and often is at variance with the other major elements of the organization. With today's high construction and interest costs, and the rapid expansion of medical knowledge and technology, the possibility of accommodating all interests by spending more dollars than originally planned is an option that has faded into history.

The goals of each group—trustees, medical staff members, the community, and hospital administration—are seen in the following way:

1. Trustees seek to maximize institutional resources, maintain a financially stable operation, deliver high quality service, and meet perceived community needs.
2. The medical staff desires a full-service hospital, with back up from a broad spectrum of physician specialists, modern equipment reflecting the latest technology, and an attractive workshop staffed by smiling and highly skilled nurses and technicians.
3. The community wants low cost hospital care available day and night, convenience, pleasant surroundings, a wide spectrum of health and social service, and prompt and courteous treatment.
4. The hospital administration shares the goals of each group, struggles to avoid confrontations, and knows that total achievement is impossible.

Divided Opinion

Before 1967, trustees did not face divided opinion as to where a hospital should be headed, only how to get there. If a serious disagreement did arise among themselves, an inner power group quietly smothered it, or the dissident trustees resigned.

Today the arena and rules for hospital leadership have changed. The dissenters do not go away; they seek refuge in regulations that require their input into institutional planning. What used to be a lackadaisical planning process is now much more complex and laced with a plethora of forms to be completed and reports to be filed.

Three years used to be the average span of time from the authorization of a new building or major program to the start-up of operations. Today that time span has grown to five years, or even seven or eight with increasing frequency. The delay arises from the greater involvement of physicians and the need for the approval of various planning agencies, state boards of health, HHS, and community agencies or action groups.

In a nutshell, institutional planning has changed in one decade from an incidental administrative and trustee activity to a task typically involving at least one fulltime staff member, continuous interaction with planning agency staffs, and a steadily rising number of reports. It also requires continual updating, as medical technology and new ideas for health care delivery change. Unanticipated approval delays and tightening regulations hinder the development of modern medical care, as the realities of external planning restrain the freedoms of yesterday.

ROLES IN ACHIEVING EFFECTIVE HOSPITAL PLANNING

Developing a master plan that promotes the delivery of quality medical care has become a real test of a trustee's understanding and leadership skills. Today the first step in understanding what it is all about is to realize that nobody has ever applied cost/benefit analysis to mandated planning. Dollars are needlessly wasted documenting trivia and recasting the same data countless times in different reporting formats for each agency.

Well-Defined Statement of Goals

An effective hospital planning process must rest on a well-defined statement of institutional goals. Statements about providing high quality care of treating the sick or caring for the needy were fine in the days of low budgets, limited technologies, inexpensive construction, and private payment of hospital bills. Today such generalized statements are not meaningful.

A hospital can no longer "be all things to all people" for health care. Delivering services to the geriatric or chronically ill in a general hospital is an inappropriate use of capital investment.

Today, with $130,000-plus per bed construction costs, mechanical systems costing 60 percent of the total cost of a building, and $600,000 CAT scanners, a hospital is no longer a physicians' workshop, but the most expensive part of medical care. The expense of acute care in modern hospitals necessitates the use of integrated systems of treatment that function at high performance levels consistently.

As medical services within a community continue to integrate, hospitals need a role and mission statement that defines their specific role in the local health care system. Levels of hospital care today must reflect the increasing subspecialization occurring in medicine. A pediatrician is not a pediatric oncologist, and an internist is not a cardiologist.

Trustees must know enough about the medical care scene to understand where their hospital fits into the spectrum of the health care system.

An inability to understand the fundamental need for an institutional statement of purpose has caused many fumbles and false starts in health care. Often a board of trustees may be upset by an HSA rejecting an 1122 request for a CAT scanner, but the board often does not realize that it did not justify the equipment with a coherent statement of mission. Too frequently trustees revert to political arm-twisting, emotional appeals, and other tactics akin to the schemes used in a political convention.

A board can only begin effective planning after developing a statement of mission. Then they need to assemble and analyze market and demand data relevant to the institution's purpose. Rather than argue the merits and intricacies of how this is done, assume that the administrative staff, consulting firm, or local HSA has prepared an adequate data base and concentrate on how to use it.

Interdependency of Physicians, Administrators, and Trustees

Modern medicine necessitates a growing interdependency of physicians, administrators, and trustees. No one element has enough knowledge to put a major hospital program into operation alone, which is why hospital staffs spend so much time in committee meetings. Initiating a new hospital service typically requires the input of at least several clinical specialists, members of the nursing staff, secretaries, engineers, finance officers, lawyers, insurance experts, housekeepers, architects, and administrators. Once conceived, a new service can take anywhere from several months to a year before a plan can be recommended to a board of trustees.

When a five- or ten-year plan for the hospital is contemplated for one project, the time span increases significantly, and the number of people involved rises geometrically.

To insist thoughtlessly on haste in planning almost invariably invites carelessness, maybe not in the total amount of dollars spent on a project, but at least in the resulting bruised feelings, emotional insecurities, lowered morale, and lack of drive among the participants to continue to strive for excellence.

Organizing Planning

Effective planning starts with the collection and analysis of data, then defining and identifying the implications of this information, and listing available alternatives. The alternatives need to spell out what the various types of clinical programs will accomplish, how they will operate, what they will cost, and how many patients will be served.

The process of organizing planning in a hospital often takes different routes through a hospital structure. When the medical staff, hospital staff, trustees, and community all need to be included, the process requires some nimble steps, if egos and interests of all parties are to be protected.

Programs can frequently arise when the administration must simultaneously deal with the medical staff and the community. Each wants to protect his or her own turf. Further, when the HSA requires community comment on a proposed plan, the previous efforts of solving problems with the medical staff can quickly come unglued, particularly if the community demands are not achievable from a medical point of view. Also, major roadblocks to future efficiencies may be established.

Premature publicity about alternatives being considered may set off a community debate, political interference at the local level, bureaucratic posturing at the state level, a medical staff boycott, or even the triggering of competitive responses by other hospitals. Further complications develop because the board of trustees, as a whole, does not usually participate in these early planning stages.

Financing

Once the administration consolidates the interests of the community and the medical staff into a proposed program, detailed calculations of dealing with the financing need to be undertaken. Construction, remodeling, and operating costs must be estimated for both the initial period and the long-range future. The financial impact must then be evaluated in terms of reimbursement formulas and the coverages of Blue Cross, Blue Shield, Medicare, and Medicaid.

At this point, the administrative staff often regrets involvement in the project because financing capabilities usually fall short of expected needs.

This is also the time when community groups and medical staff members begin to feel the promises of the administration ring false. No matter how many times a group hears that planning is only preliminary, it always senses the task is complete when the initial recommendations are adopted. Usually everyone then says no one told them the plan would be revised.

After defining financing and operating costs, and comparing them to available funds, the administration must choose either to adopt the projects in order of importance or try to take a piece out of each program. Either alternative shrinks the financial commitment, but typically, neither approach works.

Cost-cutting ideas fail because in some cases interrelationships of space requirements, medical desirability, practicalities of remodeling or construction, and mechanical systems' problems may make partial reductions almost impossible. Also, the medical staff and community groups may not want to sacrifice a proposed program to the greater need for a new boiler, expanded laundry, or space for medical records. There is no easy answer.

Recycle Proposals

Under these conditions, the next step is to recycle the total package of proposals, keeping in mind which programs should have the highest priority and why. Considerations of medical need, financing, manpower, construction sequences, and new technologies cannot be reduced to one simple answer. Additional administrative work must develop realistic probabilities of what each project will accomplish and how much it will cost.

Deciding on the Master Plan

Finally, the hospital administration must decide on the long-range plan and its financial feasibility. As the master plan is discussed by the interested parties, administrators must become advocates for a particular set of recommendations. If two programs are of equal importance, however, both should be presented to the board of trustees with supporting documentation.

Board Approval

Once a program has been decided and approved, the board of trustees begins its most responsible work. Even though a trustee committee has monitored the plan as it developed, the proposal is still an administrative document until it is placed on the agenda of the board of trustees.

When a major planning document is introduced for board consideration, it should be assigned to a committee for review and recommendation. Often it becomes difficult to decide whether it should go to a buildings and grounds committee, the finance committee, to a special committee, or to the executive committee of the board.

Hospitals allocate this responsibility differently. In some, a dominant personality directs the assignment. In others, the entire board decides to sit as a committee of the whole or the board avoids assigning the review to a committee that is not in favor of the project. If a board chairperson has been thinking ahead, he will have appointed a planning committee staffed by trustees capable of taking a broad perspective on health care issues.

Once a planning document goes to a committee, the committee's first order of business should be to check to see if the plan is consistent with the goals of the hospital. Occasionally, a goal statement may be modified when the logic of a plan compels such a review or when new areas of service suddenly become achievable and fundable.

Once a committee determines that the planning is consistent with the hospital's stated goals, it needs to review the assumptions on which market analysis and demand data are based. Then it should consider all the ramifications of the project.

When a committee has completed its work, the document should be returned to the board for adoption or modification. After discussing the committee's report and possible amendments, the finance committee should then be asked to consider the proposal and prepare recommendations on how to fund the program. The assumptions on which market demand are premised should be carefully analyzed to assure that they remain operational in the future.

After the finance committee accepts the master plan, it must be presented to the board of trustees for action. If everyone has done a competent job up to this point, the master plan should be able to withstand the board's review and be ready for final acceptance.

ISSUES IN THE 1980s

The decade ahead will be characterized by restrictive reimbursement policies, rising costs of new medical technology, high construction costs, increasing medical specialization, increasing regulation, and continuing inflation. A hospital in the eighties will no longer be able to serve all of the health care needs in its service area that were the typical hospital response in the fifties, sixties, and seventies. To act in such a fashion in the eighties will not be possible, even for a strong, well-financed, and well-managed institution.

What a hospital does, it should do well and with considerable humanity. To try to cover all the bases in acute medical care is to assume that it will either be done in a poor way or at such a high cost that the majority of the population will be excluded from its benefits.

To survive as a valued medical resource, institutional planning must be carefully done, with a new awareness of market opportunities. In this process, hospitals will need to consider modifying their traditional market approach, and thereby, they will raise physician eyebrows. Historically, hospitals and physicians have accepted five limitations in marketing techniques:

1. full support of the concept of fee for service in medical practice, even when conditions were inappropriate for its applications;

2. equal economic treatment of all members of the medical staff;
3. the provisions of service at just one location, the hospital site;
4. tacit agreement not to compete economically with physician activities;
5. competition only between hospitals, in terms of the scope of clinical services and quality of care, but not economically.

In the late seventies, leading hospitals reexamined these limitations, and, as a result, redefined their roles and missions to a broader concept of being a provider of broad-gauged, multihospital services, from prevention to rehabilitation. They also began to develop health care conglomerates. What kinds of ventures these efforts are likely to develop remains for the future to decide.

Historically, the community health care market has been the domain of the physician until the past decade. Today, all sorts of commercial ventures have entered it, from rent-a-nurse companies to fly-away laboratory analysis. These companies and other similar ones have recognized that physicians' practices are essentially small business with low capital investment, and that many small businesses in one industry will deter market domination by any one of the small firms.

In a few situations today, the local hospital has become the core of half a dozen or more corporate entities pursuing a variety of activities. The outer limits of this kind of development are unknown. They have been undertaken by nonprofit hospitals, not on the basis that bigger is better, but rather because of a deep concern to protect a high quality and level of medicine in their institutions and a recognition that restricted reimbursement practices would, sooner or later, deteriorate their present financial situation.

The successful hospital planning effort of the eighties will be accomplished only if its trustees and medical staff members understand not only the local situation, but the federal level as well. Whether people agree or disagree with the regulatory efforts focused on hospitals, they need to be able to anticipate future events and develop an institutional plan that both maximizes future opportunities and, likewise, minimizes potential institutional damage.

The traditional ways of hospitals must change and become more flexible. The stop and go lights of yesterday will be of little assistance. The challenge to achieve excellence in planning is tougher but more necessary than ever before.

Chapter 47

The Bottom Line

The general theme that has been developed in this book is that the future is likely to be much different than the past. Since the turn of the twentieth century, hospitals have been on the same road, getting better and better in caring for the patient. In following that path, hospitals have evolved from an institution focused on nursing care into a technological industry with increasing needs for capital funds. This transformation has taken place but has not yet been widely recognized.

A TURNING POINT

By the time the calendar rolls over to the twenty-first century, it will be evident that the decade of the eighties was a turning point. To those who prefer to see things as they were, it will not seem much different. Patients will still be going to surgery, and surgeons will still be operating on patients. Physicians will still be determining the diagnostic and treatment orders for patients, and hospital personnel will still be carrying them out. The episode of illness resulting in an interaction between patient and physician and hospital will look to the participants in 2000 A.D. much like it does today. Because of the increased use of ambulatory services, those patients admitted to the hospital will be more acutely ill, but this will be noticeable only in terms of the use of ancillary services and the average length of stay.

What is taking place will not affect the daily routines of a hospital because it is organizational and financial in character. The successful hospital of today will be the health care corporation of tomorrow. The hospital will not be a single corporation devoted to inpatient care, but a conglomerate of nonprofit and for-profit organizations joined together by a holding company. Instead of having two product lines—inpatient care and outpatient ancillary services—it will have several products ranging from physical fitness programs to industrial safety programs to real estate investment to prepayment. In the aggregate, it will have a sophisticated marketing arm and a strong financial orientation, and is apt to be one of the largest employers in town.

ROLE OF CHIEF EXECUTIVES

As this conglomerate evolves, it will more closely resemble large for-profit corporations with multiple product lines and multiple outlets. The tools and techniques of management will be similar to those used by corporations of similar size and complexity. The uniqueness of patient care will remain lodged in the hospital subsidiary where the traditional values will continue to be of primary concern. The linkages to the other corporate bodies will reflect the broadened range of management interests. What occurs on a daily basis will not be of overriding importance to chief executives in the holding companies who will be focusing on the long-range concerns confronting the health care corporation. Their time will be taken up with reviewing annual budgets, determining the assumptions to be used in preparing five-year rolling budgets, keeping abreast of what is happening in the money markets, reviewing space allocations and reallocations, interviewing replacements for key executives leaving the conglomerate, approving major capital expenditures, dovetailing programs and services into a strategic marketing plan, determining additional marketing opportunities requiring risk dollars, and representing the enterprise to external forces. They will have a full platter of activities determining where the organization will be in five and ten years in the future.

Administrators of today's hospital will become the vice-presidents of hospital operations in tomorrow's vertically integrated health care corporation. They will be joined at the senior executive level by a vice-president of finance along with the presidents of other subsidiaries. Chief executives of these newly emerging corporations will not necessarily be drawn from the ranks of hospital administration. Depending on the needs of the corporation, they may come from the marketing area, from finance, or from hospital operations.

ROLE OF PHYSICIANS

As the freestanding hospital of today shifts into a health care corporation, the role of physicians will remain largely unchanged. As the decision makers on diagnosis and treatment they will continue to be a primary factor in the hospital setting, but the collective voices of the medical profession will be muted at the level of the parent corporation. Because physicians are involved in a hands on activity and their efforts are devoted to clinical interests, their role remains unchanged. To a great extent they will not ever be aware that the hospital is now part of a larger system and not a system unto itself. About the only observable difference to physicians in this vertically integrated system will be their awareness that their ability to bring to bear all of the resources needed to care for their patients is much greater than that of their peers who are still functioning in a free-standing hospital. In addition, specialists who depend on referrals for economic survival will probably be unaware that the health care conglomerate has fashioned a web that protects this interest through its involvement with primary care centers, health programs provided to local industry, and fitness programs all aimed at capturing all of the health care needs in one structure.

THE FUTURE

The future belongs to those organizations of trustees, physicians, and hospital executives who come to appreciate that the ways of the past have run their course and the time has now arrived to think in more global terms and who are willing to make a commitment to the future in keeping with the emerging needs of the public. Imagination and risk taking on a massive scale are key ingredients to removing the dead hand of the past.

The need for doing so can be recognized when the amount of expenditures for personal health care expenditures are projected for the next ten years. In 1980, the aggregate spending for hospitals, nursing homes, physicians services, drugs, optometrists, and so on was $220 billion. If the rate of inflation annually averages 10 percent, the total expenditures will rise to $553 billion. If, as some medical economists are predicting, the percent of the gross national product for personal health care rises from 9.1 percent to 12 percent, the total outlay will be approximately $750 billion, of which hospitals will account for about one-third.[1]

In all likelihood, this three-time dollar increase in health care services will be provided by fewer organizational units. Even with 200,000 more physicians in active practice in 1990, this will be the case. During this decade, more of the physicians coming into practice will be joining existing groups in increasing numbers, hospitals will become larger, and fewer of them will be needed as the average number of patient days per 1,000 population declines.

New services will continue to develop, but as part of the conglomerate. These will include fitness programs, contract industrial health packages, professional office buildings, retirement homes, hospices, and multiple units of hospitals. This expansion will require capital investment and flexibility of organizational structure, and will add to the financial strength of the health care corporation because of product differentiations. As these conglomerates evolve, these annual budgets will rise significantly each year, and by the end of the decade there are apt to be several that have revenues of over $1 billion a year, with considerably more in the range of $500 million to $1 billion.

As this growth takes place, opportunities in other countries will be sought after, in much the same fashion as the investor-owned Hospital Corporation of America has begun developing hospitals in Australia. The initial wave of overseas activities will occur among the for-profit health care conglomerates. The leaders will have become multinational health care corporations.

This book is about management and governance functions in the health care field. For the past 70 years patient care has dominated the thinking of those associated with hospitals. As the future unfolds, the imperative of patient care is going to be joined with two other imperatives: organizations for health care and a major concern on financing. This will not mean that there will be less concern about patients; rather, the years ahead are going to lead to increasing complexity requiring greater sophistication in the management of these important resources. It is a challenge that is unparalleled in the history of hospitals.

NOTE

1. Robert M. Gibson and Daniel R. Waldo, "National Health Expenditures, 1980," *Health Care Financing Review*, 3, No. 1 (September 1981): 1-54.

Index

A

Abortion, 436
Access (to hospital care), 105, 206
 Gary program and, 395
 reasonable, 12-13
Accountability
 CEO and, 169, 172
 corporate structure and, 72
 cost, 103-109
 increasing, 231
 internal audit and, 303
 medical staffs and, 247
 physician-directors and, 243-44
 trustees and, 236
Accounting, merger and, 45-46
Acquisition concept (merger), 40-42
Administration graduate programs
 delegation and, 201
 emotional control as administrative
  skill and, 201-202
 the future and, 203-204
 hospital personality and, 198
 medical staff and, 199
 organizational triad and, 199-200
 personality of administrators and,
  197

reasonable expectations and, 202-
  203
 specialists and, 200
 trustees and, 198-99, 200
Administrative staff
 CEO management of, 157-59, 167
 government and, 151
 hospital resource competition and,
  27
 merger and, 43, 44
 role statement and, 28
Administrators. *See also* Chief
 executive officer (CEO)
 ambulatory care and, 381-82
 appraisal of, 274-77
 behavioral changes in, 170-71, 172
 behavior of medical staff and,
  239-40
 budget and, 252, 254-55
  as staff-control tool, 289-94
 changes in health care and, 19
 competitors/team players and, 211-
  14
 control of organizational behavior
  by, 212-14
 corporate structure and, 74-76
 family and, 170-71

N

About the Authors

EVERETT A. JOHNSON, PH.D., is professor and director of the Institute of Health Administration at Georgia State University in Atlanta, and is director of The E.J. Group, Inc., for consulting activities.

Mr. Johnson holds a Masters of Business Administration and a Ph.D. degree from the University of Chicago. He has been engaged in graduate education for hospital administration, as well as in organizing a hospital and health care consulting firm.

Mr. Johnson has served the professional society of hospital administration as regent, governor, and president; the American Hospital Association on councils, the House of Delegates, and the Nominating Committee; and has served as a director of both the Indiana and Atlanta Blue Cross plans. In addition, he has been president of the Indiana Hospital Association and a member of the Advisory Council on Nursing of the Department of Health, Education and Welfare.

In 1968, Mr. Johnson received the Tri-State Award of Merit. In 1973 and 1978, he received the Edgar C. Hayhow Award of the American College of Hospital Administrators for the article of the year.

RICHARD L. JOHNSON is president of the TriBrook Group, Inc., of Oak Brook, Illinois. After receiving a Masters of Business Administration, he was the associate director of the graduate program in hospital administration and assistant superintendent of The University of Chicago hospitals. Later he was director of The Teaching Hospitals at the University of Missouri and associate professor in the School of Medicine. Mr. Johnson served as assistant director of the American Hospital Association for a number of years and then joined the management consultant firm of A. T. Kearney and Company, where he was a vice-president and member of its board of directors. With two colleagues in 1972, he founded the firm he now heads. A fellow in the American College of Hospital Administrators since 1959, Mr. Johnson was named the Dean Conley award recipient for an article published in *Hospital Progress* in 1979. He served as chairman of the American Association of Hospital Consultants in 1979–80. In 1952, he coauthored *Hospitals Visualized* with Ray E. Brown.